Lipidology

Editor

STEPHEN J. NICHOLLS

CARDIOLOGY CLINICS

www.cardiology.theclinics.com

Consulting Editors
JORDAN M. PRUTKIN
DAVID M. SHAVELLE
TERRENCE D. WELCH
AUDREY H. WU

May 2018 • Volume 36 • Number 2

ELSEVIER

1600 John F. Kennedy Boulevard • Suite 1800 • Philadelphia, Pennsylvania, 19103-2899

http://www.theclinics.com

CARDIOLOGY CLINICS Volume 36, Number 2
May 2018 ISSN 0733-8651, ISBN-13: 978-0-323-58348-0

Editor: Stacy Eastman
Developmental Editor: Sara Watkins

Cardiology Clinics (ISSN 0733-8651) is published quarterly by Elsevier Inc., 360 Park Avenue South, New York, NY 10010-1710. Months of issue are February, May, August, and November. Business and Editorial Offices: 1600 John F. Kennedy Blvd., Ste. 1800, Philadelphia, PA 19103-2899. Customer Service Office: 3251 Riverport Lane, Maryland Heights, MO 63043. Periodicals post-age paid at New York, NY and additional mailing offices. Subscription prices are $339.00 per year for US individuals, $640.00 per year for US institutions, $100.00 per year for US students and residents, $430.00 per year for Canadian individuals, $804.00 per year for Canadian institutions, $464.00 per year for international individuals, $804.00 per year for international institutions and $220.00 per year for Canadian and international students/residents. To receive student/resident rate, orders must be accompanied by name of affiliated institution, data of term, and the *signature* of program/residency coordinator on institution letterhead. Orders will be billed at individual rate until proof of status is received. Foreign air speed delivery is included in all *Clinics* subscription prices. All prices are subject to change without notice. **POSTMASTER:** Send address changes to *Cardiology Clinics*, Elsevier Health Sciences Division, Subscription Customer Service, 3251 Riverport Lane, Maryland Heights, MO 63043. **Customer Service: 1-800-654-2452 (U.S. and Canada); 314-447-8871 (outside U.S. and Canada). Fax: 314-447-8029. E-mail: journalscustomerservice-usa@ elsevier.com (for print support); journalsonlinesupport-usa@elsevier.com (for online support).**

Reprints. For copies of 100 or more, of articles in this publication, please contact the Commercial Reprints Department, Elsevier Inc., 360 Park Avenue South, New York, NY 10010-1710. Tel.: 212-633-3874; Fax: 212-633-3820; E-mail: reprints@elsevier.com.

Cardiology Clinics is also published in Spanish by McGraw-Hill Interamericana Editores S. A., P.O. Box 5-237, 06500, Mexico D. F., Mexico; in Portuguese by Reichmann and Alfonso Editores Rio de Janeiro, Brazil; and in Greek by Dimitrios P. Lagos, 8 Pondon Street, GR115-28 Ilissia, Greece.

Cardiology Clinics is covered in *MEDLINE/PubMed (Index Medicus), Excerpta Medica, The Cumulative Index to Nursing and Allied Health Literature* (CINAHL).

Contributors

NIKHIL S. BASSI, MD
Cardiology Fellow, Section of Cardiology,
University of California, Los Angeles, UCLA
Cardiovascular Center (Westwood),
Los Angeles, California, USA

LANE B. BENES, MD
Cardiology Fellow, Section of Cardiology,
The University of Chicago Medicine, Chicago,
Illinois, USA

AREF A. BIN ABDULHAK, MD, MSc
Division of Cardiovascular Medicine,
Department of Internal Medicine, University
of Iowa Carver College of Medicine,
Department of Epidemiology, Prevention
Intervention Center, The University of Iowa,
College of Public Health, Iowa City, Iowa,
USA

ALBERICO LUIGI CATAPANO, PhD
Professor of Pharmacology, Department of
Pharmacological and Biomolecular Sciences,
University of Milan, IRCCS Multimedica, Milan,
Italy

M. JOHN CHAPMAN, PhD, DSc
INSERM Emeritus Director and Research
Professor, National Institute for Health and
Medical Research (INSERM) and University of
Pierre and Marie Curie (UPMC)–Paris 6,
Pitié-Salpêtrière University Hospital, Paris,
France

MICHAEL H. DAVIDSON, MD
Professor of Medicine, Section of Cardiology,
The University of Chicago Medicine, Chicago,
Illinois, USA

BELINDA A. DI BARTOLO, PhD
Postdoctoral Research Fellow, South
Australian Health and Medical Research
Institute, The University of Adelaide, Adelaide,
South Australia, Australia

KATRINA L. ELLIS, PhD
Research Fellow, Faculty of Medicine and
Health Sciences, School of Medicine, School
of Biomedical Sciences, The University of
Western Australia, Crawley, Western Australia,
Australia

MA FENG, BSc
Doctoral Fellow, National Institute for Health
and Medical Research (INSERM), INSERM
UMR 1166 ICAN, University of Pierre and Marie
Curie (UPMC)–Paris 6, AP-HP, Groupe
Hospitalier Pitié-Salpêtrière, Paris, France

BRIAN A. FERENCE, MD, MPhil, MSc, FACC
Benjamin Meaker Visiting Professor, Institute
for Advanced Studies, University of Bristol,
Bristol, United Kingdom; Division of
Cardiovascular Medicine, Wayne State
University School of Medicine, UHC, Detroit,
Michigan, USA

SAVVAS HADJIPHILIPPOU, BSc, MBBS
Department of Primary Care and Public Health,
Imperial College, London, United Kingdom

ARASH HAGHIKIA, MD
Department of Cardiology, Charité
Universitätsmedizin Berlin, Campus Benjamin
Franklin, German Center for Cardiovascular
Research (DZHK), Partner Site Berlin, Berlin,
Germany

SATOSHI HONDA, MD
Postdoctoral Research Fellow, South
Australian Health and Medical Research
Institute, The University of Adelaide, Adelaide,
South Australia, Australia

MOHAMAD A. KALOT, MD
Research Fellow, Department of Medicine,
American University of Beirut, Beirut, Lebanon

MAAIKE KOCKX, PhD
Atherosclerosis Laboratory, ANZAC Research
Institute, University of Sydney, Concord
Repatriation General Hospital, Concord,
New South Wales, Australia

ANATOL KONTUSH, PhD
INSERM Research Director, National Institute for
Health and Medical Research (INSERM),
INSERM UMR 1166 ICAN, University of Pierre
and Marie Curie (UPMC)–Paris 6, AP-HP, Groupe
Hospitalier Pitié-Salpêtrière, Paris, France

**LEONARD KRITHARIDES, MBBS, PhD,
FRACP, FCSANZ, FESC, FAHA**
Department of Cardiology, Concord Hospital,
Atherosclerosis Laboratory, ANZAC Research
Institute, University of Sydney, Concord,
New South Wales, Australia

ULF LANDMESSER, MD
Department of Cardiology, Charité
Universitätsmedizin Berlin, Campus Benjamin
Franklin, German Center for Cardiovascular
Research (DZHK), Partner Site Berlin,
Berlin Institute of Health (BIH), Berlin,
Germany

DIMITRI P. MIKHAILIDIS, BSc, MSc, MD
Department of Clinical Biochemistry, Royal
Free Campus, University College London
Medical School, University College London,
London, United Kingdom

ADAM J. NELSON, MBBS
Cardiology Fellow, South Australian Health
and Medical Research Institute, The University
of Adelaide, Adelaide, South Australia,
Australia

STEPHEN J. NICHOLLS, MBBS, PhD
Deputy Director, Professor, South Australian
Health and Medical Research Institute,
The University of Adelaide, Adelaide,
South Australia, Australia

ANGELA PIRILLO, PhD
Center for the Study of Atherosclerosis,
E. Bassini Hospital, IRCCS MultiMedica,
Milan, Italy

FABIANA RACHED, MD, PhD
Clinical Researcher in Atherosclerosis Unit,
Heart Institute (InCor), Medical School,
University of São Paulo, Albert Einstein
Hospital, São Paulo, Brazil

**KAUSIK K. RAY, BSc, MBChB, MD, MPhil
(Cantab)**
Department of Primary Care and Public Health,
Imperial College, London, United Kingdom

JENNIFER G. ROBINSON, MD, MPH
Division of Cardiovascular Medicine,
Department of Internal Medicine, University of
Iowa Carver College of Medicine, Prevention
Intervention Center, Professor, Department of
Epidemiology, The University of Iowa, College
of Public Health, Professor, Department of
Medicine, University of Iowa Hospitals and
Clinics, Iowa City, Iowa, USA

KERRY-ANNE RYE, PhD
School of Medical Sciences, University of
New South Wales, Sydney, New South Wales,
Australia

ANUM SAEED, MD
Clinical Postdoctoral Fellow, Section of
Cardiovascular Research, Department of
Medicine, Baylor College of Medicine, Center
for Cardiometabolic Disease Prevention,
Houston, Texas, USA

DAISUKE SHISHIKURA, MD
Postdoctoral Research Fellow, South
Australian Health and Medical Research
Institute, The University of Adelaide, Adelaide,
South Australia, Australia

KOHEI TAKATA, MD, PhD
Postdoctoral Research Fellow, South
Australian Health and Medical Research
Institute, The University of Adelaide, Adelaide,
South Australia, Australia

GERALD F. WATTS, MD, DSc
Winthrop Professor, Faculty of Medicine and
Health Sciences, School of Medicine, The
University of Western Australia, Crawley,
Western Australia, Australia; Department of
Cardiology, Lipid Disorders Clinic, Royal Perth
Hospital, Perth, Western Australia, Australia

Contents

Apolipoprotein B–containing lipoproteins and low-density lipoprotein play a key role in atherosclerotic vascular disease. Modified forms of low-density lipoprotein drive inflammation, an integral aspect of plaque progression. High-density lipoprotein particles are equipped to protect low-density lipoprotein from enzymatic and nonenzymatic modification. Under normal conditions, high-density lipoproteins facilitate cholesterol efflux from tissues, preventing its accumulation with deleterious consequences. However, the high-density lipoprotein particles characteristic of dyslipidemic states associated with premature atherosclerosis are typically dysfunctional as a result of alteration in their metabolism and consequently their structure and composition. Such an effect indirectly enhances low-density lipoprotein atherogenicity.

Mendelian randomization studies demonstrate that apolipoprotein B–containing lipoproteins have both causal and cumulative effects on the risk of atherosclerotic cardiovascular disease. The clinical benefit of lipid-lowering therapies depends on both the absolute reduction in circulating apolipoprotein B–containing lipoproteins and the total duration of exposure to these particles. Because atherosclerosis seems to be caused by the retention of apolipoprotein B–containing lipoproteins rather than by the cholesterol content carried by those lipoproteins, high-density lipoprotein–mediated efflux of cholesterol from the arterial wall may not reduce the risk of atherosclerotic cardiovascular disease.

Ischemic heart disease remains the leading cause of death worldwide. Low-density lipoprotein cholesterol (LDL-C) has proved to have a causal relationship with atherosclerotic cardiovascular disease. Lowering LDL-C improves outcomes, although some patients continue to have residual risk of cardiovascular disease. Cardiovascular risk prediction calculators are routinely used to identify patients most at risk. Research into other lipoprotein factors has suggested that they may have advantages over LDL-C and improve the ability to identify those most at risk. Although some technology is not widely available, there is potential for better risk prediction in specific groups.

Statins are essential medications in the management of patients with clinical atherosclerotic cardiovascular disease and have been supported by numerous clinical trials. Emerging evidence suggests that adding ezetimibe to statin therapy is associated with a net benefit and improved hard clinical outcomes, particularly in patients with significantly elevated atherosclerotic cardiovascular disease risk and elevated low-density lipoprotein cholesterol levels.

Statin intolerance is the inability to tolerate a dose of statin required to sufficiently reduce cardiovascular risk. With the five-step approach, more than 90% of these patients might be treated with statins. The principal approaches are to try not to discontinue statin therapy and to treat these patients as effectively as possible. New therapies with the proprotein convertase subtilisin-kexin type 9 inhibitors and bempedoic acid might be an effective response to these needs. In case of lack of achieved goal of the therapy, nutraceuticals with confirmed low-density lipoprotein cholesterol reduction properties may be considered as a part of the lipid-lowering combination therapy.

Type 2 diabetes is associated with elevated levels of triglycerides and small, dense low-density lipoprotein particles, in addition to low levels of high-density lipoprotein cholesterol. Clinical trials have demonstrated the clear cardiovascular benefit of use of statin therapy in patients with diabetes. Additional lipid-modifying agents are typically guided by the presence of additional lipid abnormalities. The optimal use of existing lipid agents and the potential for novel therapies in patients with diabetes is reviewed.

High levels of low-density lipoprotein cholesterol (LDL-C) are directly associated with an increased risk of cardiovascular disease. Reducing LDL-C levels reduces the incidence of cardiovascular events. Several lipid-lowering approaches are available to achieve the LDL-C levels recommended by current guidelines, statins being the first-line therapy. However, many patients cannot achieve the recommended LDL-C levels with current therapies. The discovery of the role of proprotein convertase subtilisin kexin 9 (PCSK9) in the regulation of plasma LDL-C levels suggested it as a potential pharmacologic target and led to the development of PCSK9 inhibitors for the management of LDL-C levels.

Although statins are first-line therapy for low-density lipoprotein cholesterol (LDL-C) reduction, many individuals on maximally tolerated statin therapy have elevated LDL-C. Bempedoic acid (ETC-1002) is a novel once-daily LDL-C–lowering agent in phase 3 clinical trials. In phase 1 and 2 studies, ETC-1002 was efficacious in lowering LDL-C when used as monotherapy and when added to statin and/or ezetimibe and was well tolerated in patients with statin intolerance. ETC-1002 also improved cardiometabolic risk factors. Ongoing phase 3 studies of ETC-1002 are evaluating its long-term efficacy and safety and effects on cardiovascular events. This article discusses current evidence and future directions for ETC-1002.

CARDIOLOGY CLINICS

ISSUE OF RELATED INTEREST

Endocrinology and Metabolism Clinics, March 2016, (Vol. 45, No. 1)
Lipidology
Edward A. Gill, Christie M. Ballantyne, and Kathleen L. Wyne, *Editors*
Available at: http://www.endo.theclinics.com/

THE CLINICS ARE AVAILABLE ONLINE!
Access your subscription at:
www.theclinics.com

Preface
Lipidology

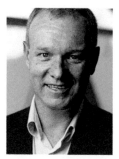

Stephen J. Nicholls, MBBS, PhD
Editor

For nearly three decades, the development of effective pharmacological approaches to targeting plasma lipoproteins has played an important role in the prevention of cardiovascular disease. The consistent observation of benefit with statins has profoundly influenced treatment of patients with high cardiovascular risk. However, there are considerable challenges to the use of these agents, and additional lipid abnormalities are unlikely to be optimally treated by statin monotherapy. Accordingly, there is a major need to identify how to most effectively use existing lipid-modifying agents and to identify new challenges, which provide the potential to develop new therapies.

This issue of *Cardiology Clinics* spans the current state of the clinical approach to lipid management. It highlights the role of existing lipid-lowering agents, their therapeutic challenges, and the development of treatment algorithms that attempt to guide their most optimal use. It then highlights the role of emerging therapies and the potential to develop new agents targeting lipoproteins not optimally managed by statin therapy. While advances in lipid management have had a profound influence on cardiovascular outcomes, there remains considerable work moving forward in order to achieve more effective reductions in risk.

Stephen J. Nicholls, MBBS, PhD
South Australian Health and
Medical Research Institute
The University of Adelaide
PO Box 11060
Adelaide, SA 5001, Australia

E-mail address:
stephen.nicholls@sahmri.com

Cardiol Clin 36 (2018) xiii
https://doi.org/10.1016/j.ccl.2017.12.015
0733-8651/18/© 2017 Published by Elsevier Inc.

Impact of Lipoproteins on Atherobiology
Emerging Insights

Ma Feng, BSc[a,b], Fabiana Rached, MD, PhD[c],
Anatol Kontush, PhD[a,b], M. John Chapman, PhD, DSc[d,*]

KEYWORDS

- LDL • HDL • Dyslipidemia • CETP • Monocyte-derived macrophage

KEY POINTS

- Modified low-density lipoproteins constitute a key driver of plaque inflammation through their interaction with monocyte-derived macrophages in the arterial intima.
- Inflammatory cytokines are central actors in amplifying the inflammatory response.
- High-density lipoprotein may inhibit the modification of both low-density lipoprotein lipids and proteins by virtue of their antioxidative biological activities.
- High-density lipoproteins are frequently dysfunctional in dyslipidemic states involving subnormal high-density lipoprotein cholesterol levels.
- Markedly elevated high-density lipoprotein cholesterol levels seem to be deleterious; under such conditions, high-density lipoprotein particles may display defective biological activities consistent with increased cardiovascular risk.

INTRODUCTION

Despite extensive basic and clinical research and prevention strategies involving efficacious therapies, atherosclerotic cardiovascular disease (ASCVD) and its clinical manifestations, such as myocardial infarction, ischemic stroke, and peripheral vascular disease, represent the leading cause of morbidity and mortality throughout the world.[1] Moreover, ASCVD constitutes a major economic burden to society; indeed, the global cost of CVD is expected to exceed US$1 billion dollars by 2030.

Atherobiology encompasses the complex processes that underlie the initiation, formation, and progression of the arterial atherosclerotic plaque, processes that can ultimately be expressed as a thrombotic event, the consequence of the formation of an occlusive or partially occlusive thrombus at the surface of an eroded or ruptured lesion.[2–4]

The key factors that act in a multiplicative and interactive manner to initiate atherosclerotic plaque formation at sites of predilection in the arterial tree are multiple, and include not only dyslipidemia, but also smoking, hypertension, hemodynamic factors, oxidative stress, and diabetic hyperglycemia, the latter possibly involving advanced glycation end products, and others.[2–5] Among these modifiable risk factors, dyslipidemia is prominent, and implies marked imbalance between elevated circulating levels of cholesterol in the form of apolipoprotein (apo)-B–containing, lipoproteins (including very low-density lipoprotein, intermediate density lipoproteins,

Disclosure: The authors have nothing to disclose.
[a] National Institute for Health and Medical Research (INSERM), INSERM UMR 1166 ICAN, University of Pierre and Marie Curie – Paris 6, 91 Boulevard de l'Hôpital, Paris 75013, France; [b] AP-HP, Groupe Hospitalier Pitié-Salpêtrière, 91 Boulevard de l'Hôpital, Paris 75013, France; [c] Heart Institute (InCor), Medical School, University of Sao Paulo, and Albert Einstein Hospital, 44, Avenida Doutor Eneas Carvalho de Aguiar, Sao Paulo 05403-000, Brazil; [d] National Institute for Health and Medical Research (INSERM) and University of Pierre and Marie Curie – Paris 6, Pitié-Salpêtrière University Hospital, 91 Boulevard de l'Hôpital, Paris 75013, France
* Corresponding author. NSFA, 13 Avenue des Arts, Saint Maur 94100, France.
E-mail address: john.chapman@upmc.fr

low-density lipoproteins [LDL] and lipoprotein [a]), versus subnormal levels of cholesterol transported in the form of high-density lipoproteins (HDL) containing apoAI.[2,5–7]

It has long been recognized that elevated levels of plasma apoB-containing particles are atherogenic, and indeed this concept has been consolidated with recent evidence attesting to the causality of LDL in the pathophysiology of ASCVD from genetic, Mendelian randomization, epidemiologic, and interventional studies.[8] By contrast, the potential atheroprotectivity of elevated levels of HDL has been brought into question by recent prospective population cohort studies.[9–11] Indeed, a reassessment of the relationship between cardiovascular risk and circulating concentrations of HDL on the one hand, and the functionality of HDL particles on the other, is ongoing. This article updates emerging insights into the atherobiology of apoB-containing particles on the one hand, and apoAI-containing HDL on the other.

FOCUS ON THE ATHEROBIOLOGY OF APOLIPOPROTEIN B–CONTAINING LIPOPROTEINS

Circulating lipoproteins, and particularly elevated levels of LDL as occurs in familial hypercholesterolemia for example, play key roles as initiating factors in atherogenesis but equally drive plaque progression.[2–8] On a mechanistic basis, substantial evidence attests to the penetration of the endothelial layer by atherogenic lipoproteins at sites of activation such as arterial branch points, and to the potential for retention within the arterial intima of all forms of such apoB100-containing particles (LDL, very low-density lipoprotein, very low-density lipoprotein remnants, and lipoprotein [a]).[12] Lipoprotein retention occurs by both particle trapping in the extracellular matrix network and by electrostatic interaction.[12] Upon retention, LDL may be modified by aggregation, lipolysis, oxidation, or proteolysis. Modified LDL, frequently containing oxidized lipids, acts as a chronic stimulator of the innate and adaptive immune response. As a consequence, both endothelial cells and smooth muscle cells are activated to express surface adhesion molecules, (eg, vascular cell adhesion molecule–1, intercellular adhesion molecule–1), chemoattractants (eg, monocyte chemoattractant protein-1), and growth factors (eg, macrophage colony-stimulating factor and granulocyte-macrophage colony-stimulating factor), which bind to receptors on circulating monocytes and stimulate their homing and migration into the intima, with subsequent differentiation into macrophages or dendritic cells.[4] Modified LDLs are taken up by intimal monocyte-derived macrophages through scavenger receptor or other pathways.[13] Macrophage foam cells filled with droplets of lipoprotein-derived cholesteryl esters (CEs) result, classically displaying a proinflammatory phenotype, an essential element not only in the early fatty streak lesion, but also in determining the progression of the lesion (**Fig. 1**).

It has now emerged that the transformation of the monocyte-macrophage to the M1 or inflammatory phenotype, together with the ultimate fate of this cell, are key determinants of the ensuing intraplaque inflammatory response.[4,13,14] Typically, the chronic inflammatory response becomes maladaptive, resulting in failure to resolve inflammation. Macrophage-derived foam cells lose mobility owing to their lipid load and are unable to exit the arterial wall. In addition, defective efferocytosis leads to an increased inflammatory response, necrotic core expansion subsequent to the accumulation of cellular debris and cholesterol, and plaque progression. Macrophage necrosis amplifies this inflammatory response in a self-perpetuating cycle. At the center of this scenario is the macrophage NLRP3 inflammasome that, under the impact of inflammatory cytokines released from several cell types, including T-helper type 1, T-helper type 2, T-regulatory lymphocytes, and mast cells, drives the production and secretion of a spectrum of factors favoring plaque progression and instability; these include matrix-degrading enzymes, reactive oxygen species, proinflammatory eicosanoids, cytokines (including interleukin-1 beta) and lipids. Importantly, it is currently believed that it is the binding of modified LDL to pattern recognition receptors such as Toll-like receptors on macrophages, which constitutes the primary trigger for secretion of these proinflammatory factors.[4,5,12–14] For further insight into these complex cellular pathways, the reader is referred to the comprehensive review by Libby and colleagues.[15]

It is of immediate relevance that the reduction in cardiovascular outcomes seen recently in the CANTOS (Canakinumab Anti-inflammatory Thrombosis Outcomes Study) trial, in which cananikumab, a human monoclonal antibody to interleukin-1 beta, was used to attenuate residual inflammation in statin-treated patients with elevated levels of highly sensitive C-reactive protein (>2 mg/dL) and incident ASCVD, attests to the key role of inflammation in plaque formation and progression, and ultimately in plaque stability and instability.[16]

Nonetheless, it is noteworthy that modified LDL is the primary ligand in macrophage foam cell formation and, as such, is the primum movens in driving inflammatory cell recruitment, foam cell formation, cellular apoptosis and necrosis, smooth muscle cell proliferation and extracellular matrix

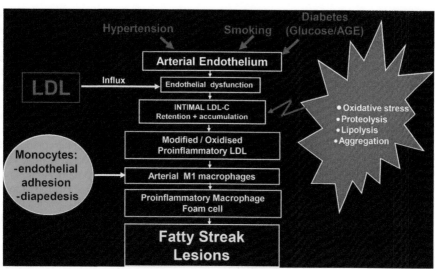

Fig. 1. Early events in atherogenesis. Modifiable risk factors impact the endothelium, inducing activation at sites of low shear stress in the arterial tree. Endothelial permeability increases, with enhanced penetration of apolipo-protein (apo)B–containing lipoproteins, including low-density lipoprotein (LDL). Intimal retention results from electrostatic binding of LDL to matrix components. Concomitantly, circulating monocytes bind to endothelial adhesion proteins and enter the intima by diapedesis, where they differentiate to macrophages. Under the impact of modified LDL, inflammatory cytokines and other factors, they transform to proinflammatory foam cell macrophages on cellular uptake of modified LDL with formation of cholesteryl ester-rich lipid droplets. The foam cell macrophage produces a spectrum of proinflammatory factors, whose production is further ampli-fied by interaction with other leukocyte cell types. AGE, advanced glycation end products.

synthesis, and in the adaptive immune response that results in amplification of the chronic inflam-matory response by lymphocyte subsets; the initial stages of atherosclerotic lesion formation are summarized schematically in **Fig. 1**, and empha-size the central actors in the development of the in-flammatory response in the arterial intima.

Finally, a new dimension in our understanding of factors that impact the atherobiology of lipopro-teins recently occurred as a result of targeted gene array analysis of genome-wide association data, and has led to the identification of arterial wall-specific mechanisms of coronary artery dis-ease involving variants in genes coding for pro-teins implicated in cellular adhesion, leukocyte migration, inflammation and coagulation, and vascular smooth muscle cell differentiation.[17]

FOCUS ON THE ATHEROBIOLOGY OF APOLIPOPROTEIN AI-CONTAINING LIPOPROTEINS

For more than 50 years, low plasma levels of HDL cholesterol (HDL-C) have represented a robust and independent marker of increased cardiovascu-lar risk. By contrast, no clear evidence has emerged that HDL particles are themselves causal in the pathophysiology of premature ASCVD. In contrast, it has been widely assumed that elevated levels of

HDL-C may afford cardioprotection.[18] It has, there-fore, come as a surprise that recent prospective population-based data have documented a U-shaped curve for the relationship between HDL-C concentrations and all-cause mortality in both males and females. The mechanistic basis for an association between markedly elevated HDL-C and cardiovascular risk seems to be predominantly genetic in origin.[9–11] The structural, metabolic, and functional dimensions that underlie these findings are the subject of intense research. Nonetheless, major insights have recently emerged regarding the relationships between the metabolism, struc-ture, chemical composition (lipidome and prote-ome), and the atheroprotective functions of HDL particles in normolipidemic healthy subjects and, in addition, between defective HDL function in low HDL-C dyslipidemic states and the characteristics of HDL particles that underlie such dysfunction.

The biology of HDL is complex. HDL are small, dense, protein-rich lipoprotein particles, with a mean size of 8 to 10 nm and are classically isolated in the density range from 1.063 to 1.210 g/mL.[18] These particles are quasispherical or discoid plurimolecular complexes composed of a diversified lipidome consisting of at least 300 molecular lipid species, and a proteome of up to 50 distinct proteins; apoAI is the predomi-nant protein component.

BIOLOGICAL ACTIVITIES OF HIGH-DENSITY LIPOPROTEIN RELEVANT TO PROTECTION OF THE ENDOTHELIUM AND ARTERIAL WALL

HDL particles possess multiple biological activities relevant to the protection of the endothelium and arterial wall. HDL can contribute to atheroprotection by effluxing cellular cholesterol, attenuating vascular constriction, reducing vascular inflammation, diminishing cell death, protecting from oxidation, neutralizing bacterial infection, attenuating platelet activation, and maintaining glucose homeostasis. Cellular cholesterol efflux to HDL acceptors is presently considered to represent the key step in the reverse cholesterol transport pathway from peripheral cells to the liver for excretion into the bile. It is relevant in the context of HDL atherobiology that these particles may remove cholesterol from arterial wall cells, primarily from macrophages and macrophage-derived foam cells. Cholesterol efflux may, therefore, constitute the clinically relevant cardioprotective characteristic of HDL that underlies the epidemiologic association between low circulating levels of HDL-C and cardiovascular risk.[19] Mechanistically, reduction of plasma HDL concentration and/or HDL particle number may accelerate the development of atherosclerosis by impairing the clearance of cholesterol from the arterial wall. Consistent with the hypothesis of Miller and Miller, rates of cholesterol efflux from murine macrophages evaluated using an in vitro assay may reflect the presence of cardiovascular disease better than HDL-C levels.[20–22] Further evidence in support of this pathway is provided by infusions of both native and reconstituted HDL that possess the capacity to remove cholesterol from atherosclerotic plaques in vivo.[23]

Additional antiatherogenic actions of HDL toward the endothelium and arterial wall also possess the potential to attenuate atherosclerosis initiation and progression.[24–28] Indeed, the beneficial actions of HDL on the endothelium primarily involve vasodilatory activity, which largely reflects the capacity of HDL to stimulate nitric oxide production by endothelial cells.[29–31] Activation of nitric oxide production by HDL involves binding to scavenger receptor type B class (SR-BI) to initiate intracellular signaling through interaction of the C-terminal PDZ-interacting domain of SR-BI with the adaptor PDZ domain-containing protein PDZK1.[32,33] HDL may equally exert vasodilatory effects via the ATP binding cassette transporter G1, which involves efflux of cholesterol and 7-oxysterols from endothelial cells. This process enhances formation of active endothelial nitric oxide synthase dimers and results in decreased production of reactive oxygen species.[33] HDL may also increase the bioavailability of nitric oxide as a result of diminished cellular production of superoxide, which inactivates nitric oxide. Indeed, HDL attenuates nicotinamide adenine dinucleotide phosphate hydrogen oxidase activity, the major cellular source of superoxide, by reducing expression of its major subunits in endothelial cells.[34]

Given the central role of intraplaque inflammation in atherogenesis, it is relevant that HDL particles display potent antiinflammatory actions, with the potential to suppress chronic inflammatory response in the arterial wall. First, HDL particles decrease adhesion molecule expression in endothelial cells activated by cytokines and thereby inhibit monocyte adhesion to the endothelium.[35–39] Second, HDLs attenuate monocyte activation, reducing expression of chemokines and chemokine receptors in monocytes through nuclear factor kappa B and peroxisome proliferator-activated receptor gamma–dependent pathways.[40–42] In addition, HDL particles exert cytoprotective actions, protecting both macrophages and endothelial cells from apoptosis induced by loading with free cholesterol or by oxidized LDL.[43,44] Equally, the survival of endothelial cells is enhanced by HDL in the presence of chylomicron remnants, tumor necrosis factor-alpha and proteins of the complement system.[45–47]

Finally, HDL inhibits production of reactive oxygen species and decreases intracellular oxidative stress.[46,48–51] Cellular antioxidative activity of HDL requires interaction with surface receptors, including SR-BI and ATP binding cassette transporter G1[51,52]; by contrast, direct contact between HDL and prooxidative agents in the extracellular compartment is not required. Reduced cellular production of superoxide and hydrogen peroxide may underlie the antioxidative effect of HDL in endothelial cells.[53]

The existence of the aforementioned atheroprotective activities of HDL has been demonstrated repeatedly in extensive experiments in vitro and in vivo in animals and man. However, clinical evidence of the impact of these activities on ASCVD is still lacking.

INTERRELATIONSHIPS BETWEEN THE BIOLOGICAL ACTIVITIES AND INTRAVASCULAR METABOLISM OF HIGH-DENSITY LIPOPROTEIN

During its intravascular metabolism, HDL interacts dynamically with cellular receptors, lipid transporters, and enzymes; equally, HDL proteins and lipids are exchangeable. A majority of human plasma HDL are spherical particles, and the principal pathway of their formation originates in lipid-free apoAI or discoid HDL produced by the liver and intestine; equally, however, surface fragments of triglyceride (TG)-rich lipoproteins sequester to the HDL pool during lipolysis.[24] Cholesterol and phospholipids from cellular membranes are readily acquired by nascent discoid HDL through an ATP-binding cassette transporter A1–mediated efflux.[24] Subsequently, small spherical HDL3 and thence large spherical HDL2 are generated from esterification of free cholesterol by the action of lecithin:cholesterol acyltransferase (LCAT). HDL2 can in turn be converted to HDL3 through several pathways, including heteroexchange of CE and TG between HDL and apoB-containing lipoproteins mediated by CE transfer protein (CETP), selective uptake of CE by hepatocytes mediated by SR-BI, and hydrolysis of phospholipid and TG by hepatic lipase.[24]

HDL particles are highly heterogeneous in their biological activities on a per particle basis, reflecting in part their complex metabolism. Across the HDL subpopulation spectrum, small, dense, protein-rich HDLs display the most potent atheroprotective properties, which can be attributed to specific clusters of proteins and lipids. Specifically, small, dense, protein-rich HDLs display elevated cholesterol efflux capacity, antioxidative activity, antiinflammatory activity and cytoprotective activity, antithrombotic activity, and antiinfectious activity, whereas large HDL seems to possess enhanced antiinfectious properties.[18]

PROTEINS AND LIPIDS IN HIGH-DENSITY LIPOPROTEIN ASSOCIATED WITH ATHEROPROTECTIVE ACTIVITIES

Proteins constitute key structural and functional components of HDL particles. HDL carries a large number of different proteins, including apolipoproteins, enzymes, lipid transfer proteins, acute phase response proteins, complement components, and proteinase inhibitors.[18] ApoAI is the major HDL protein and accounts for approximately 70% of total protein in HDL. The principal functions of apoAI involve ensuring distinct structural organization of HDL, interaction with cellular receptors, activation of LCAT, and endowing HDL with multiple antiatherogenic activities. Other functionally and structurally important apolipoproteins of HDL include apoAII, apoIV, apoE, apoCII, apoCIII, apoJ, apoD, apoF, apoL-I, and apoM.[18] HDL also carries several enzymes, such as LCAT, paraoxonase 1 and platelet-activating factor-acetyl hydrolase. LCAT catalyzes the esterification of cholesterol to CEs in plasma lipoproteins, primarily in HDL but also in apoB-containing particles. In the circulation, paraoxonase 1 is almost exclusively associated with

HDL and contributes to the antioxidative properties of the lipoprotein. Plasma platelet-activating factor-acetyl hydrolase circulates in association with LDL and HDL particles, with the majority of the enzyme bound to small, dense LDL and to lipoprotein (a).[54] Lipid transfer proteins present in HDL include CETP and phospholipid transfer protein (PLTP). CETP facilitates bidirectional transfer of CEs and TG between HDL and apoB-containing lipoproteins.[55] In addition, CETP possesses phosphatidylcholine (PC) transfer activity. PLTP converts HDL into larger and smaller particles, and plays a role in extracellular phospholipid transport. Acute phase response proteins form another family of HDL-associated proteins. The major protein of this family carried by HDL is serum amyloid A. Serum amyloid A displays cholesterol efflux and antioxidative activities. Under normal conditions, the content of such proteins in HDL is, however, much lower as compared with the apolipoproteins. HDL also carries several complement components, proteinase inhibitors, and other protein components that may play a role in its atheroprotective activities.[18]

Finally, HDL contains multiple lipids that can modulate its biological activities. Phospholipids predominate in the HDL lipidome; major HDL phospholipid classes include PC, lysoPC, phosphatidylethanolamine, plasmalogens, phosphatidylinositol, phosphatidylserine, phosphatidylglycerol, phosphatidic acid, and cardiolipin. Sphingolipids include sphingomyelin, sphingosine-1-phosphate, and ceramides, as well as neutral lipids, primarily CEs and triacylglycerides. Other minor bioactive lipids present in HDL include diacylglycerides, monoacylglycerides, and free fatty acids, which may also exert biological effects.[56] Although phosphatidylserine can enhance some atheroprotective activities of HDL, lysoPC, phosphatidic acid, and TG often decrease them.

DEFECTIVE HIGH-DENSITY LIPOPROTEIN BIOLOGICAL ACTIVITIES IN DYSLIPIDEMIAS ASSOCIATED WITH PREMATURE ATHEROSCLEROTIC CARDIOVASCULAR DISEASE

Defective biological activity of HDL particles has primarily been observed to date in association with subnormal HDL levels. One of the critical elements that links the biological functions of HDL to ASCVD centers on defective HDL function in low HDL-C dyslipidemias associated with premature atherosclerosis. The attenuated atheroprotective properties of HDL in dyslipidemias raises the potential for indirect proatherogenic effects of such dysfunction. Indeed, an attenuated cholesterol efflux capacity of HDL can result in enhanced accumulation of cholesterol in the arterial wall and reduced flux through the reverse cholesterol transport pathway. Evidence for the importance of this pathway includes impaired reverse cholesterol transport pathway associated with accelerated atherosclerosis in subjects with Tangier disease and in some cases of LCAT deficiency.[57,58]

Deficiency in the antioxidative and antiinflammatory properties of HDL may also be associated with accelerated atherosclerosis. According to the oxidation hypothesis of atherosclerosis, oxidation of lipoproteins, primarily LDL, in the arterial wall represents a key event in atherogenesis.[59] As a corollary, deficient LDL protection from oxidation may accelerate atherogenesis. Impairment of the antioxidative activity of HDL in dyslipidemias involving low HDL-C levels is associated with increased oxidative stress, which has been widely discussed as a cardiovascular risk factor and may, therefore, contribute to enhanced atherogenesis.[60–64] Indeed, dyslipidemic subjects presenting with atherogenic low HDL-C dyslipidemias are characterized by both deficient antioxidative activity of HDL and elevated systemic oxidative stress.[18] Mechanistically, deficiency of antioxidative activity of HDL can facilitate the accumulation of LDL-derived proinflammatory oxidized phospholipids in vivo, resulting in enhanced local inflammation in the arterial intima.[65]

WHICH FACTORS CAN UNDERLIE SUBNORMAL OR ELEVATED LEVELS OF HIGH-DENSITY LIPOPROTEIN CHOLESTEROL?

Hypertriglyceridemia features subnormal levels of HDL-C and elevated content of TG in HDL particles secondary to the action of CETP.[55] Subnormal HDL-C levels result from marked alterations in HDL metabolism, as typified by common dyslipidemic states such as hypertriglyceridemia, hypercholesterolemia, and mixed dyslipidemia; this is equally the case in hyperalphalipoproteinemia. Furthermore, subnormal levels of HDL-C are frequently associated with inflammatory and infectious clinical conditions. The combination of low HDL-C and hypertriglyceridemia is characteristic of metabolic diseases associated with elevated cardiovascular risk, primarily prediabetes as occurs in the metabolic syndrome and in type 2 diabetes. HDL metabolism, particle structure, composition, and function strongly depend on the activity of CETP. Both plasma HDL-C levels and HDL particle number are reduced in hypertriglyceridemic states, thereby reflecting the concerted action of several mechanisms, such as accelerated clearance of small, TG-enriched HDL, reduced stability of TG-enriched HDL possessing loosely bound apoAI,

apoAI shedding from HDL particles with subsequent clearance from the circulation, and reduced availability of surface constituents of TG-rich lipoproteins that sequester to the plasma pool of nascent HDL.[66] Indeed, increased CETP activity as typically observed in hypertriglyceridemia involves increased CE transfer from HDL to TG-rich lipoproteins, producing TG-enriched HDL and decreasing HDL-C. Conversely, CETP deficiency reduces heteroexchange of TG and CE between HDL and TG-rich lipoproteins and increases HDL-C. Increased CETP activity, therefore, frequently underlies low HDL-C phenotypes. In addition, low HDL-C concentrations may result from apoAI deficiency, elevated hepatic lipase activity, and reduced activity of LCAT or lipoprotein lipase.[58,66–70] Furthermore, abnormalities in HDL metabolism impact HDL heterogeneity and particle profile. Thus, in the metabolic syndrome and type 2 diabetes, concentrations of large, cholesterol-rich HDL decrease in parallel with decrease in HDL-C, whereas levels of small, dense, cholesterol-poor HDL particles are less affected.[63,71,72]

Other factors modifying HDL-C levels include activities of PLTP, ATP-binding cassette transporter A1, and SR-BI. Although enhanced function of PLTP tends to diminish HDL-C, elevated activities of ATP-binding cassette transporter A1 and SR-BI both favor elevation in HDL-C levels, as exemplified, for example, by genetic deficiency of SR-B1.

SUMMARY

The critical role of vascular inflammation in atherogenesis and ASCVD has been emphasized by the recent CANTOS trial involving anti–interleukin-1 beta antibody therapy. We should not, however, lose sight of the critical and fundamental role played in this process by modified LDL and by other apoB-containing particles such as chylomicron remnants and lipoprotein (a) (see **Fig. 1**). Moreover, the complete or partial loss of the capacity of HDL to protect the lipid and protein components of LDL particles from the deleterious effects of inflammation and oxidative stress in dyslipidemic states may potentially amplify the role of modified LDL itself as a key driver of intraplaque inflammation. In addition, the oxidative modification of HDL leads to the formation of numerous proatherogenic substances, translating to a "double hit" on the inflammatory process. To what degree the anomalies in HDL structure, metabolism, and function discussed herein are implicated in the increased cardiovascular risk at extreme HDL-C levels remains indeterminate.

REFERENCES

1. Mozaffarian D, Benjamin EJ, Go AS, et al. Heart disease and stroke statistics–2015 update: a report from the American Heart Association. Circulation 2015;131:e29–322.
2. Chapman MJ. From pathophysiology to targeted therapy for atherothrombosis: a role for the combination of statin and aspirin in secondary prevention. Pharmacol Ther 2007;113(1):184–96.
3. Hansson GK. Inflammation, atherosclerosis and coronary artery disease. N Engl J Med 2005;352:1185–95.
4. Fog Bentzon J, Otsuka F, Virmani R, et al. Mechanisms of plaque formation and rupture. Circ Res 2014;114:1852–66.
5. Chapman MJ, Sposito A. Hypertension and dyslipidaemia in obesity and insulin resistance: pathophysiology, impact on atherosclerotic disease and pharmacotherapy. Pharmacol Ther 2008;117:354–73.
6. Chapman MJ, Ginsberg HN, Amarenco P, et al, European Atherosclerosis Society Consensus Panel. Triglyceride-rich lipoproteins and high-density lipoprotein cholesterol in patients at high risk of cardiovascular disease: evidence and guidance for management. Eur Heart J 2011;32:1345–61.
7. Taskinen MR, Borén J. New insights into the pathophysiology of dyslipidemia in type 2 diabetes. Atherosclerosis 2015;239:483–95.
8. Ference BA, Ginsberg HN, Graham I, et al. Low-density lipoproteins cause atherosclerotic cardiovascular disease. 1. Evidence from genetic, epidemiologic, and clinical studies. A consensus statement from the European Atherosclerosis Society Consensus Panel. Eur Heart J 2017;38:2459–72.
9. Madsen CM, Varbo A, Nordestgaard BG. Extreme high high-density lipoprotein cholesterol is paradoxically associated with high mortality in men and women: two prospective cohort studies. Eur Heart J 2017;38(32):2478–86.
10. Ko DT, Alter DA, Guo H, et al. High-density lipoprotein cholesterol and cause-specific mortality in individuals without previous cardiovascular conditions. The CANHEART Study. J Am Coll Cardiol 2016;68:2073–83.
11. Bowe B, Xie Y, Xian H, et al. High density lipoprotein cholesterol and the risk of all-cause mortality among U.S. veterans. Clin J Am Soc Nephrol 2016;11:1784–93.
12. Borén J, Williams KJ. The central role of arterial retention of cholesterol-rich apolipoprotein-B-containing lipoproteins in the pathogenesis of atherosclerosis: a triumph of simplicity. Curr Opin Lipidol 2016;27: 473–83.
13. Steinberg D, Witztum JL. Oxidized low-density lipoprotein and atherosclerosis. Arterioscler Thromb Vasc Biol 2010;30:2311–6.
14. Tabas I. Macrophage death and defective inflammation resolution in atherosclerosis. Nat Rev Immunol 2010;10:36–46.
15. Libby P, Tabas I, Fredman G, et al. Inflammation and its resolution as determinants of acute coronary syndromes. Circ Res 2014;114:1867–79.
16. Ridker PM, Everett BM, Thuren T, et al, CANTOS Trial Group. Antiinflammatory therapy with canakinumab for atherosclerotic disease. N Engl J Med 2017; 377:1119–31.
17. Howson JMM, Zhao W, Barnes DR, et al. Fifteen new risk loci for coronary artery disease highlight arterial-wall-specific mechanisms. Nat Genet 2017;49:1113–9.
18. Kontush A, Chapman MJ. High-density lipoproteins: structure, metabolism, function and therapeutics. Hoboken (NJ): John Wiley & Sons; 2011.
19. von Eckardstein A, Nofer JR, Assmann G. High density lipoproteins and arteriosclerosis. Role of cholesterol efflux and reverse cholesterol transport. Arterioscler Thromb Vasc Biol 2001;21:13–27.
20. Miller GJ, Miller NE. Plasma-high-density-lipoprotein concentration and development of ischaemic heart-disease. Lancet 1975;1:16–9.
21. Khera AV, Cuchel M, de la Llera-Moya M, et al. Cholesterol efflux capacity, high-density lipoprotein function, and atherosclerosis. N Engl J Med 2011; 364:127–35.
22. Li XM, Tang WH, Mosior MK, et al. Paradoxical association of enhanced cholesterol efflux with increased incident cardiovascular risks. Arterioscler Thromb Vasc Biol 2013;33:1696–705.
23. Kingwell BA, Chapman MJ. Future of high-density lipoprotein infusion therapies: potential for clinical management of vascular disease. Circulation 2013; 128:1112–21.
24. Nofer JR, Kehrel B, Fobker M, et al. HDL and arteriosclerosis: beyond reverse cholesterol transport. Atherosclerosis 2002;161:1–16.
25. Assmann G, Nofer JR. Atheroprotective effects of high-density lipoproteins. Annu Rev Med 2003;54: 321–41.
26. Assmann G, Gotto AM Jr. HDL cholesterol and protective factors in atherosclerosis. Circulation 2004; 109:III8–14.
27. Navab M, Ananthramaiah GM, Reddy ST, et al. The oxidation hypothesis of atherogenesis: the role of oxidized phospholipids and HDL. J Lipid Res 2004;45:993–1007.
28. Kontush A, Chapman MJ. Functionally defective HDL: a new therapeutic target at the crossroads of dyslipidemia, inflammation and atherosclerosis. Pharmacol Rev 2006;3:342–74.
29. Nofer JR, van der Giet M, Tölle M, et al. HDL induces NO-dependent vasorelaxation via the lysophospholipid receptor S1P3. J Clin Invest 2004;113:569–81.
30. Drew BG, Fidge NH, Gallon-Beaumier G, et al. High-density lipoprotein and apolipoprotein AI increase endothelial NO synthase activity by protein association and multisite phosphorylation. Proc Natl Acad Sci U S A 2004;101:6999–7004.

31. Mineo C, Deguchi H, Griffin JH, et al. Endothelial and antithrombotic actions of HDL. Circ Res 2006; 98:1352–64.

32. Movva R, Rader DJ. Laboratory assessment of HDL heterogeneity and function. Clin Chem 2008;54: 788–800.

33. Saddar S, Yuhanna IS, Mineo C, et al. Abstract 1275: mutations in the C-terminal transmembrane domain of scavenger receptor class B type I (SR-BI) selectively inhibit the cholesterol sensing that is required for HDL-initiated Intracellular Signaling. Circulation 2009;120:S469a.

34. Terasaka N, Yu S, Yvan-Charvet L, et al. ABCG1 and HDL protect against endothelial dysfunction in mice fed a high-cholesterol diet. J Clin Invest 2008;118: 3701–13.

35. Van Linthout S, Spillmann F, Lorenz M, et al. Vascular-protective effects of high-density lipoprotein include the downregulation of the angiotensin II type 1 receptor. Hypertension 2009;53:682–7.

36. Shaw JA, Bobik A, Murphy A, et al. Infusion of reconstituted high-density lipoprotein leads to acute changes in human atherosclerotic plaque. Circ Res 2008;103:1084–91.

37. van Leuven SI, Birjmohun RS, Franssen R, et al. ApoAI-phosphatidylcholine infusion neutralizes the atherothrombotic effects of C-reactive protein in humans. J Thromb Haemost 2009;7:347–54.

38. Cockerill GW, Rye KA, Gamble JR, et al. High-density lipoproteins inhibit cytokine-induced expression of endothelial cell adhesion molecules. Arterioscler Thromb Vasc Biol 1995;15:1987–94.

39. Calabresi L, Franceschini G, Sirtori CR, et al. Inhibition of VCAM-1 expression in endothelial cells by reconstituted high density lipoproteins. Biochem Biophys Res Commun 1997;238:61–5.

40. Baker PW, Rye KA, Gamble JR, et al. Ability of reconstituted high density lipoproteins to inhibit cytokine-induced expression of vascular cell adhesion molecule-1 in human umbilical vein endothelial cells. J Lipid Res 1999;40:345–53.

41. Bursill CA, Castro ML, Beattie DT, et al. High-density lipoproteins suppress chemokines and chemokine receptors in vitro and in vivo. Arterioscler Thromb Vasc Biol 2010;30:1773–8.

42. Drew BG, Duffy SJ, Formosa MF, et al. High-density lipoprotein modulates glucose metabolism in patients with type 2 diabetes mellitus. Circulation 2009;119:2103–11.

43. Drew BG, Duffy SJ, Forbes JM, et al. Abstract 1273: high density lipoprotein modulates glucose metabolism by multiple mechanisms. Circulation 2009; 120:S468c–469.

44. Negre-Salvayre A, Dousset N, Ferretti G, et al. Antioxidant and cytoprotective properties of high-density lipoproteins in vascular cells. Free Radic Biol Med 2006;41:1031–40.

45. Terasaka N, Wang N, Yvan-Charvet L, et al. High-density lipoprotein protects macrophages from oxidized low-density lipoprotein-induced apoptosis by promoting efflux of 7-ketocholesterol via ABCG1. Proc Natl Acad Sci U S A 2007;104:15093–8.

46. Speidel MT, Booyse FM, Abrams A, et al. Lipolyzed hypertriglyceridemic serum and triglyceride-rich lipoprotein cause lipid accumulation in and are cytotoxic to cultured human endothelial cells. High density lipoproteins inhibit this cytotoxicity. Thromb Res 1990;58:251–64.

47. Sugano M, Tsuchida K, Makino N. High-density lipoproteins protect endothelial cells from tumor necrosis factor-alpha-induced apoptosis. Biochem Biophys Res Commun 2000;272:872–6.

48. Hamilton KK, Zhao J, Sims PJ. Interaction between apolipoproteins A-I and A-II and the membrane attack complex of complement. Affinity of the apoproteins for polymeric C9. J Biol Chem 1993;268:3632–8.

49. Suc I, Escargueil-Blanc I, Troly M, et al. HDL and ApoA prevent cell death of endothelial cells induced by oxidized LDL. Arterioscler Thromb Vasc Biol 1997;17:2158–66.

50. Robbesyn F, Garcia V, Auge N, et al. HDL counterbalance the proinflammatory effect of oxidized LDL by inhibiting intracellular reactive oxygen species rise, proteasome activation, and subsequent NF-kappaB activation in smooth muscle cells. FASEB J 2003;17:743–5.

51. Yvan-Charvet L, Pagler TA, Seimon TA, et al. ABCA1 and ABCG1 protect against oxidative stress-induced macrophage apoptosis during efferocytosis. Circ Res 2010;106:1861–9.

52. Tabet F, Lambert G, Cuesta Torres LF, et al. Lipid-free apolipoprotein A-I and discoidal reconstituted high-density lipoproteins differentially inhibit glucose-induced oxidative stress in human macrophages. Arterioscler Thromb Vasc Biol 2011;31:1192–200.

53. de Souza JA, Vindis C, Nègre-Salvayre A, et al. Small, dense HDL 3 particles attenuate apoptosis in endothelial cells: pivotal role of apolipoprotein A-I. J Cell Mol Med 2010;14:608–20.

54. Tselepis AD, Dentan C, Karabina SA, et al. PAF-degrading acetylhydrolase is preferentially associated with dense LDL and VHDL-1 in human plasma. Catalytic characteristics and relation to the monocyte-derived enzyme. Arterioscler Thromb Vasc Biol 1995;15:1764–73.

55. Chapman MJ, Le Goff W, Guerin M, et al. Cholesteryl ester transfer protein: at the heart of the action of lipid-modulating therapy with statins, fibrates, niacin, and cholesteryl ester transfer protein inhibitors. Eur Heart J 2010;31:149–64.

56. Lhomme M, Camont L, Chapman MJ, et al. Lipidomics in lipoprotein biology. In: Ekroos K, editor. Lipidomics: technologies and applications. Weinheim (Germany): Wiley-VCH; 2012. p. 197–231.

57. Oram JF. Tangier disease and ABCA1. Biochim Biophys Acta 2000;1529:321–30.

58. Kuivenhoven JA, Pritchard H, Hill J, et al. The molecular pathology of lecithin: cholesterol acyltransferase (LCAT) deficiency syndromes. J Lipid Res 1997;38:191–205.

59. Steinberg D, Parthasarathy S, Carew TE, et al. Beyond cholesterol. Modifications of low-density lipoprotein that increase its atherogenicity. N Engl J Med 1989;320:915–24.

60. Schwedhelm E, Bartling A, Lenzen H, et al. Urinary 8-iso-prostaglandin F2alpha as a risk marker in patients with coronary heart disease: a matched case-control study. Circulation 2004;109:843–8.

61. Meisinger C, Baumert J, Khuseyinova N, et al. Plasma oxidized low-density lipoprotein, a strong predictor for acute coronary heart disease events in apparently healthy, middle-aged men from the general population. Circulation 2005;112:651–7.

62. Hansel B, Giral P, Nobecourt E, et al. Metabolic syndrome is associated with elevated oxidative stress and dysfunctional dense high-density lipoprotein particles displaying impaired antioxidative activity. J Clin Endocrinol Metab 2004;89:4963–71.

63. Kontush A, de Faria EC, Chantepie S, et al. A normotriglyceridemic, low HDL-cholesterol phenotype is characterised by elevated oxidative stress and HDL particles with attenuated antioxidative activity. Atherosclerosis 2005;182:277–85.

64. Nobécourt E, Jacqueminet S, Hansel B, et al. Defective antioxidative activity of small dense HDL3 particles in type 2 diabetes: relationship to elevated oxidative stress and hyperglycaemia. Diabetologia 2005;48:529–38.

65. Ansell BJ, Navab M, Hama S, et al. Inflammatory/antiinflammatory properties of high-density lipoprotein distinguish patients from control subjects better than high-density lipoprotein cholesterol levels and are favorably affected by simvastatin treatment. Circulation 2003;108:2751–6.

66. Lamarche B, Rashid S, Lewis GF. HDL metabolism in hypertriglyceridemic states: an overview. Clin Chim Acta 1999;286:145–61.

67. Ng DS, Vezina C, Wolever TS, et al. Apolipoprotein A-I deficiency. Biochemical and metabolic characteristics. Arterioscler Thromb Vasc Biol 1995;15:2157–64.

68. Tato F, Vega GL, Grundy SM. Bimodal distribution of cholesteryl ester transfer protein activities in normotriglyceridemic men with low HDL cholesterol concentrations. Arterioscler Thromb Vasc Biol 1995;15:446–51.

69. Hovingh GK, Hutten BA, Holleboom AG, et al. Compromised LCAT function is associated with increased atherosclerosis. Circulation 2005;112:879–84.

70. Blades B, Vega GL, Grundy SM. Activities of lipoprotein lipase and hepatic triglyceride lipase in postheparin plasma of patients with low concentrations of HDL cholesterol. Arterioscler Thromb 1993;13:1227–35.

71. Syvänne M, Ahola M, Lahdenperä S, et al. High density lipoprotein subfractions in non-insulin-dependent diabetes mellitus and coronary artery disease. J Lipid Res 1995;36:573–82.

72. Blatter Garin MC, Kalix B, Morabia A, et al. Small, dense lipoprotein particles and reduced paraoxonase-1 in patients with the metabolic syndrome. J Clin Endocrinol Metab 2005;90:2264–9.

Causal Effect of Lipids and Lipoproteins on Atherosclerosis
Lessons from Genomic Studies

Brian A. Ference, MD, MPhil, MSc*

KEYWORDS

- Genomics • Mendelian randomization • Lipids • LDL • Apolipoprotein B • VLDL • Triglycerides
- HDL

KEY POINTS

- The causal effect of apolipoprotein B–containing lipoproteins on the risk of atherosclerotic cardiovascular disease (ASCVD) depends on both the absolute magnitude and total duration of exposure to those particles.
- The clinical benefit of lowering low-density lipoproteins (LDLs) is determined by the absolute reduction in circulating LDL particles (measured by apolipoprotein B [apoB]) rather than the reduction in cholesterol carried by those particles (measured by LDL cholesterol).
- The clinical benefit of lowering triglycerides is determined by the absolute reduction in circulating very low-density lipoproteins (VLDLs) and remnant particles (measured by apoB) rather than the reduction in triglycerides carried by those particles.
- Because atherosclerosis is caused by the retention of apoB-containing lipoproteins within the artery wall rather than the cholesterol content carried by those particles, high-density lipoprotein–mediated efflux of cholesterol from the artery wall may not reduce the risk of atherosclerosis.

INTRODUCTION

The apolipoprotein B (apoB)-100–containing lipoproteins, the vast majority of which are low-density lipoproteins (LDLs), carry cholesterol esters from the liver to the peripheral cells, whereas apolipoprotein A1-containing high-density lipoproteins (HDLs) carry excess cholesterol from the peripheral cells back to the liver.[1] The apoB-containing non-HDLs less than 70 nm in diameter freely flux across the arterial wall endothelial membrane, where they may interact with proteoglycans to become retained within the arterial wall, leading to the initiation and progression of atherosclerotic plaques.[2] By contrast, the apolipoprotein A1-containing HDL particles do not become retained but instead can efflux cholesterol from lipid-laden macrophages within the arterial wall and, therefore, can potentially decrease the progression of atherosclerosis and reduce the risk of atherosclerotic events.[3]

Consistent with this proposed mechanism for atherosclerosis, numerous epidemiologic studies have reported a strong, consistent, and dose-dependent association between increasing concentrations of plasma LDL cholesterol (LDL-C) and an increasing risk of atherosclerotic cardiovascular disease (ASCVD) and a similarly strong, consistent, and dose-dependent inverse association between increasing concentrations of plasma HDL cholesterol (HDL-C) and a decreasing risk of ASCVD.[4]

Disclosure: The author has nothing to disclose.
Institute for Advanced Studies, University of Bristol, 3rd Floor, Senate House, Bristol BS8 1UH, UK
* Division of Cardiovascular Medicine, Wayne State University School of Medicine, UHC, 4H-34, Detroit, MI 48202.
E-mail address: bference@med.wayne.edu

Cardiol Clin 36 (2018) 203–211
https://doi.org/10.1016/j.ccl.2017.12.001
0733-8651/18/© 2017 Elsevier Inc. All rights reserved.

cardiology.theclinics.com

Multiple randomized trials have demonstrated that lowering LDL-C by reducing LDL particles through up-regulation of hepatic LDL receptors with statins, ezetimibe, and PCSK9 inhibitors reduces the risk of atherosclerotic events proportional to the absolute reduction in LDL-C concentration.[5–7] By contrast, therapies that reduce LDL-C through mechanisms other than up-regulation of the LDL receptors have failed to consistently demonstrate a reduction in clinical events in randomized trials, thus raising the possibility that the clinical benefit of lowering LDL-C may depend on how LDL-C is lowered.[8,9] Similarly, therapies that predominantly lower triglyceride levels or increase HDL-C levels have also failed to consistently reduce the risk of cardiovascular events in randomized trials, thus raising the possibility that these lipids may not be causally related to the development of atherosclerosis.[10–15]

In this article, evidence from mendelian randomization studies is evaluated to assess the causal effect of various lipids and lipoproteins on the risk of ASCVD to help inform the interpretation of randomized trials and to make inferences about which therapies are most likely to reduce the risk of ASCVD events.

MENDELIAN RANDOMIZATION

A mendelian randomization study is an explicit attempt to introduce a randomization scheme into an observational study to assess whether an observed association between an exposure and an outcome is likely to be causal.[16] These studies use genetic variants that are associated with the exposure of interest as a proxy for higher or lower levels of the exposure. Because allocation of genetic variants is approximately random and occurs at conception, this study design should be less susceptible to confounding, reverse causation, and other forms of bias that can limit the validity of observational studies, thus permitting inferences to be made about causality.

Perhaps the most intuitive way to explain the concept of mendelian randomization is by way of analogy with a randomized trial. For example, numerous genetic variants are associated with lower LDL-C. Each of these variants is inherited approximately randomly at the time of conception in a process sometimes referred to as mendelian randomization. Therefore, inheriting an LDL-C–lowering allele is analogous to being randomly allocated to an LDL-C–lowering therapy whereas inheriting the other allele is analogous to being randomly allocated to usual care. If allocation is random and if the variant under study is associated only with LDL-C, but not with other

pleiotropic effects, then the only difference between the groups being compared should be their plasma LDL-C level. Therefore, measuring the association between LDL-C–lowering variants and the risk of risk of cardiovascular disease should provide an unconfounded estimate of the causal effect of lifelong exposure to lower LDL-C on the risk of cardiovascular disease in a manner analogous to a long-term randomized trial.[17,18]

LOW-DENSITY LIPOPROTEIN CHOLESTEROL

Numerous genetic variants are associated with lower LDL-C.[19] Nearly all these variants are also associated with a corresponding lower risk of ASCVD, thus providing powerful naturally randomized evidence that LDL is causally associated with the risk of ASCVD.[20] There is a dose-dependent log-linear relationship between the absolute magnitude of lifelong exposure to lower LDL-C and the corresponding risk of ASCVD. This relationship is similar to the dose-dependent log-linear relationship between the absolute reduction in LDL-C and the corresponding proportional reduction in cardiovascular events observed in the statin trials. The slope of these log-linear relationships, however, is much steeper for lifelong genetically determined exposure to lower LDL-C compared with short-term pharmacologically mediated lower LDL-C, thus implying that LDL has both causal and cumulative effects on the risk of ASCVD (**Fig. 1**).[21]

The magnitude of the cumulative effect of LDL-C on the risk of ASCVD can be estimated by adjusting the effect of each genetic variant on ASCVD for a standard decrement in LDL-C and then meta-analyzing the adjusted effect estimates, using the same methods for meta-analyzing a group of statin trials. Using this method of creating a genetic LDL score, long-term exposure to each unit lower LDL-C is associated with an approximately 3-fold greater reduction in the risk of ASCVD (on the log scale) compared with short-term exposure to LDL-C started later in life. More specifically, long-term exposure to each millimole per liter lower LDL-C is associated with up to a 55% reduction in the relative risk of ASCVD whereas each millimole per liter short-term reduction in LDL-C during treatment with a statin is associated with an approximately 20% reduction in risk.[21] This finding has important public health implications because it suggests that, for lowering LDL-C, both "lower is better" and "earlier is better." The apparent reduced efficacy of short-term exposure compared with long-term exposure to lower LDL-C may explain much of the residual risk of ASCVD among persons treated with a statin or other lipid-lowering therapy. This observation implies that the

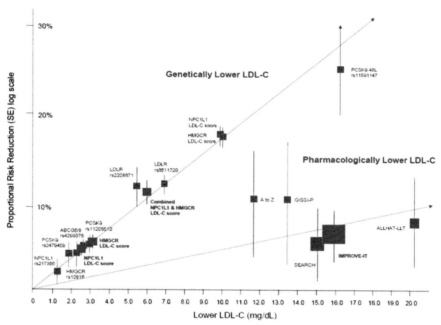

Fig. 1. Causal and cumulative effect of LDLs. Plot of absolute magnitude of genetically mediated lifetime and pharmacologically mediated short-term exposure to lower LDL. ABCG5/8, ATP-binding cassette sub-family G member 5/8; ALLHAT-LLT, the Lipid-Lowering Trial component of the Antihypertensive and Lipid-Lowering Treatment to Prevent Heart Attack Trial; A to Z, the A to Z randomized trial; GISSI-P, the GISSI-Prevenzione trial; HMGCR, HMG-CoA reductase; IMPROVE-IT, the IMProved Reduction of Outcomes: Vytorin Efficacy International Trial; LDLR, LDL receptor; NPC1L1, Niemann-Pick C1-Like 1; PCSK9, proprotein convertase subtilisin/kexin type 9; SEARCH, the Study of the Effectiveness of Additional Reductions in Cholesterol and Homocysteine trial.

most effective strategy to reduce the residual risk among persons treated with an LDL-C–lowering therapy is to initiate the LDL-C lowering earlier in the atherosclerotic disease process.

What is the Causal Effect of Lowering Low-Density Lipoprotein Cholesterol by Inhibiting HMG-CoA Reductase?

Several variants in the gene that encodes for HMG-CoA reductase, the target of statins, are independently associated with lower LDL-C.[18] These genetic variants have a remarkably similar metabolomic profile compared with statins, thus providing naturally randomized evidence that LDL-C–lowering variants in the HMG-CoA reductase gene (*HMGCR*) mimic the biological effects of statins.[22]

Furthermore, LDL-C–lowering variants in *HMGCR* are associated with a corresponding lower risk of ASCVD, thus demonstrating that lower LDL-C due to HMG-CoA inhibition is causally associated with a lower risk of ASCVD.[23] *HMGCR* variants are associated with a similar proportional reduction in multiple different composite cardiovascular events in all subgroups evaluated, just as statins reduce the risk of multiple composite cardiovascular events by approximately the same amount per millimole per liter reduction in LDL-C in all subgroups

studied.[23,24] Together, the agreement between the naturally randomized genetic evidence and the randomized trial data provide strong evidence that the effect of treatment with a statin on the risk of cardiovascular events is due, at least in part, to the corresponding reduction in LDL-C from inhibiting HMG-CoA reductase.

What is the Causal Effect of Lowering Low-Density Lipoprotein Cholesterol by Inhibiting NPC1L1?

LDL-C–lowering variants in the gene that encodes NPC1L1, the target of ezetimibe, are also associated with a lower risk of ASCVD, thus providing naturally randomized evidence that lowering LDL-C by inhibiting NPC1L1 is causally associated with a lower risk of ASCVD.[23] Variants in the *NPC1L1* and *HMGCR* genes have a nearly identical effect on the risk of ASCVD per unit lower LDL-C. This finding anticipates that lowering LDL-C by inhibiting NPC1L1 with ezetimibe should reduce the risk of cardiovascular events by the same amount as lowering LDL-C by inhibiting HMG-CoA reductase with a statin, when measured per unit change in LDL-C.

This results is precisely what the IMPROVE-IT trial showed. In the IMPROVE-IT trial, 6 years of treatment with ezetimibe reduced LDL-C by 12.5 mg/dL and reduced the risk of major vascular events by 6.5%. The magnitude of this risk reduction is nearly exactly what would have been anticipated for the same absolute reduction in LDL-C and the same duration of treatment with a statin.[6] The agreement between the naturally randomized genetic evidence and the randomized trial data suggests that lowering LDL-C with ezetimibe, a statin, or a combination of both should reduce the risk of ASCVD events proportional to the absolute reduction in LDL-C, regardless of which therapy is used. This finding challenges the orthodoxy that the statin dose should be maximized prior to adding additional LDL-C–lowering agents. Instead, these data suggest that the combination of a low-dose to moderate-dose statin plus ezetimibe should produce the same reduction in LDL-C and, therefore, should produce the same corresponding reduction in the risk of ASCVD events but has the potential to minimize the dose-dependent statin-induced side effects, thus offering a safer but equally efficacious alternative to treatment with a high-dose statin.

What is the Causal Effect of Lowering Low-Density Lipoprotein Cholesterol by Inhibiting PCSK9?

Loss of function mutations in the PCSK9 gene were originally reported to be associated with 0.5-mmol/L lower lifetime exposure to LDL-C and a large corresponding 50% proportional reduction in the lifetime risk of ASCVD.[25] This finding motivated the discovery and development of monoclonal antibodies and other therapies directed against PCSK9. Because LDL-C has both causal and cumulative effects on the risk of ASCVD events, however, the effect of these loss-of-function mutations seem to have substantially overestimated the potential clinical benefit of PCSK9 inhibitor therapies and may have created a somewhat exaggerated expectation about what to expect from PCSK9 inhibition.

Like NPC1L1 variants, variants in the PCSK9 gene have the same effect on the risk of ASCVD per unit lower LDL-C compared with variants in the HMGCR gene.[24] This finding implies that variants that mimic the effect of PCSK9 inhibitors and statins have biologically equivalent effects on the risk of ASCVD per unit lower LDL-C, and therefore statins and PCSK9 inhibitors should have therapeutically equivalent effects on the risk of cardiovascular events per unit lower LDL-C.

In the FOURIER trial, 2 years of treatment with the monoclonal antibody evoloculmab reduced LDL-C by 1.4 mmol/L and reduced the risk of major cardiovascular events by 17%.[7] The magnitude of this risk reduction was nearly exactly what would have been anticipated for the same absolute reduction in LDL-C after 2 years of treatment with a statin, precisely as anticipated by the naturally randomized genetic evidence.[26] The remarkable agreement between naturally randomized genetic evidence and the apparently equivalent effects of PCSK9 inhibitors and statins on the risk of major vascular events per unit change in LDL-C during each year of treatment in the FOURIER trial emphasizes that the clinical benefit of lowering LDL-C seems to be determined by both the absolute reduction in LDL-C and the total duration of exposure to lower LDL-C.

Does the Mechanism of Lowering Low-Density Lipoprotein Cholesterol Matter?

Genetic variants that mimic the effect of statins, ezetimibe, and PCSK9 inhibitors all have approximately the effect on the risk of ASCVD per unit lower LDL-C. Nearly all genetic variants that are associated primarily with LDL-C seem to have similar effects on the risk of ASCVD when measured per unit lower LDL-C.[27] This finding implies that the clinical benefit of lower LDL-C may be independent of the mechanism by which LDL-C is lowered.

This conclusion is consistent with a meta-analysis of more than 50 randomized trials, involving more than 350,000 subjects and 50,000 major cardiovascular events that compared the effect of therapies that lower LDL-C by 8 different mechanisms. Nearly all therapies evaluated (including statins, fibrates, niacin, bile resins, diet, and ileal bypass surgery) were associated with a similar 20% to 25% relative reduction in the risk of cardiovascular events per millimole per liter reduction in LDL-C.[28] The notable exception to this observation was the cholesterol ester transfer protein (CETP) inhibitors.

In the ACCLERATE trial, 2 years of treatment with evacetrapib plus a statin reduced LDL-C by 29 mg/dL (0.75 mmol/L) compared with treatment with a statin alone but did not significantly reduce the risk of cardiovascular events.[8] The result of this trial caused some investigators to question the causal effect of LDL-C on the risk of ASCVD and raises the possibility that the clinical benefit of lowering LDL-C may depend on how LDL-C is lowered.

Genetic variants in the CETP gene that are associated with lower CETP activity are associated with a higher HDL-C, lower LDL-C, and corresponding lower risk of ASCVD, thus demonstrating that lower CETP activity is causally associated with a lower risk of ASCVD.[29–32] The effect of genetic CETP inhibition on the risk of ASCVD seems to be proportional to the absolute decrease in LDL-C rather than to changes in HDL-C.[32] *CETP* variants have a nearly identical effect on the risk of ASCVD per unit lower LDL-C compared with other genetic variants that are associated with lower LDL-C. If this is true, then how could treatment with evacetrapib robustly lower LDL-C by 29 mg/dL in the ACCELERATE trial but fail to reduce cardiovascular events?

Is Atherosclerosis Caused by Low-Density Lipoprotein Cholesterol or Low-Density Lipoprotein Particles?

Plasma LDL-C levels are used to estimate the concentration of circulating LDL particles. Under most circumstances, LDL-C and LDL particle (or apoB) concentrations are highly correlated and therefore provide essentially the same information. It is only when LDL-C and LDL particle concentrations become discordant that the differential causal effect on the risk of ASCVD of the cholesterol content carried by LDL particles (estimated by LDL-C) and the concentration of circulating particles themselves (estimated by apoB concentration) can be compared.

When considered alone, genetic variants that mimic CETP inhibitors are associated with concordant changes in LDL-C and apoB. When combined with variants that mimic statins, genetic variants that mimic CETP inhibitors are associated with the same decrease in LDL-C but a substantially attenuated decrease in apoB and a corresponding attenuated effect on ASCVD that is proportional to the attenuated decrease in apoB but substantially less than expected per unit LDL-C. This finding strongly suggests that the causal effect of LDL on ASCVD is determined by the circulating concentration of apoB particles rather than by the cholesterol content carried by those particles.[32]

Consistent with the genetic evidence, a similar discordance between the observed reduction in LDL-C and apoB has been noted whenever any CETP inhibitor is added to a statin and seems to explain the results of both the ACCELERATE trial and the recently reported REVEAL trial.[8,9,32–34] In the ACCELERATE trial, treatment with evacetrapib plus a stain reduced LDL-C by 29 mg/dL but only reduced apoB by 13 mg/dL. After 2 years of treatment, this absolute reduction in LDL-C should have reduced the risk of cardiovascular death, nonfatal myocardial infarction, or stroke by 12.5% but only reduced the risk of this composite outcome by 3% (hazard ratio [HR] 0.97; 95% CI, 0.91–1.04), which is exactly what would have been anticipated based on the 13 mg/dL absolute reduction in apoB.[8] Similarly, in the recently completed 30,000 participant REVEAL trial,

treatment with anacetrapib plus a statin reduced LDL-C by 24 mg/dL but only reduced apoB by 12 mg/dL. After 4 years of treatment, this absolute reduction in LDL-C should have reduced the risk of cardiovascular death, nonfatal myocardial infarction, or stroke by 15.5% but only reduced the risk of this composite outcome by 6.8% (HR 0.932; 95% CI, 0.86–1.00), which is exactly what would have been anticipated based on the 12-mg/dL absolute reduction in apoB.[9]

The striking agreement between the naturally randomized genetic evidence and the randomized trials evaluating the effect of CETP inhibitors added to a statin strongly implies that the causal effect of LDL on ASCVD is determined by the concentration of circulating LDL particles (as estimated by apoB) rather than by the cholesterol content carried by the LDL particles (as estimated by LDL-C). Therefore, therapies that lower LDL-C by lowering LDL particles via up-regulation of hepatic LDL receptors should reduce the risk of ASCVD proportional to the absolute change in either LDL-C or apoB, because these changes are concordant. By contrast, therapies that lower LDL-C by a mechanism other than up-regulation of hepatic LDL receptors, for example, by altering the lipid content of LDL particles, may not reduce LDL-C and apoB proportionally. These therapies are likely to reduce the risk of ASCVD proportional to the absolute change in apoB, which may be less than expected per unit change in LDL-C, depending on the degree of discordance between the observed absolute reductions in LDL-C and apoB.

TRIGLYCERIDE-RICH VERY LOW-DENSITY LIPOPROTEINS AND THEIR REMNANTS

Just as the measurement of plasma LDL-C is used to estimate the concentration of circulating LDL particles, plasma triglyceride levels are used to estimate the concentration of VLDL particles and their remnants. Because VLDL particles and their remnants are apoB-containing lipoproteins, they can be retained within the arterial wall and may therefore increase the risk of ASCVD.

Observational epidemiologic studies have consistently demonstrated that increasing plasma triglyceride levels are associated with an increasing risk of ASCVD.[4] In addition, non–HDL-C, which is an estimate of the concentration of all circulating apoB-containing particles, including both LDL and VLDL, is strongly associated with the risk of ASCVD and has approximately the same effect on ASCVD risk as LDL-C.[4]

Mendelian randomization studies of genetic variants associated with triglyceride levels are confounded by pleiotropy, because nearly all variants associated with triglycerides are also associated with HDL-C, LDL-C or both.[19] Therefore, the causal effect of changes in triglycerides mediated by these variants cannot be independently assessed. Multivariable mendelian randomization analysis suggests, however, that triglyceride levels are likely causally associated with the risk of ASCVD and seem to have the same magnitude of effect as LDL-C, thus implying that the effect of triglycerides on ASCVD is mediated by the circulating concentration of VLDL and its remnant particles rather than by the triglyceride content carried by those particles.[35,36]

By contrast, randomized trials of triglyceride-lowering therapies, primarily the fibrates, have failed to consistently demonstrate that lowering triglycerides reduces the risk of ASCVD events.[10–13] This failure can be explained by the modest reduction in triglycerides observed in these studies. The circulating concentration of VLDL and its remnant particles is estimated by dividing the triglyceride concentration by 5 (on the milligram per deciliter scale). Therefore, if the apoB-containing LDL and VLDL particles have the same atherogenic effect when measured on the same scale as suggested by the mendelian randomization studies, then to achieve the same effect as a 40-mg/dL reduction in LDL-C, triglyceride levels would have to be reduced by 5-fold this quantity, or 200 mg/dL, to achieve the same proportional reduction in the risk of ASCVD. The mean reduction in triglyceride levels in the fibrate trials was only 20 mg/dL to 25 mg/dL, a fraction of what would be needed to significantly reduce the risk of major vascular events within a short-term trial.

The observation that large absolute reductions in plasma triglyceride levels of 200 mg/dL must be achieved to produce the same reduction in apoB-containing particles as a 40-mg/dL reduction in LDL-C (a reduction in LDL-C that has consistently resulted in a 20% relative risk reduction in ASCVD events within randomized trials) suggests that only very potent triglyceride-lowering therapies will likely be clinically useful and that these therapies are likely to reduce the risk of ASCVD only among persons with very high triglyceride levels. This finding has important implications for the design of randomized trials evaluating a new generation of therapies designed to lower triglycerides by blocking inhibition of the lipoprotein lipase pathway.[37] Because the causal effect of apoB-containing lipoproteins seems determined by the circulating concentration of these particles rather than by their lipid content, the clinical benefit of these novel therapies in development likely will be determined by the achieved absolute reductions in apoB rather than by the observed changes in trigylcerides, LDL-C, or non-HDL-C (**Fig. 2**).

HIGH-DENSITY LIPOPROTEINS

Plasma HDL particles can efflux cholesterol from lipid-laden macrophages within the arterial wall in the process of reverse cholesterol transport and, therefore, may decrease the development and progression of atherosclerotic lesions. The inverse association between HDL-C and the risk of ASCVD is among the most consistent and reproducible associations in observational epidemiology.

By contrast, evidence from mendelian randomization studies does not provide compelling evidence that HDL-C is causally associated with the risk of ASCVD.[38–40] Most genetic variants associated with HDL-C, however, are also associated with directionally opposite changes in triglycerides, LDL-C, or both, thus making unconfounded causal estimates of the effect of HDL-C on the risk of ASCVD difficult using the mendelian randomization study design.

Similarly, most therapies that raise HDL-C (including niacin, fibrates, and CETP inhibitors) also lower triglycerides, LDL-C, or both.[8–14] As a result, it can be argued that the clinical benefit of raising HDL-C has not been robustly and directly tested in randomized trials. In the dal-OUTCOMES trial, however, treatment with the CETP inhibitor dalcetrapib increased HDL-C by 12 mg/dL and increased cholesterol efflux but did not have any effect on LDL-C or apoB and did not reduce the risk of major cardiovascular events.[15] In addition, in the ACCLERATE and REVEAL trials, treatment with potent CETP inhibitors more than doubled HDL-C levels (by 43–58 mg/dL) but did not seem to reduce the risk of ASCVD events beyond that expected from the modest reductions in apoB levels. Furthermore, several randomized trials have shown that directly infused HDL mimetics can increase HDL-C concentration and measures of cholesterol efflux but have not reduced the progression of atherosclerosis as measured by intravascular ultrasound.[41,42]

Together the naturally randomized genetic studies and the randomized trials suggest that, as with the apoB-containing lipoproteins, the cholesterol content of HDL particles does not seem causally associated with the risk of ASCVD. Therefore, therapies that simply increase plasma HDL-C concentration by increasing the cholesterol content carried by those particles are unlikely to reduce the risk of ASCVD events. Whether therapies that potently increase cholesterol efflux or alter the function of HDL particles will reduce the risk of ASCVD is unknown. If the risk of atherosclerosis is determined by the concentration of circulating apoB-containing particles, however, which become retained within the artery wall rather than by the cholesterol content carried by those

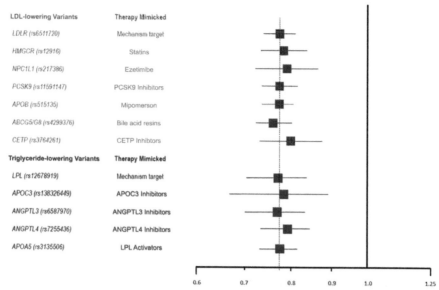

Fig. 2. Effect of genetic variants that mimic LDL and triglyceride-lowering therapies on the risk of cardiovascular disease per unit change in apoB-containing lipoproteins. Boxes represent point estimate of effect of each variant on the risk of cardiovascular disease per 10 mg/dL lower apoB. Lines represent 95% CIs. The dotted line represents mean effect for variants that lower LDL cholesterol (LDL-C) by reducing LDL particles through up-regulating the LDL receptor on the risk of cardiovascular disease per 10 mg/dL lower apoB. The figure demonstrates that genetic variants that mimic LDL-C and triglyceride-lowering therapies seem to have the same effect on the risk of cardiovascular disease per unit change in apoB despite being associated with very different corresponding reductions in LDL-C and triglycerides, indicating that the causal effect of these variants (and therapies) is determined by the absolute reduction in apoB-containing particles rather than by the changes in lipid content carried by those particles. ABCG5/8, ATP-binding cassette sub-family G member 5/8; ANGPTL3, Angiopoietin-like 3; ANGPTL4, Angiopoietin-like 4; APOA5, apolipoprotein A-V; APOB, apolipoprotein B; APOC3, Apolipoprotein C-III; CETP, cholesterol ester transfer protein; HMGCR, HMG-CoA reductase; LDLR, LDL receptor; LPL, lipoprotein lipase; NPC1L1, Niemann-Pick C1-Like 1; PCSK9, proprotein convertase subtilisin/kexin type 9.

particles, as suggested by the naturally randomized genetic evidence, then effluxing cholesterol from the macrophages within the arterial wall may not have any effect on the risk of ASCVD, thus challenging the role of reverse cholesterol transport in the development of atherosclerosis.

LIPOPROTEIN(A)

Lipoprotein(a) (Lp[a]) is an LDL particle with an apolipoprotein(a) [apo(a)] moiety covalently bound to the its apoB component.[43] Because it is an apoB-containing lipoprotein less than 70 nm in diameter, Lp(a) can freely flux across endothelial membranes and become retained within the arterial wall and thus may increase the risk of ASCVD.

Observational epidemiologic studies have reported that increased plasma Lp(a) concentration is associated with an increased risk of ASCVD but that it seems a much weaker risk factor for most people than LDL-C.[44] By contrast, mendelian randomization studies have consistently demonstrated that lifelong exposure to higher Lp(a) levels due to variants in the LPA gene is strongly and

causally associated with an increased risk of ASCVD.[45,46]

Some mendelian randomization studies have suggested that the risk of ASCVD is linearly proportional to log-transformed changes in Lp(a) levels.[47] A 1-unit log-transformed decrease represents a 63% reduction in Lp(a) levels, implying that a reduction Lp(a) from 100 mg/dL to 37 mg/dL (63 mg/dL) would have the same effect on the risk of ASCVD as an Lp(a) reduction from 10 mg/dL to 3.7 mg/dL (6.3 mg/dL), a 10-fold difference in the absolute change in Lp(a) levels. This is extremely unlikely because Lp(a) is an apoB-containing LDL-like particle. Instead, like other aopB-containing particles, the effect of Lp(a) on the risk of ASCVD is more likely proportional to the absolute change in Lp(a) levels.

Several trials of therapies that lower Lp(a) by 20% to 30% (including niacin, CETP inhibitors, and PCSK9 inhibitors) have not provided any evidence that lowering Lp(a) reduces the risk of ASCVD. Because the median Lp(a) among participants enrolled in these trials was only 12 mg/dL to 20 mg/dL, however, the observed 20% to 30%

reduction in Lp(a) translated into only very small absolute decreases in Lp(a) levels of 2.5 mg/dL to 4.5 mg/dL.[7–9,13,14] These data imply that large absolute reductions in Lp(a) may be needed to reduce the risk of atherosclerotic events and, therefore, only persons with very high baseline Lp(a) levels are likely to benefit from potent Lp(a)-lowering agents currently in development.

SUMMARY

Mendelian randomization studies clearly demonstrate that apoB-containing lipoproteins, the vast majority of which are LDL particles, have both causal and cumulative effects on the risk of ASCVD. The remarkable agreement between the mendelian randomization studies and the results of randomized trials demonstrate that the clinical benefit of lipid-lowering therapies depends on both the absolute reduction in circulating apoB-containing lipoproteins (rather than the corresponding reduction in plasma LDL-C or triglyceride levels) and the total duration of exposure to lower LDL and other apoB-containing lipoproteins. Is possible that much of the residual risk of ASCVD events experienced by patients treated with a statin or other lipid-lowering agent may be because lipid-lowering therapy was initiated too late in the atherosclerotic disease process. Furthermore, because mendelian randomization studies suggest that atherosclerosis seems to be caused by the retention of apoB-containing lipoproteins rather than by the cholesterol content carried by those lipoproteins, HDL-mediated efflux of cholesterol from the arterial wall may not reduce the risk of ASCVD.

REFERENCES

1. Goldstein JL, Brown MS. A century of cholesterol and coronaries: from plaques to genes to statins. Cell 2015;161:161–72.
2. Skålén K, Gustafsson M, Rydberg EK, et al. Subendothelial retention of atherogenic lipoproteins in early atherosclerosis. Nature 2002;417:750–4.
3. Chapman MJ, Le Goff W, Guerin M, et al. Cholesteryl ester transfer protein: at the heart of the action of lipid-modulating therapy with statins, fibrates, niacin, and cholesteryl ester transfer protein inhibitors. Eur Heart J 2010;31:149–64.
4. Emerging Risk Factors Collaborators. Lipid-related markers and cardiovascular disease prediction. JAMA 2012;307:2499–506.
5. Cholesterol Treatment Trialists' (CTT) Collaboration. Efficacy and safety of more intensive lowering of LDL cholesterol: a meta-analysis of data from 170 000 participants in 26 randomised trials. Lancet 2010;376:1670–81.
6. Cannon CP, Blazing MA, Giugliano RP, et al. Ezetimibe added to statin therapy after acute coronary syndromes. N Engl J Med 2015;372:2387–97.
7. Sabatine MS, Giugliano RP, Keech AC, et al. Evolocumab and clinical outcomes in patients with cardiovascular disease. N Engl J Med 2017;376:1713–22.
8. Lincoff AM, Nicholls SJ, Riesmeyer JS, et al. Evacetrapib and cardiovascular outcomes in high-risk vascular disease. N Engl J Med 2017;376:1933–42.
9. HPS3/TIMI55–REVEAL Collaborative Group. Effects of anacetrapib in patients with atherosclerotic vascular disease. N Engl J Med 2017;377:1217–27.
10. Keech A, Simes RJ, Barter P, et al, FIELD study investigators. Effects of long-term fenofibrate therapy on cardiovascular events in 9795 people with type 2 diabetes mellitus (the FIELD study): randomised controlled trial. Lancet 2005;366:1849–61.
11. Ginsberg HN, Elam MB, Lovato LC, et al, ACCORD Study Group. Effects of combination lipid therapy in type 2 diabetes mellitus. N Engl J Med 2010; 362(17):1563–74.
12. Rubins HB, Robins SJ, Collins D, et al. Gemfibrozil for the secondary prevention of coronary heart disease in men with low levels of high-density lipoprotein cholesterol. Veterans Affairs High-Density Lipoprotein Cholesterol Intervention Trial Study Group. N Engl J Med 1999;341:410–8.
13. AIM-HIGH Investigators. Niacin in patients with low HDL cholesterol levels receiving intensive statin therapy. N Engl J Med 2011;365:2255–67.
14. HPS2-THRIVE Collaborative Group. Effects of extended-release niacin with laropiprant in high-risk patients. N Engl J Med 2014;371:203–12.
15. Schwartz GG, Olsson AG, Abt M, et al. Effects of dalcetrapib in patients with a recent acute coronary syndrome. N Engl J Med 2012;367:2089–99.
16. Davey Smith G, Hemani G. Mendelian randomization: genetic anchors for causal inference in epidemiological studies. Hum Mol Genet 2014;23(R1):R89–98.
17. Ference BA. Mendelian randomization studies: using naturally randomized genetic data to fill evidence gaps. Curr Opin Lipidol 2015;26:566–71.
18. Ference BA. How to use Mendelian randomization to anticipate the results of randomized trials. Eur Heart J 2017. https://doi.org/10.1093/eurheartj/ehx462.
19. Global Lipids Genetics Consortium. Discovery and refinement of loci associated with lipid levels. Nat Genet 2013;45:1274–83.
20. CARDIoGRAMplusC4D Consortium.. A comprehensive 1000 genomes-based genome-wide association meta-analysis of coronary artery disease. Nat Genet 2015;47: 1121–30.
21. Ference BA, Yoo W, Alesh I, et al. Effect of long-term exposure to lower low-density lipoprotein cholesterol beginning early in life on the risk of coronary heart disease: a Mendelian randomization analysis. J Am Coll Cardiol 2012;60:2631–9.

22. Würtz P, Wang Q, Soininen P, et al. Metabolomic profiling of statin use and genetic inhibition of HMG-CoA reductase. J Am Coll Cardiol 2016;67:1200–10.

23. Ference BA, Majeed F, Penumetcha R, et al. Effect of naturally random allocation to lower low-density lipoprotein cholesterol on the risk of coronary heart disease mediated by polymorphisms in NPC1L1, HMGCR, or both: a 2 x 2 factorial Mendelian randomization study. J Am Coll Cardiol 2015;65:1552–61.

24. Ference BA, Robinson JG, Brook RD, et al. Variation in PCSK9 and HMGCR and risk of cardiovascular disease and diabetes. N Engl J Med 2016;375:2144–53.

25. Cohen JC, Boerwinkle E, Mosley TH Jr, et al. Sequence variations in PCSK9, low LDL, and protection against coronary heart disease. N Engl J Med 2006;354(12):1264–72.

26. Ference BA, Cannon CP, Landmesser U, et al. Reduction of low density lipoprotein-cholesterol and cardiovascular events with proprotein convertase subtilisin-kexin type 9 (PCSK9) inhibitors and statins: an analysis of FOURIER, SPIRE, and the Cholesterol Treatment Trialists Collaboration. Eur Heart J 2017. https://doi.org/10.1093/eurheartj/ehx450.

27. Ference BA, Ginsberg HN, Graham I, et al. Low-density lipoproteins cause atherosclerotic cardiovascular disease. 1. Evidence from genetic, epidemiologic, and clinical studies. A consensus statement from the European Atherosclerosis Society Consensus Panel. Eur Heart J 2017;38:2459–72.

28. Silverman MG, Ference BA, Im K, et al. Association between lowering LDL-C and cardiovascular risk reduction among different therapeutic interventions: a systematic review and meta-analysis. JAMA 2016;316:1289–97.

29. Thompson A, Di Angelantonio E, Sarwar N, et al. Association of cholesteryl ester transfer protein genotypes with CETP mass and activity, lipid levels, and coronary risk. JAMA 2008;299:2777–88.

30. Johannsen TH, Frikke-Schmidt R, Schou J, et al. Genetic inhibition of CETP, ischemic vascular disease and mortality, and possible adverse effects. J Am Coll Cardiol 2012;60:2041–8.

31. Ridker PM, Paré G, Parker AN, et al. Polymorphism in the CETP gene region, HDL cholesterol, and risk of future myocardial infarction: genomewide analysis among 18 245 initially healthy women from the Women's Genome Health Study. Circ Cardiovasc Genet 2009;2:26–33.

32. Ference BA, Kastelein JJP, Ginsberg HN, et al. Association of genetic variants related to CETP inhibitors and statins with lipoprotein levels and cardiovascular risk. JAMA 2017;318(10):947–56.

33. Hovingh GK, Kastelein JJ, van Deventer SJ, et al. Cholesterol ester transfer protein inhibition by TA-8995 in patients with mild dyslipidaemia (TULIP): a randomised, double-blind, placebo-controlled phase 2 trial. Lancet 2015;386:452–60.

34. Cannon CP, Shah S, Dansky HM, et al. Safety of anacetrapib in patients with or at high risk for coronary heart disease. N Engl J Med 2010;363:2406–15.

35. Burgess S, Freitag DF, Khan H, et al. Using multivariable Mendelian randomization to disentangle the causal effects of lipid fractions. PLoS One 2014;9(10):e108891.

36. White J, Swerdlow DI, Preiss D, et al. Association of lipid fractions with risks for coronary artery disease and diabetes. JAMA Cardiol 2016;1:692–9.

37. Gaudet D, Alexander VJ, Baker BF, et al. Antisense inhibition of apolipoprotein C-III in patients with hypertriglyceridemia. N Engl J Med 2015;373:438–47.

38. Frikke-Schmidt R, Nordestgaard BG, Stene MC, et al. Association of loss-of-function mutations in the ABCA1 gene with high-density lipoprotein cholesterol levels and risk of ischemic heart disease. JAMA 2008;299:2524–32.

39. Voight BF, Peloso GM, Orho-Melander M, et al. Plasma HDL cholesterol and risk of myocardial infarction: a mendelian randomisation study. Lancet 2012;380:572–80.

40. Holmes MV, Asselbergs FW, Palmer TM, et al. Mendelian randomization of blood lipids for coronary heart disease. Eur Heart J 2015;36:539–50.

41. Andrews J, Janssan A, Nguyen T, et al. Effect of serial infusions of reconstituted high-density lipoprotein (CER-001) on coronary atherosclerosis: rationale and design of the CARAT study. Cardiovasc Diagn Ther 2017;7(1):45–51.

42. Tardif JC, Ballantyne CM, Barter P, et al. Effects of the high-density lipoprotein mimetic agent CER-001 on coronary atherosclerosis in patients with acute coronary syndromes: a randomized trial. Eur Heart J 2014;35(46):3277–86.

43. Nordestgaard BG, Langsted A. Lipoprotein(a) as a cause of cardiovascular disease: insights from epidemiology, genetics, and biology. J Lipid Res 2016;57:1953–75.

44. Emerging Risk Factors Collaboration. Lipoprotein(a) concentration and the risk of coronary heart disease, stroke, and nonvascular mortality. JAMA 2009;302:412–23.

45. Clarke R, Peden JF, Hopewell JC, et al. Genetic variants associated with Lp(a) lipoprotein level and coronary disease. N Engl J Med 2009;361:2518–28.

46. Kamstrup PR, Tybjaerg-Hansen A, Steffensen R, et al. Genetically elevated lipoprotein(a) and increased risk of myocardial infarction. JAMA 2009;301:2331–9.

47. Emdin CA, Khera AV, Natarajan P, et al. Phenotypic characterization of genetically lowered human lipoprotein(a) levels. J Am Coll Cardiol 2016;68(25):2761–72.

Lipids and Lipoproteins in Risk Prediction

Savvas Hadjiphilippou, BSc, MBBS*, Kausik K. Ray, BSc, MBChB, MD, MPhil (Cantab)

KEYWORDS

- Lipids • Low-density lipoprotein cholesterol • Atherosclerotic coronary artery disease
- Lipoproteins

KEY POINTS

- Low-density lipoprotein cholesterol (LDL-C) is causal in the development of atherosclerotic cardiovascular disease, and treatment has been shown to improve coronary artery disease mortality.
- Despite treatment of LDL-C, a proportion of patients continue to experience clinical events, known as residual risk, despite reductions.
- Research into other lipid factors that may be associated with risk has identified lipid and apolipoprotein parameters, which may offer advantages when used in conjunction with existing lipid risk prediction models.
- Studies measuring lipoprotein concentration using nuclear magnetic resonance spectroscopy are promising; however, the technology is not widely available, which limits its current use.

INTRODUCTION

Globally, ischemic heart disease remains the leading cause of death.[1] With such a significant burden on the public health system, much work has been undertaken in improving the ability to predict and subsequently reduce the risk of future coronary artery disease. The Framingham study was among the first to establish cholesterol as a risk factor for cardiovascular disease.[2] Cholesterol metabolism is a complex process (**Fig. 1**) and decades of research have demonstrated that the cholesterol cargo transported principally by low-density lipoprotein (LDL) particles initiates atherogenesis and is a causal factor in the development of atherosclerotic cardiovascular

disease.[3–6] Although elevated total cholesterol (TC) and low high-density lipoprotein cholesterol (HDL-C) are associated with increased cardiovascular risk, to this date given its proven causal nature, lowering LDL cholesterol (LDL-C) has been the main therapeutic target.[7] Reducing LDL-C results in reductions in major coronary and vascular events. A meta-analysis quantified that a 1 mmol/L reduction in LDL-C was associated with a 10% reduction in all-cause mortality, a 20% reduction in coronary artery disease–related mortality, and a reduction of 21% to 23% in fatal and nonfatal events.[8]

Risk prediction calculators incorporate recognized causal associations between risk factors and cardiovascular disease in an attempt to

Disclosures: Dr S. Hadjiphilippou has nothing to disclose. Dr K.K. Ray reports personal fees from Medicines Company, during the conduct of the study; grants from Sanofi, grants from Regeneron, grants from Amgen, grants from Pfizer, grants from MSD, personal fees from Sanofi, personal fees from Amgen, personal fees from Regeneron, personal fees from Pfizer, personal fees from Kowa, personal fees from Algorithm, personal fees from IONIS, personal fees from Esperion, personal fees from Novo Nordisk, personal fees from Takeda, personal fees from Boehringer Ingelheim, personal fees from Resverlogix, personal fees from Abbvie, personal fees from Cerenis, personal fees from Cipla, personal fees from Mylan, personal fees from Janssen, personal fees from Lilly, outside the submitted work.
Department of Primary Care and Public Health, School of Public Health, Imperial College, Imperial Centre for Cardiovascular Disease Prevention, Reynolds Building, St. Dunstan's Road, London W6 8RP, UK
* Corresponding author.
E-mail address: s.hadjiphilippou@nhs.net

cardiology.theclinics.com

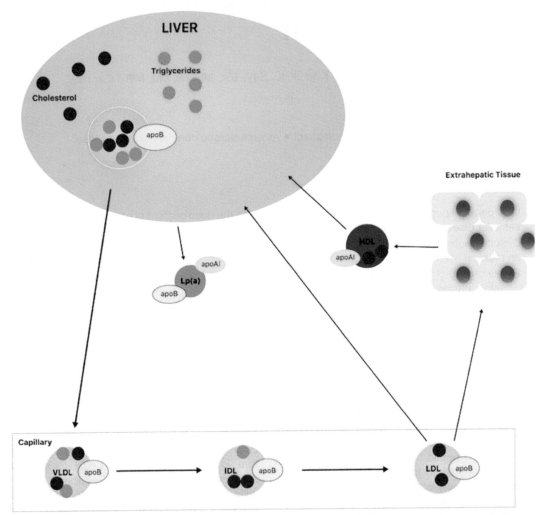

Fig. 1. The cholesterol pathway. Endogenous cholesterol synthesis occurs via the mevalonate pathway. In the liver, cholesterol esters, triglycerides (TGs), and phospholipids are packaged with apoB100, into very-low-density lipoproteins (VLDLs), which are released into the circulation. Apolipoproteins are proteins that bind to lipids to form lipoproteins and they are a key part of lipid metabolism. Apolipoprotein A-I (apoA-I) is the largest component of high-density lipoprotein (HDL), which additionally acts as a mediator in transferring cholesterol from cells to HDL. ApoB100 is present in LDL, intermediate-density lipoproteins (IDLs), VLDLs, and chylomicrons. It is important in binding the lipoprotein to specific tissue receptors, as well as for transporting cholesterol to peripheral cells. Most of the TGs in VLDL are hydrolyzed by lipoprotein lipase (LPL) in extrahepatic tissues, generating TG-depleted IDL, which is either cleared or converted to LDL by further depletion of TGs. LDL particles are the main carriers of cholesterol within the blood and are cleared from the circulation primarily by hepatic LDL receptors on hepatocytes that recognize apoB100 as a ligand. HDL is a class of lipoprotein synthesized by the liver, packaged with apolipoproteins as a complex, whose function is to transport cholesterol from extrahepatic tissues to the liver for excretion. Lipoprotein(a) (Lp[a]) is an LDL-like particle consisting of a variable repeat apolipoprotein(a) particle bound to an LDL particle that exists mainly in the circulation. apoA1, apolipoprotein A-I; apoB, apolipoprotein B100; HDL, high-density lipoprotein; IDL, intermediate-density lipoprotein; LDL, low- density lipoprotein; Lp(a), lipoprotein(a); VLDL, very-low-density lipoprotein.

identify individuals most at risk and hence most likely to benefit from lipid-lowering therapies.[9–11] However, even among those treated with LDL-C–lowering therapies, residual cardiovascular risk remains.[12] In the Scandinavian Simvastatin Survival Study (4S), 19% of subjects in the simvastatin group experienced 1 or more major coronary events despite treatment.[13] This has prompted research into other factors that may be contributory toward atherosclerotic cardiovascular disease aside from LDL-C. There is evidence that incorporating other measures of atherogenic lipoproteins, such as apolipoprotein B100 (apoB100) or non-HDL-C, even if not for widespread use, may offer advantages,[11,14] particularly in specific subpopulations. Whether newer lipid markers can better predict future cardiovascular risk than traditional lipid measures do remains unclear. There is considerable debate as to whether the cholesterol content of different lipoproteins, particle number, or size may be more appropriate measures of risk; however, uncertainty remains on the cost-benefits of routine use of these measures in addition to current practice in general populations free from cardiovascular disease.

TRADITIONAL LIPID RISK FACTORS
Non–High-Density Lipoprotein Cholesterol

Non-HDL-C is the TC in atherogenic lipoproteins after HDL-C has been subtracted and includes LDL, VLDL, IDL, and Lp(a). There is increasing evidence that non-HDL-C is more strongly associated with cardiovascular risk than LDL-C alone, including in statin-treated patients[15–19] (**Table 1**). At a genetic level, the non-HDL-C genetic risk score is strongly associated with coronary artery disease and conferred a risk of coronary artery disease beyond that of LDL-C.[20] This becomes particularly relevant for patients with low LDL-C levels (<2.6 mmol/L) who under other circumstances would have been considered to have

met their target LDL-C levels with treatment. Despite the low LDL-C levels, those with a non-HDL-C greater than 3.4 mmol/L have been shown to have a hazard ratio (HR) for further coronary heart disease of 1.84 (95% CI 1.12–3.04) when compared with those with non-HDL-C levels less than 3.4 mmol/L.[21]

However, why should non-HDL-C be more strongly associated with risk of coronary artery disease than LDL-C? Perhaps this relates to non-HDL-C more accurately representing the total content of cholesterol in all atherogenic particles rather than the fraction with LDL alone. There has, as a result, been a shift in dyslipidemia guidance toward an increasing role in using non-HDL-C as measure of therapeutic efficacy and atherogenic risk. In the United Kingdom, guidelines now recommend the use of non-HDL-C rather than LDL-C as a primary prevention target given that it is a better cardiovascular disease risk predictor, its measurement is more accurate and cost-effective, and it does not require a fasting sample to be taken.[22] The 2016 Canadian guidance recommends the use of non-HDL as an alternate target to LDL-C to evaluate risk in adults and anticipates a shift to this as a primary target as clinicians become more familiar with its use. In addition, it recommends use of non-HDL-C as the treatment target of choice in patients with elevated TG levels (>1.5 mmol/L) because it is not affected by eating or by TG levels.[23]

Triglycerides

Guidance on using TG levels is less clear. The PROVE-IT TIMI 22 (The Pravastatin or Atorvastatin Evaluation and Infection Therapy–Thrombolysis in Myocardial Infarction 22) trial, demonstrated that low on-treatment TG levels (<1.69 mmol/L) were associated with reduced coronary heart disease risk compared with higher TG levels (HR 0.73, CI 0.62–0.87; P<.001).[24] In addition, for each 0.11 mmol/L decrement in on-treatment TG levels, the incidence of death, myocardial infarction, and recurrent acute coronary syndrome was lower by 1.6% or 1.4% after adjustment for LDL-C or non-HDL. The strength of association seems to be attenuated after adjusting for established risk factors.[25] Moreover, a population-based study by the Emerging Risk Factors Collaboration (ERFC) found that the association between TG levels and coronary artery disease risk was lost after adjusting for HDL-C, non-HDL-C, and standard risk factors.[4] Given the findings of this study, it has been postulated that remnant cholesterol may more likely be the etiologic reason for atherosclerotic

Table 1
Adjusted hazard ratios for risk of major cardiovascular events for individual lipids and lipoprotein markers

	Boekholdt et al,[19] 2012[a]	Kastelein et al,[15] 2008[b]	Ridker et al,[16] 2005[c]
LDL-C	1.13	1.15	1.62
Non-HDL-C	1.16	1.19	2.51
apoB100	1.14	1.19	2.50
apoB100/ apoA-I ratio	—	1.24	3.01
TC/HDL ratio	—	1.21	3.81
apoA	—	—	1.75
HDL-C	—	—	2.32

[a] Hazard ratios for risk of major cardiovascular events adjusted for established risk factors.
[b] Individual relationships between on-treatment levels and major cardiovascular events in TNT (Treating to New Targets) trial and IDEAL (the Incremental Decrease in Events through Aggressive Lipid Lowering) study. Calculated by a Cox proportional hazard model with adjustment for the effects of study, age, and sex.
[c] Hazard ratios of future cardiovascular events among individuals in the extreme quintiles of each measured variable.

cardiovascular disease. Remnant cholesterol is the cholesterol found in TG-rich lipoproteins (VLDL, IDL) and TG levels are a surrogate marker of remnant cholesterol.[26] A 1 mmol/L increase in remnant cholesterol is associated with a 2.8-fold causal risk for ischemic heart disease independent of reduced HDL-C.[26]

Although the ERFC 2009 study did not demonstrate an association, that does not preclude a causal relationship between TG and cardiovascular risk. Further investigating a polymorphism of apolipoprotein A5, a genetic determinant of TG concentrations, revealed that this was related to the risk of coronary heart disease in a dose-dependent manner.[27] Heterozygous loss-of-function genetic mutations resulting in lower TG levels were also found to be associated with reduced risk of atherosclerotic cardiovascular disease.[28,29] Although currently no national dyslipidemia guidelines recommend TG as a treatment target because no randomized trials have convincingly demonstrated benefit from TG lowering, they do still represent a good marker of increased cardiovascular risk.

High-Density Lipoprotein Cholesterol

Since the original Framingham study report demonstrating that low HDL-C levels were associated with increased cardiovascular risk, low HDL-C is has been suggested to be an independent risk marker for coronary heart disease.[30–32] The association between HDL-C and cardiovascular risk, however, is not as straightforward as occasionally portrayed to patients in the clinical setting. The JUPITER trial analysis demonstrated that residual risk after aggressive statin therapy is not related to HDL-C concentrations.[33] Further analysis of JUPITER (The Justification for the Use of Statins in Prevention: an Intervention Trial Evaluating Rosuvastatin) trial participants with LDL-C less than 3.4 mmol/L identified that this on-treatment residual risk was likely to be related to other lipid parameters, such as apoB100 and VLDL.[34] Additionally, genetic polymorphisms related to HDL-C were not associated with the risk of myocardial infarction, suggesting that raising HDL-C levels may not reduce the risk of myocardial infarction.[35]

Total Cholesterol to High-Density Lipoprotein Cholesterol Ratio

The TC to HDL-C (TC/HDL-C) ratio does, however, have a clearer association with cardiovascular risk. The imbalance between the atherogenic and protective lipoprotein seems to correlate with cardiovascular risk. In an analysis of 32,826 subjects from the Nurses' Health Study, the TC/HDL-C ratio

was found to be independently associated with risk of coronary heart disease events among postmenopausal women (relative risk [RR] 1.6).[36] In addition, the study suggested that the single TC/HDL-C ratio may be more useful than its separate values. Baseline TC/HDL-C ratio was also predictive of coronary events in other studies[37–39] and has since been incorporated into many risk prediction tools. However, a major limitation is that the relationship between HDL-C and risk is not linear. Hence, at higher levels, the protective effects of higher HDL-C may be overestimated.

EMERGING RISK FACTORS
Apolipoproteins

Apolipoproteins are proteins that bind to lipids to form lipoproteins. Within HDL, the main apolipoprotein is apoA-I, whereas within LDL the main apolipoprotein is apoB100. Measured apolipoprotein levels give an indication of the concentration of lipoproteins rather than the cholesterol content of lipoproteins. Given that apoB100 is present not only in LDL but also in VLDL and IDL, its level gives a better estimate of the concentration of atherogenic particles.[40] ApoB100 and apoA-I have been shown to have similar strengths of associations with coronary heart disease as non-HDL-C and HDL-C, respectively.[4,16]

ApoB100 is associated with the risk of coronary heart disease independent of other traditional risk factors.[41] In the Air Force/Texas Coronary Atherosclerosis Prevention Study (AFCAPS/TexCAPS) study,[37] only apoB100 was a predictor of cardiovascular risk both at baseline and at 1-year follow-up, whereas LDL-C was not ($P<.001$). Similarly, only apoA-I achieved statistical significance as a predictor of outcome at 1-year follow-up, whereas HDL-C did not. The association between apoB100 and cardiovascular risk is recognized within national guidance[23,42,43] with treatment targets (Table 2). More recently, a causal role for apoB100 in the development of atherosclerotic cardiovascular disease has been suggested following studies on cholesterol ester transfer protein inhibition.[44,45] Based on what is already known from the Cholesterol Treatment Trialists'

Table 2 Secondary target levels for patients with a Framingham Risk Score greater than 20%		
	ApoB100	Non-HDL-C
Canada[23]	<0.0016 mmol/L	<2.6 mmol/L
European[42]	<0.0016 mmol/L	<2.6 mmol/L
USA[43]	<0.0016 mmol/L	<2.6 mmol/L

Regression Line,[8] reductions in cardiovascular risk seem to be proportional to changes in the concentration of apoB100 lipoproteins rather than LDL-C or HDL-C.[44,45]

Although the concentration of apoA-I on HDL-C is variable and therefore limits its clinical utility as an isolated biomarker, the same is not true of the apoB100/apoA-I ratio, which is significantly associated with future cardiovascular risk.[15,46] In the AFCAPS/TexCAPS study[37] the apoB100/apoA-I ratio was associated with coronary events at both baseline and 1-year follow-up unlike the TC/HDL ratio, which only predicted outcomes at baseline and not at 1-year follow-up. In a further prospective cohort study, the apoB100/apoA-I ratio demonstrated an HR of 3.18 (95% CI 2.12–4.75). This association was independent of nonlipid covariates.[16] In the INTERHEART (The Effect of Potentially Modifiable Risk Factors Associated with Myocardial Infarction) study,[47] the apoB100/apoA-I ratio was associated with the strongest effect on the RR (3.58, 95% CI 2.08–6.19). To date, the European Society of Cardiology and European Atherosclerosis Society (EAS) dyslipidemia guidelines[42] recommend that the TC/HDL-C ratio and the apoB100/ApoA-I ratio are useful in risk estimation but not for diagnosis or treatment targets.

Lipoprotein(a)

Lp(a) is an LDL-like particle that consists of a variable repeat apolipoprotein(a) particle bound to an LDL particle. Elevated levels of Lp(a) are associated with increased cardiovascular risk.[48] The Lp(a) gene is noted to be the strongest monogenetic risk factor for coronary artery disease regardless of race.[49] Although Lp(a) demonstrates a weak correlation with known risk factors, including TC, non-HDL-C, and apoB100, there is a continuous correlation between Lp(a) and risk of coronary heart disease.[50] The RR for coronary heart disease does not vary by sex, non-HDL-C, or HDL-C, suggesting that Lp(a) is an independent risk factor for coronary heart disease.[50] Genome-wide studies have further supported a causal role for Lp(a) in the development of coronary disease.[51]

In 2010, the EAS recommended screening for elevated Lp(a) in individuals at intermediate or high coronary heart disease risk,[52] whereas Canadian guidelines recommend the use of Lp(a) in risk assessment of individuals at intermediate risk or with a family history of premature coronary artery disease.[23]

Lipoprotein Particles

To date, measurement of the cholesterol content of lipids, such as LDL-C, has been the main measure of cardiovascular risk; however, the cholesterol content of LDL particles is known to vary among individuals,[53] which may result in discrepancies between cholesterol content and particle numbers. It was, therefore, postulated that particle size and concentration represent a more accurate marker of future cardiovascular risk. These can be measured using techniques such as ultracentrifugation, gel electrophoresis, or nuclear magnetic resonance (NMR) spectroscopy and values are expressed as particles per liter (concentration) or nanometers (particle size).

Using NMR in a cohort of healthy women, measured lipoproteins were significantly associated with incident cardiovascular disease and comparable with that of standard lipids or apolipoproteins but not superior.[54] The association between LDL particle concentration and coronary artery disease events seems to remain even after accounting for LDL-C.[55,56] Additionally, lipoprotein particle number and size has been shown to be more strongly associated with vascular structure and function than other traditional lipid measurements.[57] Considering the associations, does addition of lipoprotein particle size and concentration improve the risk prediction capability? The Bogalusa Heart Study has not demonstrated that advanced lipoprotein variables predict increased carotid intimamedia thickness better than traditional lipoproteins, albeit lipoprotein particles were measured using ultracentrifugation and subjects were young (20–38 years) asymptomatic adults.[58] More importantly, in discordant subjects (ie, those with a difference between LDL-C and LDL particle concentration >12%), only LDL particle concentration was associated with incident cardiovascular disease (HR 1.45).[59]

Although showing promise, national dyslipidemia guidance does not currently recommend using lipoprotein particle size for risk estimation due to their heterogeneous nature and contributory effect on future risk, as well as the unclear causal relation of subclasses to atherosclerosis. In addition, the technology and expertise required for measuring particle size and number is not widely available.

SUMMARY

Since identifying LDL-C as a causal factor in developing atherosclerotic cardiovascular disease and evidence that despite reductions in LDL-C residual risk remains, there has been an increasing emphasis on identifying other lipids, apolipoproteins, and their ratios to improve risk prediction. With the discovery and increasing use of other measures, such as non-HDL-C and apoB100, coupled with techniques to measure these, which are standardized and less influenced by diet, there will undoubtedly be a drive to include these within future risk prediction models after their cost-effectiveness over traditional markers has been assessed. Already, the UK National Institute for Health and Care Excellence recommends the use of non-HDL-C rather than LDL-C as a primary target, and European and Canadian guidelines have introduced non-HDL-C, apoB100, and their ratios as alternative measures to LDL-C in specific circumstances. Lipid particle concentration and size has sparked considerable interest and, although there is an association with cardiovascular risk, practical difficulties in using this for routine clinical practice limits its use for now.

Ultimately, among the main decisions to be made for any clinician is whether to treat or not to treat. In cases in which there is no uncertainty, newer lipid measures may not add much value beyond traditional measures. By contrast, in the future, in those individuals in whom the decision to treat is less clear, such as those at low or intermediate risk, the addition of further lipid and apolipoprotein measurements where available may provide clarity and help with earlier identification.

REFERENCES

1. Global Health Estimates 2015: Deaths by cause, age, sex, by country and by region, 2000–2015. Geneva: World Health Organization; 2016. Available at: http://www.who.int/healthinfo/global_burden_disease/estimates/en/index1.html. Accessed January 11, 2018.
2. Castelli WP. Cholesterol and lipids in the risk of coronary artery disease–the Framingham Heart Study. Can J Cardiol 1988;4(Suppl A):5A–10A.
3. Ference BA, Robinson JG, Brook RD, et al. Variation in *PCSK9* and *HMGCR* and risk of cardiovascular disease and diabetes. N Engl J Med 2016;375(22): 2144–53.
4. Emerging Risk Factors Collaboration. Major lipids, apolipoproteins, and risk of vascular disease. JAMA 2009;302(18):1993–2000.
5. Ference BA, Ginsberg HN, Graham I, et al. Low-density lipoproteins cause atherosclerotic cardiovascular disease. 1. Evidence from genetic, epidemiologic, and clinical studies. A consensus statement from the European Atherosclerosis Society Consensus Panel. Eur Heart J 2017;1–14. https://doi.org/10.1093/eurheartj/ehx144.
6. Baigent C, Keech A, Kearney PM, et al. Efficacy and safety of cholesterol-lowering treatment: prospective meta-analysis of data from 90 056 participants in 14 randomised trials of statins. Lancet 2005;366(9493): 1267–78.
7. Stone NJ, Robinson JG, Lichtenstein AH, et al. American College of Cardiology/American Heart Association Task Force on Practice Guidelines. 2013 ACC/AHA guideline on the treatment of blood cholesterol to reduce atherosclerotic cardiovascular risk in adults: a report of the American College of Cardiology/American Heart Association Task Force on Practice Guidelines. Circulation 2014; 129(25 Suppl 2):S1–45.
8. Cholesterol Treatment Trialists' (CTT) Collaboration, Baigent C, Blackwell L, Emberson J, et al. Efficacy and safety of more intensive lowering of LDL cholesterol: a meta-analysis of data from 170 000 participants in 26 randomised trials. Lancet 2010; 376(9753):1670–81.
9. Hippisley-Cox J, Coupland C, Vinogradova Y, et al. Predicting cardiovascular risk in England and Wales: prospective derivation and validation of QRISK2. BMJ 2008;336(7659):1475–82.
10. D'Agostino RB, Vasan RS, Pencina MJ, et al. General cardiovascular risk profile for use in primary care: the Framingham heart study. Circulation 2008;117(6):743–53.
11. Ridker PM, Buring JE, Rifai N, et al. Development and validation of improved algorithms for the assessment of global cardiovascular risk in women: the Reynolds risk score. JAMA 2007; 297(6):611–9.
12. Sampson UK, Fazio S, Linton MF. Residual cardiovascular risk despite optimal LDL-cholesterol reduction with statins: the evidence, etiology, and therapeutic challenges. Curr Atheroscler Rep 2012;14(1):1–10.
13. Randomised trial of cholesterol lowering in 4444 patients with coronary heart disease: the Scandinavian Simvastatin Survival Study (4S). Lancet 1994; 344(8934):1383–9.
14. Di Angelantonio E, Gao P, Pennells L, et al. Lipid-related markers and cardiovascular disease prediction. JAMA 2012;307(23):2499–506.
15. Kastelein JJP, Van Der Steeg WA, Holme I, et al. Lipids, apolipoproteins, and their ratios in relation to cardiovascular events with statin treatment. Circulation 2008;117(23):3002–9.
16. Ridker PM, Rifai N, Cook NR, et al. Non-HDL cholesterol, apolipoproteins A-I and B100, standard lipid measures, lipid ratios, and CRP as risk factors for cardiovascular disease in women. JAMA 2005; 294(3):326–33.
17. Rallidis LS, Pitsavos C, Panagiotakos DB, et al. Non-high density lipoprotein cholesterol is the best discriminator of myocardial infarction in young individuals. Atherosclerosis 2005;179(2): 305–9.

18. Farwell WR, Sesso HD, Buring JE, et al. Non-high-density lipoprotein cholesterol versus low-density lipoprotein cholesterol as a risk factor for a first nonfatal myocardial infarction. Am J Cardiol 2005; 96(8):1129–34.

19. Boekholdt SM, Arsenault BJ, Mora S, et al. Association of LDL cholesterol, non–HDL cholesterol, and apolipoprotein B levels with risk of cardiovascular events among patients treated with statins. JAMA 2012;307(12):1302.

20. Helgadottir A, Gretarsdottir S, Thorleifsson G, et al. Variants with large effects on blood lipids and the role of cholesterol and triglycerides in coronary disease. Nat Genet 2016;48(6):634–9.

21. Arsenault BJ, Rana JS, Stroes ESG, et al. Beyond low-density lipoprotein cholesterol respective contributions of non–high-density lipoprotein cholesterol levels, triglycerides, and the total cholesterol/high-density lipoprotein cholesterol ratio to coronary heart disease risk in apparently health. J Am Coll Cardiol 2010;55:35–41.

22. NICE guidelines. Cardio cardiovascular disease: risk assessment vascular disease: risk assessment and reduction, including lipid and reduction, including lipid modification modification. NICE Guidel; 2014. Available at: nice.org.uk/guidance/cg181.

23. Anderson TJ, Grégoire J, Pearson GJ, et al. 2016 Canadian Cardiovascular Society guidelines for the management of dyslipidemia for the prevention of cardiovascular disease in the adult. Can J Cardiol 2016;32(11):1263–82.

24. Miller M, Cannon CP, Murphy SA, et al. Impact of triglyceride levels beyond low-density lipoprotein cholesterol after acute coronary syndrome in the PROVE IT-TIMI 22 trial. J Am Coll Cardiol 2007. https://doi.org/10.1016/j.jacc.2007.10.038.

25. Sarwar N, Danesh J, Eiriksdottir G, et al. Triglycerides and the risk of coronary heart disease 10 158 incident cases among 262 525 participants in 29 western prospective studies. Circulation 2007; 115(4):450–9.

26. Varbo A, Benn M, Tybjærg-Hansen A, et al. Remnant cholesterol as a causal risk factor for ischemic heart disease. J Am Coll Cardiol 2013; 61(4):427–36.

27. Sarwar N, Sandhu MS, Ricketts SL, et al. Triglyceride-mediated pathways and coronary disease: collaborative analysis of 101 studies. Lancet 2010; 375(9726):1634–9.

28. Dewey FE, Gusarova V, Dunbar RL, et al. Genetic and pharmacologic inactivation of ANGPTL3 and cardiovascular disease. N Engl J Med 2017; 377(3):211–21.

29. Jørgensen AB, Frikke-Schmidt R, Nordestgaard BG, et al. Loss-of-function mutations in APOC3 and risk of ischemic vascular disease. N Engl J Med 2014; 371(1):32–41.

30. Gordon T, Castelli WP, Hjortland MC, et al. High-density lipoprotein as a protective factor against coronary heart disease. The Framingham Study. Am J Med 1977;62(5):707–14.

31. Abbott RD, Wilson PW, Kannel WB, et al. High-density lipoprotein cholesterol, total cholesterol screening, and myocardial infarction. The Framingham Study. Arterioscler Thromb Vasc Biol 1988; 8(3):207–11.

32. Barter P, Gotto AM, LaRosa JC, et al. HDL cholesterol, very low levels of LDL cholesterol, and cardiovascular events. N Engl J Med 2007; 357(13):1301–10.

33. Ridker PM, Genest J, Boekholdt SM, et al. HDL cholesterol and residual risk of first cardiovascular events after treatment with potent statin therapy: an analysis from the JUPITER trial. Lancet 2010; 376(9738):333–9.

34. Lawler PR, Akinkuolie AO, Chu AY, et al. Atherogenic lipoprotein determinants of cardiovascular disease and residual risk among individuals with low low-density lipoprotein cholesterol. J Am Heart Assoc 2017;6(7):e005549.

35. Voight BF, Peloso GM, Orho-Melander M, et al. Plasma HDL cholesterol and risk of myocardial infarction: a mendelian randomisation study. Lancet 2012;380(9841):572–80.

36. Shai I, Rimm EB, Hankinson SE, et al. Multivariate assessment of lipid parameters as predictors of coronary heart disease among postmenopausal women: potential implications for clinical guidelines. Circulation 2004;110(18):2824–30.

37. Gotto AM, Whitney E, Stein EA, et al. Relation between baseline and on-treatment lipid parameters and first acute major coronary events in the Air Force/Texas Coronary Atherosclerosis Prevention Study (AFCAPS/TexCAPS). Circulation 2000;101(5):477–84.

38. Baseline risk factors and their association with outcome in the west of Scotland coronary prevention study. The west of Scotland coronary prevention study group. Am J Cardiol 1997;79(6):756–62.

39. Pedersen TR, Olsson AG, F'rgeman O, et al. Lipoprotein changes and reduction in the incidence of major coronary heart disease events in the Scandinavian Simvastatin Survival Study (4S). Atheroscler Suppl 2004;5(3):99–106.

40. Ganda OP. Refining lipoprotein assessment in diabetes: apolipoprotein B makes sense. Endocr Pract 2009;15(4):370–6.

41. Lamarche B, Moorjani S, Lupien PJ, et al. Apolipoprotein A-I and B levels and the risk of ischemic heart disease during a five-year follow-up of men in the Québec Cardiovascular Study. Circulation 1996;94(3):273–8.

42. Catapano AL, Graham I, De Backer G, et al. 2016 ESC/EAS guidelines for the management of dyslipidaemias: the task force for the management of dyslipidaemias of the European Society of Cardiology (ESC) and European Atherosclerosis Society (EAS) developed with the special contribution of the Europea. Atherosclerosis 2016;253:281–344.

43. Brunzell JD, Davidson M, Furberg CD, et al. Lipoprotein management in patients with cardiometabolic risk. Consensus conference report from the American Diabetes Association and the American College of Cardiology Foundation. J Am Coll Cardiol 2008;51(15):1512–24.

44. Ference BA, Kastelein JJP, Ginsberg HN, et al. Association of genetic variants related to CETP inhibitors and statins with lipoprotein levels and cardiovascular risk. JAMA 2017. https://doi.org/10.1001/jama.2017.11467.

45. HPS3/TIMI55-REVEAL Collaborative Group. Effects of Anacetrapib in patients with atherosclerotic vascular disease. N Engl J Med 2017. https://doi.org/10.1056/NEJMoa1706444.

46. Walldius G, Jungner I, Holme I, et al. High apolipoprotein B, low apolipoprotein A-I, and improvement in the prediction of fatal myocardial infarction (AMORIS study): a prospective study. Lancet 2001;358(9298):2026–33.

47. Talmud PJ, Hawe E, Miller GJ, et al. Nonfasting apolipoprotein B and triglyceride levels as a useful predictor of coronary heart disease risk in middle-aged UK men. Arterioscler Thromb Vasc Biol 2002;22(11):1918–23.

48. Craig WY, Neveux LM, Palomaki GE, et al. Lipoprotein(a) as a risk factor for ischemic heart disease: metaanalysis of prospective studies. Clin Chem 1998;44(11):2301–6.

49. Tsimikas S. A test in context: lipoprotein(a): diagnosis, prognosis, controversies, and emerging therapies. J Am Coll Cardiol 2017;69(6):692–711.

50. Emerging Risk Factors Collaboration. Lipoprotein (a) concentration and the risk of coronary heart disease, stroke, and nonvascular mortality. JAMA 2009;302(4):412–23.

51. Clarke R, Peden JF, Hopewell JC, et al. Genetic variants associated with Lp(a) lipoprotein level and coronary disease. N Engl J Med 2009;361(26):2518–28.

52. Nordestgaard BG, Chapman MJ, Ray K, et al. Lipoprotein(a) as a cardiovascular risk factor: current status. Eur Heart J 2010;31(23):2844–53.

53. Cromwell WC, Otvos JD, Keyes MJ, et al. LDL particle number and risk of future cardiovascular disease in the Framingham Offspring Study - implications for LDL management. J Clin Lipidol 2007;1(6):583–92.

54. Mora S, Otvos JD, Rifai N, et al. Lipoprotein particle profiles by nuclear magnetic resonance compared with standard lipids and apolipoproteins in predicting incident cardiovascular disease in women. Circulation 2009;119(7):931–9.

55. Toth PP, Grabner M, Punekar RS, et al. Cardiovascular risk in patients achieving low-density lipoprotein cholesterol and particle targets. Atherosclerosis 2014;235(2):585–91.

56. Shiffman D, Louie JZ, Caulfield MP, et al. LDL subfractions are associated with incident cardiovascular disease in the Malmö Prevention Project Study. Atherosclerosis 2017;263:287–92.

57. Urbina EM, McCoy CE, Gao Z, et al. Lipoprotein particle number and size predict vascular structure and function better than traditional lipids in adolescents and young adults. J Clin Lipidol 2017;11(4):1023–31.

58. Tzou WS, Douglas PS, Srinivasan SR, et al. Advanced lipoprotein testing does not improve identification of subclinical atherosclerosis in young adults: the Bogalusa Heart Study. Ann Intern Med 2005;142(9):742–50.

59. Otvos JD, Mora S, Shalaurova I, et al. Clinical implications of discordance between LDL cholesterol and LDL particle number. J Clin Lipidol 2011;5(2):105–13.

Optimizing Statins and Ezetimibe in Guideline-Focused Management

Aref A. Bin Abdulhak, MD, MSc[a,b,c],
Jennifer G. Robinson, MD, MPH[a,c,d,e],*

KEYWORDS

- Statin • Ezetimibe • Hyperlipidemia • Cholesterol • Atherosclerotic cardiovascular diseases
- Diabetes mellitus • Polyvascular disease

KEY POINTS

- Statins are the cornerstone of cholesterol management in patients with atherosclerotic cardiovascular disease.
- Certain groups of patients may remain at significantly elevated risk of cardiovascular events, and may benefit from adding nonstatin agents in addition to statin therapy.
- Low-density lipoprotein cholesterol (LDL-C) thresholds based on a patient's risk category may guide selection of patients who may benefit the most from nonstatin therapy.
- Ezetimibe is a nonstatin LDL-C lowering agent that has been shown to further reduce cardiovascular risk when added to background statin therapy.

INTRODUCTION

Statins are one of the most commonly used medications in the management of atherosclerotic cardiovascular diseases (ASCVDs). Statins lower blood cholesterol through competitive inhibition of 3-hydroxy-3-methylglutaryl-CoA and, ultimately, inhibition of cholesterol synthesis, as well as through lowering low-density lipoprotein cholesterol (LDL-C) concentration. Many large randomized clinical trials have demonstrated that statins significantly reduce several important cardiovascular outcomes, including myocardial infarction, stroke, and mortality, as well as revascularizations.[1–4]

The 2013 American College of Cardiology (ACC) and American Heart Association (AHA) blood cholesterol guideline[5] has recommended, as a class IA recommendation, use of statins as first-line therapy to lower serum LDL-C among 3 groups of patients: (1) those with clinical ASCVD, including patients with acute coronary syndrome, stroke, peripheral vascular disease; (2) diabetic patients age 40 to 75 years; and (3) patients with LDL-C levels

Disclosure: J.G. Robinson has received grants from Amarin, Amgen, AstraZeneca, Eli Lilly, Esai, Esperion, GlaxoSmithKline, Merck, Pfizer, Regeneron, Sanofi, and Takeda. She is also a consultant for Akcea/Ionis, Amgen, Dr Reddy, Eli Lilly, Esperion, Merck, Pfizer, and Regeneron/Sanof. A.A. Bin Abdulhak has nothing to disclose.
 a Division of Cardiovascular Medicine, Department of Internal Medicine, University of Iowa Carver College of Medicine, 200 Hawkins Drive, Iowa City, IA 52242, USA; b Department of Epidemiology, University of Iowa, College of Public Health, 200 Hawkins Drive, Iowa City, IA 52242, USA; c Prevention Intervention Center, University of Iowa, College of Public Health, 200 Hawkins Drive, Iowa City, IA 52242, USA; d Department of Epidemiology, University of Iowa, College of Public Health, 145 North Riverside Drive, S455 CPHB, Iowa City, IA 52242, USA; e Department of Medicine, University of Iowa Hospitals and Clinics, 200 Hawkins Drive, Iowa City, IA 52242, USA
* Corresponding author. Department of Epidemiology, University of Iowa, College of Public Health, 145 North Riverside Drive, S455 CPHB, Iowa City, IA 52242.
E-mail address: jennifer-g-robinson@uiowa.edu

greater than or equal to 190 mg/dL (as a class IB recommendation). Nonetheless, certain groups of patients may remain at significantly elevated risk of atherosclerotic cardiovascular events despite maximally tolerated statin therapy, and may benefit from adding nonstatin lipid-lowering agents in addition to statin therapy.[6] The nonstatin lipid-lowering agent, ezetimibe, inhibits the Niemann-Pick C1-like 1 protein, thereby reducing cholesterol absorption in the small intestine and, subsequently, the LDL-C level in the blood. A randomized clinical trial has shown that ezetimibe reduces cardiovascular events when added to simvastatin.[7] This article discusses optimization of statin and ezetimibe in guideline-focused management.

DISCUSSION

The 2013 ACC/AHA cholesterol guideline[5] has moved away from treat-to-target LDL-C goals, and strongly recommends statin therapy to reduce cardiovascular risk, regardless of LDL-C, based on an extensive body of clinical trial evidence. Statin therapy was given a strong class I recommendation in the following groups of patients:

1. Clinical ASCVD, including patients with coronary artery disease, stroke, transient ischemic attack, peripheral vascular diseases presumed to be of atherosclerotic origin, and patients with coronary or other arterial revascularization (class IA)
2. Individuals with an LDL-C greater than or equal to 190 mg/dL (class IB)
3. Diabetic individuals between 40 to 75 years old with LDL-C of 70 to 189 mg/dL (class IA)
4. Individuals 40 to 75 years old with LDL-C between 70 and 189 mg/dL or diabetes who have a 10-year ASCVD risk of greater than or equal to 7.5% (class IA).

High-intensity statins are preferred up to age 75 years in groups 1 to 3, and may be considered in group 4; moderate intensity statin initiation is otherwise recommended. On average, high-intensity statins reduce LDL-C by 50%; however, response is variable and patients may be unable to tolerate the recommended dose of statin. An additional LDL-C lowering agent may be desirable for some patients who remain at high risk of ASCVD despite maximally tolerated statin therapy.[6] As such, a shared decision-making discussion between the patient and the clinician is suggested whenever adding a nonstatin lipid-lowering agent is considered.[5,8] Shared decision-making should include consideration of the potential for further reduction in cardiovascular risk, potential for harms, and consideration of patient preferences for therapy. To determine the potential for benefit, the concept of net benefit was introduced in the 2013 ACC/AHA cholesterol guideline. When extended to include the concept of LDL-C thresholds, introduced by Robinson and colleagues,[9] this can inform the decision-making process of whether to add nonstatin agents. The net benefit approach was emphasized in the ACC consensus clinical expert decision pathway for nonstatins released in 2016[8] and an updated document[10] in 2017 that aimed to inform clinicians about adding nonstatin lipid-lowering agents for LDL reduction in addition to statin therapy.

The pathway identified certain factors needing special consideration if a nonstatin therapy is being contemplated, including

1. Percent LDL-C reduction from baseline while on guideline-directed statin therapy
2. Baseline ASCVD risk of patients with ASCVD with and without comorbidities on guideline-directed statin therapy
3. Patients' predicted 10-year ASCVD risk without clinical ASCVD, or LDL-C greater than or equal to 190 while not on statin therapy
4. Additional percentage of LDL-C reduction desirable beyond those achieved with maximally tolerated statin therapy
5. Presence of supportive evidence of ASCVD risk reduction with addition of nonstatin therapy to statins.

Furthermore, potential drug–drug interactions, cost, availability, route of administration, and (most important) patient preference are variables that need attention when nonstatin agents are under consideration for cholesterol management.

Based on ASCVD risk while on statin therapy, several groups of patients have been identified from a review of statin arms of clinical trials or the ACC pathways.[6,8,10] These groups of patients may have a net benefit from adding nonstatin therapy to statins, depending on their on-treatment LDL-C level.

The high-risk group (20%–29% 10-year ASCVD risk) despite maximal statin therapy, includes:

1. Patients with clinical ASCVD without high-risk characteristics (see later discussion)
2. Untreated primary LDL-C greater than or equal to 190 mg/dL, suggesting familial hypercholesterolemia.

Primary prevention patients are those on statin therapy with greater than or equal to 10% 5-year or greater than or equal to 20% 10-year ASCVD risk (without or with diabetes mellitus). Very high-risk groups (≥30% 10-year ASCVD risk) despite maximal statin therapy include clinical ASCVD patients with the following additional high-risk characteristics:

1. Diabetes mellitus
2. Familial hypercholesterolemia
3. Recent acute coronary syndrome
4. Chronic kidney disease (glomerular filtration rate 30–90 mL/min/1.73 m^2)
5. Poorly controlled risk factors
6. Polyvascular disease
7. Age greater than or equal to 65 years
8. Recurrent events
9. Elevated lipoprotein(a).

A thoughtful approach of incorporating patients' risk group and LDL-C thresholds (if not achieved by adherent patients following a period of guideline-directed statin therapy) has been suggested to guide use of nonstatin therapy in addition to statins in patients who potentially have a net benefit from adding either proprotein convertase subtilisin-like/kexin type 9 or ezetimibe.[8–10] Ezetimibe is, or soon will be, generic in most countries, which will reduce barriers to its use based on cost alone. However, given that ezetimibe lowers LDL-C 20% to 25% when added to background statin therapy, there is less cardiovascular risk reduction when baseline LDL-C levels are low. Therefore, the number-needed-to-treat (NNT) to prevent 1 event is greater than 50 patients over 5 years for most high-risk patients regardless of LDL-C levels. However, over 10 years, the NNTs are less than 50 for high-risk patients with LDL-C greater than or equal to 130 mg/dL.[11] Accordingly, high-risk patients with LDL-C greater than or equal to 130 mg/dL, very high-risk patients with LDL-C greater than or equal to 100 mg/dL, and selected extremely high-risk patients with LDL-C 70 to 99 mg/dL could benefit from ezetimibe therapy in addition to maximally tolerated statin therapy.

SUMMARY

Statins are the mainstay for the primary and secondary prevention of ASCVDs. However, several groups of patients may remain at significantly elevated risk of ASCVD events despite being on the maximally tolerated intensity of statin therapy. Therefore, a discussion about adding nonstatin agents should be undertaken between the patient and the clinician. Ezetimibe may provide a net benefit in terms of further reduction of ASCVD events when added to statin therapy in high-risk patients, which may be based on patients' risk profiles and LDL-C levels on maximally tolerated statin therapy.

REFERENCES

1. Randomised trial of cholesterol lowering in 4444 patients with coronary heart disease: the Scandinavian Simvastatin Survival Study (4S). Lancet 1994; 344(8934):1383–9.
2. Ridker PM, Danielson E, Fonseca FA, et al. Rosuvastatin to prevent vascular events in men and women with elevated C-reactive protein. N Engl J Med 2008;359(21):2195–207.
3. Schwartz GG, Olsson AG, Ezekowitz MD, et al. Effects of atorvastatin on early recurrent ischemic events in acute coronary syndromes: the MIRACL study: a randomized controlled trial. JAMA 2001;285(13):1711–8.
4. Shepherd J, Cobbe SM, Ford I, et al. Prevention of coronary heart disease with pravastatin in men with hypercholesterolemia. West of Scotland Coronary Prevention Study Group. N Engl J Med 1995;333(20):1301–7.
5. Stone NJ, Robinson JG, Lichtenstein AH, et al. 2013 ACC/AHA guideline on the treatment of blood cholesterol to reduce atherosclerotic cardiovascular risk in adults: a report of the American College of Cardiology/American Heart Association Task Force on Practice Guidelines. J Am Coll Cardiol 2014; 63(25 Pt B):2889–934.
6. Robinson JG, Huijgen R, Ray K, et al. Determining when to add nonstatin therapy: a quantitative approach. J Am Coll Cardiol 2016;68(22):2412–21.
7. Eisen A, Cannon CP, Blazing MA, et al. The benefit of adding ezetimibe to statin therapy in patients with prior coronary artery bypass graft surgery and acute coronary syndrome in the IMPROVE-IT trial. Eur Heart J 2016;37(48):3576–84.
8. Writing C, Lloyd-Jones DM, Morris PB, et al. 2016 ACC expert consensus decision pathway on the role of nonstatin therapies for LDL-cholesterol lowering in the management of atherosclerotic cardiovascular disease risk: a report of the American College of Cardiology task force on clinical expert consensus documents. J Am Coll Cardiol 2016;68(1):92–125.
9. Robinson JG, Ray K. Counterpoint: low-density lipoprotein cholesterol targets are not needed in lipid treatment guidelines. Arterioscler Thromb Vasc Biol 2016;36(4):586–90.
10. Lloyd-Jones DM, Morris PB, Ballantyne CM, et al. 2017 focused update of the 2016 ACC expert consensus decision pathway on the role of nonstatin therapies for LDL-cholesterol lowering in the management of atherosclerotic cardiovascular disease risk: a report of the American College of Cardiology task force on expert consensus decision pathways. J Am Coll Cardiol 2017;70(14):1785–822.
11. Robinson J, Stone N. The 2013 ACC/AHA guideline on the treatment of blood cholesterol to reduce atherosclerotic cardiovascular disease risk: a new paradigm supported by more evidence. Eur Heart J 2015;36:2110–8.

Statin Intolerance
Some Practical Hints

Maciej Banach, MD, PhD, FNLA, FESC[a,b,c],*, Dimitri P. Mikhailidis, BSc, MSc, MD[d]

KEYWORDS

- Adverse effects • Cardiovascular disease • Statins • Statin-associated muscle symptoms
- Therapy

KEY POINTS

- Statin intolerance is a worldwide problem concerning the inability to tolerate a dose of statin required to sufficiently reduce cardiovascular risk.
- Muscle symptoms are the most common statin-associated adverse effects.
- New therapies with the proprotein convertase subtilisin-kexin type 9 (PCSK9) inhibitors and bempedoic acid might be an effective response.

DEFINITION AND PREVALENCE

Statin intolerance is the inability to tolerate a dose of statin required to sufficiently reduce cardiovascular (CV) risk.[1] This limits the effective treatment of patients at risk of, or with, CV disease. Statin intolerance refers not only to the lack of statin treatment because of clinical or biochemical symptoms (so-called complete intolerance) but also to the treatment with insufficiently high statin doses or with insufficiently potent statins in relation to the CV risk level.[1,2]

Statin intolerance is a worldwide problem but interest in this phenomenon was intensified with the appearance of the proprotein convertase subtilisin-kexin type 9 (PCSK9) inhibitor studies in 2009.[3] Since 1994 and the Scandinavian Simvastatin Survival Study (4S) trial, in most of the available statin trials individuals with statin-associated adverse effects (SAAE) were excluded and therefore they did not show differences in drug safety between the statin and placebo groups, or between low/moderate and intense statin therapy.[2] The data on statin intolerance patients came from epidemiologic and observational studies, and the authors suggested that usually 15% to 20% of all patients on statin might suffer from different SAAE.[4]

The European Society of Cardiology/European Atherosclerosis Society consensus suggested that 29% of all patients treated with statins might present with statin-associated muscle symptoms (SAMS), but this number seems to be overestimated.[5] However, it is worth emphasizing that with the five-step approach (four diagnostic steps + therapy) for patients with statin intolerance, after excluding all conditions and risk factors that might increase this risk, and after introducing different methods of management (dose reduction, change of statin formulation, alternate-day therapy, combination therapy) more than 90% of these patients might be treated with statins and complete statin intolerance concerns only less than 5% of

Disclosure: M. Banach is on the Speakers Bureau for Abbott/Mylan, Abbott Vascular, Actavis, Akcea, Amgen, Biofarm, KRKA, MSD, Sanofi-Aventis, and Valeant; is a consultant to Abbott Vascular, Akcea, Amgen, Daichii Sankyo, Esperion, Lilly, MSD, Pfizer, Resverlogix, and Sanofi-Aventis; and receives grants from Sanofi-Aventis and Valeant. D.P. Mikhailidis has given talks and attended conferences sponsored by MSD, AstraZeneca, and Libytec.
[a] Department of Hypertension, WAM University Hospital in Lodz, Medical University of Lodz (MUL), 113 Zeromskiego Street, Lodz 90-549, Poland; [b] Polish Mother's Memorial Hospital Research Institute (PMMHRI), 281/289 Rzgowska Street, Lodz 93-338, Poland; [c] Cardiovascular Research Centre, University of Zielona Gora, 28 Zyty Street, Zielona Gora 65-046, Poland; [d] Department of Clinical Biochemistry, Royal Free Campus, University College London Medical School, University College London (UCL), Pond Street, London NW3 2QG, UK
* Corresponding author. Department of Hypertension, Medical University of Lodz, Zeromskiego 113, Lodz 90-549, Poland.
E-mail address: maciejbanach@aol.co.uk

Cardiol Clin 36 (2018) 225–231
https://doi.org/10.1016/j.ccl.2017.12.004
0733-8651/18/© 2017 Elsevier Inc. All rights reserved.

cardiology.theclinics.com

subjects (usually 1%–3%).[6] The principal approach should be to try not to discontinue statin therapy. This is a real challenge for lipidologists and those taking care of patients with dyslipidemia. Not discontinuing treatment is especially important for those with a high and very high CV risk. Statin discontinuation, which might concern even 50% to 60% of patients on statins after 2 years, is one reason why these patients often do not achieve their recommended goals of therapy (**Box 1**).[7–9]

SYMPTOMS AND CAUSALITY

SAMS are the most common adverse effects observed in patients on statins.[5] They might range from muscle weakness, muscle aches, soreness, stiffness, tenderness, and muscle cramps (but not nocturnal cramping; not necessarily with creatine kinase [CK] increase) to muscle myositis (with CK increase) and rhabdomyolysis (very rare at 1.6 per 100,000 patient-years), which is usually associated with genetic predisposition or other risk factors present during statin therapy (eg, kidney or liver disease, extensive exercise, or concomitant medication).[10,11]

It needs to be emphasized that one should always ask patients about the tolerability of muscle symptoms. If patients can tolerate the symptoms (with lack or slight CK increase) one should continue the treatment because the symptoms may be temporary and resolve after 2 to 4 weeks.[2] However, close follow-up should be maintained in case the symptoms and biochemical changes are progressive. It is important that patients should be fully aware about all the benefits of statin therapy and the CV risk increase caused by statin discontinuation or not taking a suitable statin dose.[8,9] Unfortunately, most patients usually know much more about SAAEs than the benefits associated with statin therapy. According to available data, there is several times more information on the Internet regarding side effects than on the benefits of statin use.[12] Because of this there are more and more patients with so-called nocebo effect, which is defined (despite completely different original definition of

this phenomenon) as the appearance of statin-related side effects caused by patients' knowledge (eg, from media, Internet) and expectations and not by statin therapy.[1] The first strong data on the existence of this phenomenon are based on the recent subanalysis of the Anglo-Scandinavian Cardiac Outcomes Trial-Lipid-Lowering Arm (ASCOT-LLA) trial. In the nonrandomized phase there was a 41% significant increase of the rate of SAMS in patients treated with atorvastatin in comparison with the blinded phase, where there was no significant difference between groups.[13]

SAMS, statin-related new-onset diabetes, and alanine aminotransferase (ALT) elevation are the only side effects with confirmed causality.[1,2] There are also several other possible side effects after statin therapy, including highly debatable neurocognitive disorders[14] or erectile dysfunction[2] or sleep disorders, for which the causality has not been confirmed so far; there are also data that suggest a lack of such associations.[15]

From the clinical point of view it is important to clearly present the current recommendations on the association between statin therapy and liver diseases. First of all it is crucial to remember that ALT elevation greater than three times the upper limit of normal (ULN) occurs in less than 0.5% for moderate-dose statins and rosuvastatin at all doses, and about 1% for 80 mg of atorvastatin or simvastatin (usually <3% all together),[2] and usually returns to normal after a dose reduction without the need for statin discontinuation; in most cases it is possible to return to the initial doses of statins after 2 to 4 weeks.[2,10] Because of this most of the current recommendations suggest ALT measurement only before statin therapy and thereafter in case of side effects occurrence (without necessity of regular monitoring).[2,16,17] Finally, the risk of statin-related serious liver disease is 1 per 1,000,000 with the number needed to harm at 1 million. In comparison, use of statins prevents about 33% of major CV disease events when compared with placebo; the number needed to treat is 3. Unfortunately the percentage of patients who fail to receive statins because of fear of hepatotoxicity ranges between 10% and 30%.[2,18] Furthermore, available studies indicate that statin therapy should be continued and benefits are achieved in all patients with chronic liver diseases, and therapy should be stopped only in case of acute conditions.[2] The available data suggest that even in patients with hepatitis B and C viruses, although not in acute and active forms of the disease, statins significant decrease the risk of hepatocellular carcinoma (by <30%) and reduce in the incidence of hepatitis C virus in the blood by inhibiting its replication.[2,19] They might also be beneficial in patients with

---

Box 1
Practical hints on definition and prevalence of statin intolerance

- More than 90% of patients with statin intolerance might be treated with statins and complete statin intolerance only concerns less than 5% of subjects.

- The principal approach to patients with statin intolerance should be to try not to discontinue statin therapy.

primary biliary cirrhosis in terms of improved course of the disease but primarily in terms of CV risk reduction, and even greater therapeutic benefits is noted in patients with nonalcoholic fatty liver disease and nonalcoholic steatohepatitis (almost 30% higher CV morbidity reduction in comparison with those with nonalcoholic fatty liver disease without statin therapy) (**Box 2**).[2,20,21]

FOUR-STEP DIAGNOSIS

There are doubts as to whether there are suitable and effective tools to diagnose statin intolerance (**Box 3**). The step-by-step approach to diagnosis (and then to treatment) is probably a suitable solution.[6] Described next are some useful tools on how to diagnose patients with statin intolerance:

1. *Ask when statin therapy was initiated or whether there was a dose increase in the last several weeks.* It is important because most of the symptoms (>75%) usually appear within the first 12 weeks and almost 90% in the first 6 months, so it is less likely to have statin intolerance in patients on statin therapy for a few years (unless a new external factor might be the cause).[2,10]
2. *Obtain a family history and check for conditions that might increase statin intolerance risk.* There are five important conditions/risk factors that might cause SAMS: (1) new intensive exercise (eg, with the initiation of statin therapy when there is also a recommendation for lifestyle changes), (2) hypothyroidism/hyperthyroidism (mainly hypothyroidism), (3) vitamin D deficiency (especially in countries with limited sun access annually), (4) concomitant therapy (especially with some antifungal medications;

antibiotics; human immunodeficiency virus protease inhibitors; calcium antagonists; and such drugs as cyclosporine, danazol, amiodarone, and ranolazine), and (5) family history (genetic predisposition).[1,2,6,17,22]
3. *Exclude nocebo effect and confirm whether muscle symptoms are caused by statin therapy.* It is crucial to perform a detailed subjective and objective patient examination with special attention to the character of muscle pain. SAMS manifest with large muscle symmetric (eg, bilateral) aches or bilateral aches of the smaller distal or proximal musculature, whereas nonstatin-related myalgia is associated with more diverse symptoms, such as whole-body fatigue and groin pain.[2,6,23] To confirm whether muscle pain is statin-related one should use the SAMS-Clinical Index.[6,24]
4. *Ask about the tolerability of the symptoms and always clearly emphasize the benefits of statin therapy and the risk on statin discontinuation.* Check for CK (no other predictors have been confirmed to be effective and possible to use in every-day clinical practice),[25] and remember the following principal rules based on recent guidelines[5,16,17]: (1) if the patient reports muscle pain at CK greater than or equal to 4 ULN, statin treatment should be discontinued for 4 to 6 weeks until the regression of pain and CK normalization; (2) if the patient reports tolerable muscle pain at CK less than 4 ULN, a reduction in statin dose and treatment continuation with close monitoring of CK may be considered; if clinical symptoms are exacerbated and/or the CK concentration is increased, statin treatment should be discontinued for 4 to 6 weeks until the regression of pain and CK normalization; and (3) if the patient reports intolerable muscle pain at CK less than 4 ULN, statin treatment should be discontinued for 2 to 4 weeks until the regression of pain and CK normalization.

Box 2
Practical hints on statin intolerance symptoms and causality

- Muscle symptoms are the most common adverse effects observed in patients on statins (95% of all SAAE); they might range from muscle weakness, muscle aches, soreness, stiffness, and muscle cramps to muscle myositis and rhabdomyolysis (1.6 per 100,000 patient-years).

- ALT elevation after statin therapy is rare (<3%) and ALT usually returns to normal without the need for statin discontinuation; in most cases, it is possible to return to the initial doses of statins after 2 to 4 weeks.

- Statin therapy is effective and safe and should be continued in all patients with chronic liver diseases.

Box 3
Four-step diagnosis of statin intolerance

- Ask when statin therapy was initiated or whether there was a dose increase in the last several weeks.

- Obtain a family history and check for conditions that might increase statin intolerance risk.

- Exclude nocebo effect and confirm whether muscle symptoms are caused by statin therapy.

- Ask about the tolerability of the symptoms and always clearly emphasize the benefits of statin therapy and the risk of statin discontinuation.

TREATMENT CHALLENGES

The effective therapy for patients with statin intolerance is critical,[26] especially because there is evidence suggesting that patients with statin intolerance, compared with those with good adherence, are associated with a significant increase in the risk of recurrent myocardial infarction (hazard ratio, 1.50; 95% confidence interval [CI], 1.30–1.73) and coronary diseases events (hazard ratio, 1.51; 95% CI, 1.34–1.70).[27]

The current recommendations[5,17] only present suggestions on how to manage patients after complete discontinuation of statin therapy for 2 to 6 weeks and do not provide any suggestions on how to treat patients with tolerable symptoms and a slight increase of CK (<4 ULN). It is especially critical for high-and very-high-risk patients, for whom all the options should be tried to continue effective lipid-lowering therapy. For such patients one might also change statin (eg, use another potent statin with the corresponding dose) or reduce statin dose (usually another one; eg, having intolerance for atorvastatin 80 mg, one might try to reduce the dose of another potent statin, still at the recommended dose for the patients at the highest risk [ie, rosuvastatin, 20 mg]).[6,17] One might also consider alternate-day statin therapy, especially because the recent meta-analysis from the Lipid and Blood Pressure Meta-analysis Collaboration (LBPMC) Group confirmed no statistically significant difference between alternate-day and daily regimens of atorvastatin and rosuvastatin in terms of change in low-density lipoprotein cholesterol (LDL-C; mean difference [MD], 6.79 mg/dL; 95% CI, -1.59 to 15.17; $P = .11$; and 10.51 mg/dL; 95% CI, -0.23 to 21.26; $P = .06$, respectively) and triglyceride (MD, 6.43 mg/dL; 95% CI, −5.75 to 18.61; $P = .30$; and 9.20 mg/dL; 95% CI, −2.78 to 21.19; $P = .13$, respectively). Both regimens of statins were generally well tolerated with good adherence.[28] Finally, it is important to consider combination therapy (or monotherapy in case of complete statin intolerance) with ezetimibe (and try to introduce it as quickly as possible in very-high-risk patients).[29] This treatment is effective in the reduction of atheroma plaque volume and CV events as demonstrated by trial-based evidence when administered with a statin.[30–32] Using PCSK9 inhibitors is another option.[33,34] Alirocumab and evolocumab confirmed a large LDL-C reduction effectiveness and safety in several studies with statin-intolerant patients,[35,36] and evolocumab has trial-based evidence for CV benefit when administered with a statin.[37] Probably one also should wait for the results of the Evaluation of Major Cardiovascular Events in Patients With, or at High Risk for, Cardiovascular Disease Who Are Statin Intolerant Treated With Bempedoic Acid (ETC-1002) or Placebo (CLEAR-Outcomes) trial (NCT02993406) with bempedoic acid, the first CV outcomes trial in patients with statin intolerance,[38] because the first data suggest on the high efficacy of this agent in LDL-C reduction.[39]

There are also data suggesting the possible role of coenzyme Q10 (CoQ10) and vitamin D supplementation as alternative methods to treat/prevent statin intolerance (mainly muscle symptoms).[4,6] Based on a recent meta-analysis,[40] statin therapy significantly lowers circulating CoQ10 levels (weighted MD [WMD], −0.44 mol/L; 95% CI, −0.52 to −0.37; $P<.001$). Therefore, in 2005 the hypothesis was raised that CoQ10 supplementation might improve symptoms (statin-related myalgia) and decrease CK levels.[41] However, the two largest meta-analyses on this issue carried out by the LBPMC Group did not confirm the suggested association.[42,43] The first meta-analysis[42] included the available randomized controlled trials with CoQ10 supplementation up to 400 mg/d; when compared with the control groups, there was no significant change in plasma CK activity after CoQ10 supplementation (MD, 11.69 U/L; 95% CI, −14.25 to 37.63 U/L; $P = .38$). Also, there was no significant effect on muscle pain (standardized MD, −0.53; 95% CI, −1.33 to 0.28; $P = .20$). In the updated meta-analysis[43] with CoQ10 doses up to 600 mg/d the authors obtained similar results: lack of evidence as to a significant effect of CoQ10 supplementation in reducing either the severity of myopathic pain (standardized MD, −0.36; 95% CI, −0.82 to 0.09; $P = .117$) or plasma CK activity (WMD, 3.47 U/L; 95% CI, −2.32 to 9.26; $P = .240$). Does this mean that CoQ10 supplementation is not effective? There is no clear answer to this question, because there has not been data on the efficacy of CoQ10 supplementation with the doses greater than 1000 mg (as used in some of neurologic disorders), and some practical experience showed that CoQ10 supplementation might be effective especially in patients with high deficiency of CoQ10 at the diagnosis of statin intolerance. However, it needs to be emphasized that there might be a problem with this CoQ10 therapy, both with compliance (the highest dose of CoQ10 in Poland is 100 mg and in Europe 300 mg; this would mean two to six tablets per day) and cost (from 40 to 100 Euro/month).[6,17,40–43]

Vitamin D deficiency might increase the risk of SAMS (vitamin D deficiency is a common problem in many countries and might concern 50%–60% of the population), and vitamin D supplementation might be useful in reduction of statin-related myalgia.[1,6,44] However, the meta-analysis of data from seven studies did not indicate any significant effect of statins treatment on plasma vitamin D levels.[45] The largest meta-analysis on this issue from the LBPMC Group[46] revealed a significantly lower plasma concentration of vitamin D in those with statin-associated myalgia compared with the asymptomatic subgroup (WMD, −9.41 ng/mL; 95% CI, −10.17 to −8.64; P<.00001). Furthermore, Khayznikov and colleagues[47] showed that statin intolerance associated with low serum vitamin D is safely resolved by its supplementation (50,000–100,000 units/week) in 88% to 95% cases. In a recent study Taylor and colleagues[48] suggested that low vitamin D levels are related to transient increases in muscle pain and damage, and that the damage may be exacerbated by statin therapy. Because of the previously mentioned data it is recommended to measure vitamin D levels in all patients with statin intolerance but there is no clear recommendation regarding vitamin D supplementation in SAMS.[6]

Patients with statin intolerance (partial and especially complete) are at very high risk to not achieve their LDL-C goal.[6,17,35,36] Most of them, taking into account data from trials with alirocumab and evolocumab, have very high LDL-C levels, and even combination therapy of tolerated doses of statins with ezetimibe and PCSK9 inhibitors (or monotherapy) might not be effective enough.[35,36] Therefore, there is a need to look for nonstatin agents with considerable LDL-C reduction efficacy.[49] In this context, it is important to consider the role of nutraceuticals, especially because they might have not only lipid-lowering properties, but also act as anti-inflammatory and antioxidant agents.[50] In the recent recommendations on lipid-lowering properties of nutraceuticals by the International Lipid Expert Panel, the authors for the first time summarized the available knowledge and suggested the nutraceuticals with the highest potency in lipid-lowering therapy.[51] They emphasized that the level of knowledge is still limited regarding efficacy and safety.[51] Despite this, such nutraceuticals as berberine (active daily doses, 500–1500 mg; expected LDL-C reduction of 15%–20%); plant sterols and stanols (active daily doses, 400–3000 mg; expected LDL-C reduction of 8%–12%); soluble fibers including beta-glucan, psyllium, and glucomannan (active daily doses, 5–15 g; expected LDL-C reduction of 5%–15%); garlic (active daily doses, 5–6 g; expected LDL-C reduction of 5%–10%); and green tea extracts (active daily doses, 25–100 g; expected LDL-C reduction of 5%) received the level of recommendation IA or IIaA and may be considered as an option for lipid-lowering therapy in patients with statin intolerance (**Box 4**).[51]

Box 4
Practical hints on statin intolerance therapy

- The effective therapy for statin intolerance is critical because these patients, compared with those with good adherence, are at high risk of myocardial infarction and coronary diseases events.

- For patients with statin intolerance change statin formulation, reduce dose, consider alternate-day statin therapy, and combination therapy with ezetimibe and PCSK9 inhibitors.

- PCSK9 inhibitors also confirmed large effectiveness and safety in statin-intolerant patients in monotherapy.

- Despite some data available, there is still no clear recommendation on the supplementation of CoQ10 and vitamin D in patients with statin intolerance.

- In patients with statin intolerance not at the goal of the therapy nutraceuticals with confirmed LDL-C reduction properties may be considered as part of the lipid-lowering combination therapy.

SUMMARY

Despite a large amount of data available on statin intolerance diagnosis and management there is still a large debate and need for further well-designed analyses on the suitable definition (which is easy to understand and use for primary care physicians), diagnosis (with sensitive biomarkers, with suitable clinical approach to avoid overestimation and in the consequence statin discontinuation), and therapy with effective agents in monotherapy and combination therapy with confirmed effect on CV outcomes.

REFERENCES

1. Patel J, Martin SS, Banach M. Expert opinion: the therapeutic challenges faced by statin intolerance. Expert Opin Pharmacother 2016;17: 1497–507.

2. Banach M, Rizzo M, Toth PP, et al. Statin intolerance: an attempt at a unified definition. Position paper from an International Lipid Expert Panel. Arch Med Sci 2015;11:1–23.

3. Chan JC, Piper DE, Cao Q, et al. A proprotein convertase subtilisin/kexin type 9 neutralizing antibody reduces serum cholesterol in mice and nonhuman primates. Proc Natl Acad Sci U S A 2009;106(24): 9820–5.

4. Banach M, Aronow WS, Serban C, et al. Lipids, blood pressure and kidney update 2014. Pharmacol Res 2015;95-96:111–25.

5. Stroes ES, Thompson PD, Corsini A, et al. Statin-associated muscle symptoms: impact on statin therapy. European Atherosclerosis Society consensus panel statement on assessment, aetiology and management. Eur Heart J 2015;36:1012–22.

6. Rosenson RS, Baker S, Banach M, et al. Optimizing cholesterol treatment in patients with muscle complaints. J Am Coll Cardiol 2017;70:1290–301.

7. Hobbs FD, Banach M, Mikhailidis DP, et al. Is statin-modified reduction in lipids the most important preventive therapy for cardiovascular disease? A pro/con debate. BMC Med 2016;14:4.

8. Banach M, Serban MC. Discussion around statin discontinuation in older adults and patients with wasting diseases. J Cachexia Sarcopenia Muscle 2016;7:396–9.

9. Booth JN 3rd, Colantonio LD, Chen L, et al. Statin discontinuation, reinitiation, and persistence patterns among Medicare beneficiaries after myocardial infarction: a cohort study. Circ Cardiovasc Qual Outcomes 2017;10(10):e003626.

10. Banach M, Rizzo M, Toth PP, et al. Statin intolerance: an attempt at a unified definition. Position paper from an International Lipid Expert Panel. Expert Opin Drug Saf 2015;14:935–55.

11. McClure DL, Valuck RJ, Glanz M, et al. Systematic review and meta-analysis of clinically relevant adverse events from HMG CoA reductase inhibitor trials worldwide from 1982 to present. Pharmacoepidemiol Drug Saf 2007;16:132–43.

12. Matthews A, Herrett E, Gasparrini A, et al. Impact of statin related media coverage on use of statins: interrupted time series analysis with UK primary care data. BMJ 2016;353:i3283.

13. Gupta A, Thompson D, Whitehouse A, et al, ASCOT Investigators. Adverse events associated with unblinded, but not with blinded, statin therapy in the Anglo-Scandinavian cardiac outcomes trial-lipid-lowering arm (ASCOT-LLA): a randomised double-blind placebo-controlled trial and its non-randomised non-blind extension phase. Lancet 2017;389:2473–81.

14. Banach M, Rizzo M, Nikolic D, et al. Intensive LDL-cholesterol lowering therapy and neurocognitive function. Pharmacol Ther 2017;170:181–91.

15. Broncel M, Gorzelak-Pabiś P, Sahebkar A, et al, Lipid and Blood Pressure Meta-analysis Collaboration (LBPMC) Group. Sleep changes following statin therapy: a systematic review and meta-analysis of randomized placebo-controlled polysomnographic trials. Arch Med Sci 2015;11:915–26.

16. Banach M, Jankowski P, Jóźwiak J, et al. PoLA/CFPiP/PCS guidelines for the management of dyslipidaemias for family physicians 2016. Arch Med Sci 2017;13:1–45.

17. Catapano AL, Graham I, De Backer G, et al. 2016 ESC/EAS guidelines for the management of dyslipidaemias: the task force for the management of dyslipidaemias of the European Society of Cardiology (ESC) and European Atherosclerosis Society (EAS) developed with the special contribution of the European Association for Cardiovascular Prevention and Rehabilitation (EACPR). Atherosclerosis 2016;253:281–344.

18. Bays H, Cohen DE, Chalasani N, et al, The National Lipid Association's Statin Safety Task Force. An assessment by the statin liver safety task force: 2014 update. J Clin Lipidol 2014;8:S47–57.

19. Wang C, Gale M Jr, Keller BC, et al. Identification of FBL2 as a geranyl geranylated cellular protein required for hepatitis C virus RNA replication. Mol Cell 2005;18:425–34.

20. Athyros VG, Alexandrides TK, Bilianou H, et al. The use of statins alone, or in combination with pioglitazone and other drugs, for the treatment of non-alcoholic fatty liver disease/non-alcoholic steatohepatitis and related cardiovascular risk. An Expert Panel Statement. Metabolism 2017;71:17–32.

21. Athyros VG, Tziomalos K, Gossios TD, et al, GREACE Study Collaborative Group. Safety and efficacy of long-term statin treatment for cardiovascular events in patients with coronary heart disease and abnormal liver tests in the Greek Atorvastatin and Coronary Heart Disease Evaluation (GREACE) study: a post-hoc analysis. Lancet 2010;376:1916–22.

22. Parker BA, Capizzi JA, Grimaldi AS, et al. Effect of statins on skeletal muscle function. Circulation 2013;127:96–103.

23. Rosenson RS, Miller K, Bayliss M, et al. The Statin-Associated Muscle Symptom Clinical Index (SAMS-CI): revision for clinical use, content validation, and inter-rater reliability. Cardiovasc Drugs Ther 2017;31(2):179–86.

24. Muntean DM, Thompson PD, Catapano AL, et al. Statin-associated myopathy and the quest for biomarkers: can we effectively predict statin-associated muscle symptoms? Drug Discov Today 2017;22:85–96.

25. Gluba-Brzozka A, Franczyk B, Toth PP, et al. Molecular mechanisms of statin intolerance. Arch Med Sci 2016;12:645–58.

26. Banach M, Stulc T, Dent R, et al. Statin non-adherence and residual cardiovascular risk: there is need for substantial improvement. Int J Cardiol 2016;225:184–96.

27. Serban MC, Colantonio LD, Manthripragada AD, et al. Statin intolerance and risk of coronary heart events and all-cause mortality following myocardial infarction. J Am Coll Cardiol 2017;69:1386–95.

28. Awad K, Mikhailidis DP, Toth PP, et al, Lipid and Blood Pressure Meta-analysis Collaboration (LBPMC) Group. Efficacy and safety of alternate-day versus daily dosing of statins: a systematic review and meta-analysis. Cardiovasc Drugs Ther 2017;31:419–31.

29. Serban MC, Banach M, Mikhailidis DP. Clinical implications of the IMPROVE-IT trial in the light of current and future lipid-lowering treatment options. Expert Opin Pharmacother 2016;17:369–80.

30. Tsujita K, Sugiyama S, Sumida H, et al, PRECISE–IVUS Investigators. Impact of dual lipid-lowering strategy with ezetimibe and atorvastatin on coronary plaque regression in patients with percutaneous coronary intervention: the multicenter randomized controlled PRECISE-IVUS trial. J Am Coll Cardiol 2015;66:495–507.

31. Banach M, Nikolic D, Rizzo M, et al. IMPROVE-IT: what have we learned? Curr Opin Cardiol 2016; 31(4):426–33.

32. Cannon CP, Blazing MA, Giugliano RP, et al, IMPROVE-IT Investigators. Ezetimibe added to statin therapy after acute coronary syndromes. N Engl J Med 2015;372(25):2387–97.

33. Banach M, Rizzo M, Obradovic M, et al. PCSK9 inhibition: a novel mechanism to treat lipid disorders? Curr Pharm Des 2013;19:3869–77.

34. Dragan S, Serban MC, Banach M. Proprotein convertase subtilisin/kexin 9 inhibitors: an emerging lipid-lowering therapy? J Cardiovasc Pharmacol Ther 2015;20:157–68.

35. Moriarty PM, Thompson PD, Cannon CP, et al, ODYSSEY ALTERNATIVE Investigators. Efficacy and safety of alirocumab vs ezetimibe in statin-intolerant patients, with a statin rechallenge arm: the ODYSSEY ALTERNATIVE randomized trial. J Clin Lipidol 2015;9:758–69.

36. Nissen SE, Stroes E, Dent-Acosta RE, et al, GAUSS-3 Investigators. Efficacy and tolerability of evolocumab vs ezetimibe in patients with muscle-related statin intolerance: the GAUSS-3 randomized clinical trial. JAMA 2016;315:1580–90.

37. Sabatine MS, Giugliano RP, Keech AC, et al, FOURIER Steering Committee and Investigators. Evolocumab and clinical outcomes in patients with cardiovascular disease. N Engl J Med 2017;376:1713–22.

38. Evaluation of major cardiovascular events in patients with, or at high risk for, cardiovascular disease who are statin intolerant treated with bempedoic acid (ETC-1002) or placebo (CLEAR-Outcomes) trial. Available at: https://clinicaltrials.gov/ct2/show/NCT02993406. Accessed November 5, 2017.

39. Penson P, McGowan M, Banach M. Evaluating bempedoic acid for the treatment of hyperlipidaemia. Expert Opin Investig Drugs 2017;26:251–9.

40. Banach M, Serban C, Ursoniu S, et al, Lipid and Blood Pressure Meta-analysis Collaboration (LBPMC) Group. Statin therapy and plasma coenzyme Q10 concentrations: a systematic review and meta-analysis of placebo-controlled trials. Pharmacol Res 2015;99:329–36.

41. Hargreaves IP, Duncan AJ, Heales SJ, et al. The effect of HMG-CoA reductase inhibitors on coenzyme Q10: possible biochemical/clinical implications. Drug Saf 2005;28:659–76.

42. Banach M, Serban C, Sahebkar A, et al, Lipid and Blood Pressure Meta-analysis Collaboration Group. Effects of coenzyme Q10 on statin-induced myopathy: a meta-analysis of randomized controlled trials. Mayo Clin Proc 2015;90:24–34.

43. Banach M, Serban C, Sahebkar A, et al. Futility of supplementation with CoQ10 for statin-induced myopathy: an updated (2015) meta-analysis of randomized controlled trials. Eur Heart J 2015; 36(Suppl.1):1047.

44. Ahmed W, Khan N, Glueck CJ, et al. Low serum 25 (OH) vitamin D levels (<32 ng/mL) are associated with reversible myositis-myalgia in statin-treated patients. Transl Res 2009;153:11–6.

45. Sahebkar A, Reiner Z, Simental-Mendia LE, et al. Impact of statin therapy on plasma vitamin D levels: a systematic review and meta-analysis. Curr Pharm Des 2017;23:861–9.

46. Michalska-Kasiczak M, Sahebkar A, Mikhailidis DP, et al, Lipid and Blood Pressure Meta-analysis Collaboration (LBPMC) Group. Analysis of vitamin D levels in patients with and without statin-associated myalgia: a systematic review and meta-analysis of 7 studies with 2420 patients. Int J Cardiol 2015;178:111–6.

47. Khayznikov M, Hemachrandra K, Pandit R, et al. Statin intolerance because of myalgia, myositis, myopathy, or myonecrosis can in most cases be safely resolved by vitamin D supplementation. N Am J Med Sci 2015;7:86–93.

48. Taylor BA, Lorson L, White CM, et al. Low vitamin D does not predict statin associated muscle symptoms but is associated with transient increases in muscle damage and pain. Atherosclerosis 2017; 256:100–4.

49. Sahebkar A, Serban MC, Gluba-Brzózka A, et al. Lipid-modifying effects of nutraceuticals: an evidence-based approach. Nutrition 2016;32:1179–92.

50. Patti AM, Toth PP, Giglio RV, et al. Nutraceuticals as an important part of combination therapy in dyslipidaemia. Curr Pharm Des 2017;23:2496–503.

51. Cicero AFG, Colletti A, Bajraktari G, et al. Lipid lowering nutraceuticals in clinical practice: position paper from an International Lipid Expert Panel. Arch Med Sci 2017;13:965–1005.

Treating Dyslipidemia in Type 2 Diabetes

Adam J. Nelson, MBBS, Stephen J. Nicholls, MBBS, PhD*

KEYWORDS

• Diabetes • Lipids • Cardiovascular risk • Clinical trials

KEY POINTS

- Atherosclerotic cardiovascular disease (ASCVD) presents an ongoing major public health challenge.
- There is an urgent need to identify and develop the most effective preventive strategies for reducing cardiovascular risk in patients with diabetes.
- Targeting dyslipidemia in patients with diabetes forms a cornerstone of approaches to cardiovascular prevention.

INTRODUCTION

Randomized controlled trials have demonstrated that lowering cholesterol and blood pressure has a beneficial effect on cardiovascular event rates in the primary and secondary prevention settings.[1–5] Although implementation of these therapies in clinical practice have contributed to reductions in attributed mortality, atherosclerotic cardiovascular disease (ASCVD) presents an ongoing major public health challenge. The global increase in obesity and diabetes are likely to underscore a considerable part of this challenge and associate with a greater risk of adverse outcomes in those patients whose ASCVD has become clinically manifest. Accordingly, there is an urgent need to identify and develop the most effective preventive strategies to reducing cardiovascular risk in patients with diabetes. Targeting dyslipidemia in these patients forms a cornerstone of approaches to cardiovascular prevention.

DYSLIPIDEMIA IN DIABETES

In association with insulin resistance, type 2 diabetes is typically accompanied by a specific lipid phenotype, characterized by elevated triglycerides, low levels of high-density lipoprotein cholesterol (HDL-C) and the observation that low-density lipoprotein cholesterol (LDL-C) levels are often within the normal range.[6] Activity of lipoprotein lipase, a major factor implicated in the metabolism of triglyceride-rich lipoproteins, is impaired in the setting of hyperglycemia.[7,8] The resulting increase in circulating concentration of triglyceride-rich lipoproteins activates other lipid metabolism factors that tend to decrease HDL-C levels.[9] Many lines of evidence suggest that low-density lipoprotein (LDL) per se is not normal in most patients with diabetes.[10] However, elevated LDL-C levels are encountered in 25% of patients[11] and diabetes is typically accompanied by elevated levels of small, dense LDL particles.[12,13] Accordingly, in patients in whom LDL-C levels are considered to be

Disclosure: Nicholls disclosures are research support from AstraZeneca, Amgen, Anthera, Eli Lilly, Esperion, Novartis, Cerenis, The Medicines Company, Resverlogix, InfraReDx, Roche, Sanofi-Regeneron and LipoScience and a consultant for AstraZeneca, Eli Lilly, Anthera, Omthera, Merck, Takeda, Resverlogix, Sanofi-Regeneron, CSL Behring, Esperion, Boehringer Ingelheim. Other authors have no disclosures.
South Australian Health and Medical Research Institute, University of Adelaide, PO Box 11060, Adelaide, SA 5001, Australia
* Corresponding author.
E-mail address: Stephen.Nicholls@sahmri.com

Cardiol Clin 36 (2018) 233–239
https://doi.org/10.1016/j.ccl.2017.12.005

normal, the LDL profile remains associated with increased atherogenicity.[14–18] Each of these findings presents considerable opportunity for targeting dyslipidemia, which can reduce cardiovascular risk in patients with type 2 diabetes.

STATINS AND DIABETES

Randomized controlled trials have consistently demonstrated that lowering LDL-C with statins reduces cardiovascular morbidity and mortality.[19,20] More recent studies comparing intensive and moderate statin therapy has supported the concept of benefits with more aggressive lipid lowering.[21–25] Within each of these studies, investigation of the subgroup of patients with diabetes has failed to demonstrate any evidence of heterogeneity, suggesting that statins afford a similar degree of clinical benefit in the setting of diabetes. This has been subsequently confirmed by pooled analyses of the statin trials.[3] The only placebo-controlled clinical trial performed exclusively in subjects with diabetes demonstrated a reduction in cardiovascular risk with atorvastatin.[26] These findings have underscored the consistent emphasis in treatment guidelines to assume that patients with diabetes should be considered to be at high cardiovascular risk and require treatment with a statin, regardless of the presence of clinically manifest ASCVD or baseline LDL-C levels.

In parallel, it has become apparent that statins, particularly when administered as intensive doses, are associated with a greater incidence of diagnoses of diabetes within those studies. Observations from Mendelian randomization show that polymorphisms are associated with low activity of either hydroxyl-methyl-glutaryl coenzyme A reductase[27] or proprotein convertase subtilisin kexin type 9 (PCSK9)[28] not only with low LDL-C levels but also with an elevated risk of diabetes. When combined with reports of a lower prevalence of diabetes in patients with familial hypercholesterolemia,[29] it would seem that the observation of new-onset diabetes in the statin trials is more likely a function of the lipid lowering than of the statin itself.[30,31] Nevertheless, given the cardiovascular benefits of statin therapy in patients with type 2 diabetes, these observations have not altered clinical practice in patients at high risk for ASCVD who require intensive lipid lowering with a statin.

ADDITIONAL LOW-DENSITY LIPOPROTEIN CHOLESTEROL-LOWERING AGENTS AND DIABETES

Ezetimibe is a cholesterol absorption inhibitor that reduces LDL-C by up to 20%.[32] In addition, it lowers the inflammatory marker C-reactive protein (CRP) when administered in combination with statins.[33] When added to simvastatin in patients with a recent acute coronary syndrome, ezetimibe produced a modest reduction in clinical events on long-term follow-up.[34] Subgroup analysis revealed that this clinical benefit was largely observed in patients with diabetes. Although this is likely to reflect a greater modifiability of risk in the presence of diabetes and acute coronary syndromes, it remains to be further characterized. The findings do suggest that patients with diabetes who experience an acute coronary syndrome should be treated intensively with the combination of statin and ezetimibe with a view to achieving an LDL-C less than 50 mg/dL.

PCSK9 plays an important role in regulating hepatic expression of the LDL receptor. Inhibitory monoclonal antibodies directed against circulating PCSK9 have been demonstrated to decrease LDL-C by up to 60% when administered as either monotherapy or in combination with statins.[20] Similar lipid effects have been reported in trials exclusively performed with subjects with diabetes.[35] Recent trials have demonstrated that treatment with evolocumab in addition to statins reduce LDL-C to less than 40 mg/dL and produce both regression of coronary atherosclerosis[36] and a reduction in cardiovascular events.[37] There is no evidence of heterogeneity in subgroup analysis, suggesting that patients with diabetes are likely to derive a clinical benefit from this therapy. Further analysis from the FOURIER (Further Cardiovascular Outcomes Research with PCSK9 Inhibition in Subjects with Elevated Risk) trial demonstrated higher placebo event rates in patients with diabetes and a greater absolute risk reduction with evolocumab, suggesting a lower number needed to treat.[38] Although there was no evidence in FOURIER of an increase in diagnoses of new-onset diabetes with evolocumab,[38] the Mendelian randomization data suggest that such an effect may ultimately be observed if a sufficiently high number of patients are treated for long enough.

Bempedoic acid is a liver-specific inhibitor of advanced treatment panel citrate lyase, which reduces hepatic cholesterol biosynthesis and upregulates LDL receptor expression in a similar fashion to statins. In contrast, the factor required for conversion of its prodrug to the active form is not present in skeletal muscle, underscoring its potential development for patients with statin intolerance. Lipid efficacy studies have demonstrated dose-dependent lowering of LDL-C by up to 30% and CRP by up to 40% in patients with and without diabetes.[39] A large clinical outcomes trial is currently evaluating the impact of bempedoic acid in patients with a high risk for

ASCVD with statin intolerance. Given the need to intensively lower LDL-C in patients with diabetes, this agent may prove to play an important role in cardiovascular prevention.

FIBRIC ACID DERIVATIVES

Fibrates are modest pharmacologic agonists of the peroxisome proliferator-activated receptor (PPAR)-α that raise HDL-C and lower triglycerides,[40] small dense LDL, and CRP levels.[41] Early studies using gemfibrozil demonstrated cardiovascular benefit in both primary and secondary prevention studies.[42,43] Importantly, raising levels of small high-density lipoprotein (HDL) particles is independently associated with cardiovascular benefit, whereas triglyceride lowering is not.[43] An elevated rate of myalgia with the combination of gemfibrozil and statin therapy has led to increasing use of fenofibrate as the preferred fibric acid derivative in clinical practice.[44] Serial angiographic studies demonstrated that administration of micronized fenofibrate slowed progression of obstructive disease in a cohort of subjects with coronary artery disease and diabetes.[45] This did not, however, translate to cardiovascular benefit of fenofibrate in large outcomes trials. Two randomized controlled trials performed in subjects with type 2 diabetes, 1 before widespread statin use[46] and the other on a background of statin therapy,[47] failed to demonstrate favorable reductions of the primary composite cardiovascular endpoints. Of interest, benefit was observed in the subgroups with elevated triglyceride and low HDL-C levels at baseline. This was subsequently confirmed in a meta-analysis of all fibrate trials performed to date.[48] These findings have influenced clinical practice, in which the patient with this atherogenic dyslipidemic phenotype, commonly encountered in type 2 diabetes, are primarily treated with a fibrate as part of their approach to cardiovascular risk reduction.

In parallel, development of PPAR-γ agonists produced highly prescribed glucose-lowering agents for use in diabetes. Clinical trials with pioglitazone demonstrated slowing of progression of coronary atherosclerosis.[49] In a large outcome study, the composite primary endpoint was not reduced, although there was a decrease in the combination of death, myocardial infarction, and stroke.[50] Of particular interest, favorable effects on the triglyceride to HDL-C ratio independently associated with the ability of pioglitazone to slow disease progression.[51] Whether this reflects some minor PPAR-α activity is uncertain. Although these agents were widely used in patients with diabetes, the subsequent concerns of a risk of myocardial infarction with rosiglitazone has limited their use.[52]

Considerable interest has focused on attempts to refine pharmacologic approaches to targeting various PPAR receptors. Potent PPAR-α and dual PPAR-α/γ agonists have been developed, although all of these agents have proven to be disappointing in terms of efficacy and are associated with considerable toxicity issues. Pemafibrate is a selective peroxisome proliferator activator modulator, designed with altered receptor affinity, to potentially target enhanced metabolic efficacy, while reducing tissue activity and, therefore, toxicity.[53] This agent is now being evaluated in a large cardiovascular outcomes trial conducted in statin-treated subjects with diabetes and associated hypertriglyceridemia and low HDL-C.[54]

ADDITIONAL TRIGLYCERIDE-LOWERING STRATEGIES

Omega-3 fatty acids have received considerable attention as a potential approach to preventing cardiovascular events for more than 2 decades, yet there continues to be uncertainty about their optimal clinical use. At high doses, omega-3 fatty acids have proven to be highly effective in their ability to lower triglyceride levels.[55] However, most clinical studies investigating atherosclerotic, arrhythmic, or heart failure events have been disappointing. In many of these studies, relatively low doses of omega-3 fatty acids were administered or the subject population was relatively diverse. The most compelling evidence of potential clinical benefit has been derived from a large outcome trial using relatively high doses in a Japanese cohort.[56] This finding has stimulated efforts to evaluate the cardiovascular effects of high dose (4 g daily) of eicosapentaenoic acid, as monotherapy or in combination with docosahexanoic acid, in high-risk patients with hypertriglyceridemia and low HDL-C levels. It is likely that both of these outcome trials will include a considerable number of subjects with diabetes and will provide important additional information with regard to effective cardiovascular prevention.

Elucidating the factors involved in regulation of metabolism of triglyceride-rich lipoproteins has yielded important new targets for drug development. Apolipoprotein C-III and angiopoietin-like proteins 3 and 4 inhibit activity of lipoprotein lipase, the main factor involved in triglyceride hydrolysis. Genetic studies have demonstrated that loss of function mutations of these factors associate with low levels of both triglycerides and cardiovascular risk.[57–60] These findings implicate triglycerides in the causal pathway of ASCVD[61] and have led to the development of antisense and antibody approaches for treatment of hypertriglyceridemia.[62] Given the need to comprehensively evaluate the safety profile of these agents, they will need to be subjected to large clinical trials, which will involve a considerable number of subjects with type 2 diabetes.

HIGH-DENSITY LIPOPROTEIN TARGETED THERAPIES

Epidemiology and animal studies suggest that HDL plays a protective role against the development of ASCVD.[63] This is further supported by observations that HDL is a central player in the facilitation of reverse cholesterol transport and favorably modifies inflammatory, oxidative, and thrombotic mediators of atherosclerosis.[64,65] Given that small degrees of HDL-C raising contribute to the benefit of statins and fibrates, there has been major interest in developing new approaches to targeting HDL function. Nicotinic acid is the most potent HDL-C–raising agent currently used in clinical practice. Although early studies before the use of statins suggested cardiovascular benefit,[66] and subsequent angiographic studies demonstrated regression in the setting of statin therapy with immediate release niacin,[67] considerable issues with tolerance have limited its use. Attempts to limit intolerance by extending formulation of release[68] or administration in combination with a prostanoid antagonist[69] have failed to reduce cardiovascular events in the setting of contemporary statin use. This disappointment was associated with a range of adverse effects, of which worsening glycemic control in patients with diabetes is commonly encountered. Accordingly, empirical use of niacin is not currently advocated for use in patients with diabetes. It is likely to be reserved for patients with dyslipidemia that is difficult to treat despite use of other lipid-modifying agents.

Two major strategies have dominated the approach to targeting HDL functionality. Infusing delipidated HDL mimetics received early support by a small proof of concept imaging study demonstrating early regression of coronary atherosclerosis in subjects following an acute coronary syndrome.[70] However, several recent studies performed in the setting of high intensity statin therapy have not been able to replicate these findings.[71] No mimetic, to date, has been evaluated with regard to its ability to reduce cardiovascular event rates. Cholesteryl ester transfer protein (CETP) inhibitors have been developed primarily based on their ability to substantially raise HDL-C

levels. However, the field has been limited by reports of toxicity[72] and futility with several agents.[73,74] Although a recent trial suggested modest cardiovascular benefit with long-term administration of a potent CETP inhibitor,[75] this may have resulted from the ability of this agent to also reduce LDL-C levels. It remains to be determined whether any CETP inhibitor will reach clinical practice. An optimistic finding from each of the trials on CETP inhibitors is their ability to exert favorable effects on either glycemic control or the rate of diagnoses of new-onset diabetes.[76] Although the mechanism underlying this potential benefit is uncertain, it may indicate that these agents may be of potential use in higher risk patients with either established type 2 diabetes or insulin resistance. Clinical trials need to be performed to further evaluate how this translates to potential clinical benefit.

SUMMARY

Diabetes is associated with both a classic dyslipidemic phenotype and increased risk of adverse cardiovascular events. Evidence to date suggests that patients with diabetes should be considered high risk, regardless of the clinical manifestation of ASCVD, warranting use of statin therapy and intensive LDL-C lowering. The presence of additional lipid targets in diabetes highlights the need for use of additional agents. The development of an exciting range of new therapies has the potential to modulate cardiovascular outcomes in patients with diabetes. Completion of pivotal clinical trials will determine which of these approaches will become important in clinical practice.

REFERENCES

1. Baigent C, Keech A, Kearney PM, et al. Efficacy and safety of cholesterol-lowering treatment: prospective meta-analysis of data from 90,056 participants in 14 randomised trials of statins. Lancet 2005;366: 1267–78.
2. Blood Pressure Lowering Treatment Trialists' Collaboration. Blood pressure-lowering treatment based on cardiovascular risk: a meta-analysis of individual patient data. Lancet 2014;384:591–8.
3. Cholesterol Treatment Trialists' (CTT) Collaboration, Baigent C, Blackwell L, Emberson J, et al. Efficacy and safety of more intensive lowering of LDL cholesterol: a meta-analysis of data from 170,000 participants in 26 randomised trials. Lancet 2010;376: 1670–81.
4. Ettehad D, Emdin CA, Kiran A, et al. Blood pressure lowering for prevention of cardiovascular disease

and death: a systematic review and meta-analysis. Lancet 2016;387:957–67.

5. Yusuf S, Lonn E, Pais P, et al. Blood-pressure and cholesterol lowering in persons without cardiovascular disease. N Engl J Med 2016;374:2032–43.

6. Kannel WB. Lipids, diabetes, and coronary heart disease: insights from the Framingham Study. Am Heart J 1985;110:1100–7.

7. Knudsen P, Eriksson J, Lahdenpera S, et al. Changes of lipolytic enzymes cluster with insulin resistance syndrome. Botnia Study Group. Diabetologia 1995;38:344–50.

8. Taskinen MR. Lipoprotein lipase in diabetes. Diabetes Metab Rev 1987;3:551–70.

9. Chan DC, Watts GF. Dyslipidaemia in the metabolic syndrome and type 2 diabetes: pathogenesis, priorities, pharmacotherapies. Expert Opin Pharmacother 2011;12:13–30.

10. Malave H, Castro M, Burkle J, et al. Evaluation of low-density lipoprotein particle number distribution in patients with type 2 diabetes mellitus with low-density lipoprotein cholesterol <50 mg/dl and non-high-density lipoprotein cholesterol <80 mg/dl. Am J Cardiol 2012;110:662–5.

11. Jacobs MJ, Kleisli T, Pio JR, et al. Prevalence and control of dyslipidemia among persons with diabetes in the United States. Diabetes Res Clin Pract 2005;70:263–9.

12. Feingold KR, Grunfeld C, Pang M, et al. LDL subclass phenotypes and triglyceride metabolism in non-insulin-dependent diabetes. Arterioscler Thromb 1992;12:1496–502.

13. Garvey WT, Kwon S, Zheng D, et al. Effects of insulin resistance and type 2 diabetes on lipoprotein subclass particle size and concentration determined by nuclear magnetic resonance. Diabetes 2003;52: 453–62.

14. Austin MA, King MC, Vranizan KM, et al. Atherogenic lipoprotein phenotype. A proposed genetic marker for coronary heart disease risk. Circulation 1990;82:495–506.

15. Chapman MJ, Guerin M, Bruckert E. Atherogenic, dense low-density lipoproteins. Pathophysiology and new therapeutic approaches. Eur Heart J 1998;19(Suppl A):A24–30.

16. Taskinen MR. Diabetic dyslipidaemia: from basic research to clinical practice. Diabetologia 2003;46: 733–49.

17. Tozer EC, Carew TE. Residence time of low-density lipoprotein in the normal and atherosclerotic rabbit aorta. Circ Res 1997;80:208–18.

18. Verges B. New insight into the pathophysiology of lipid abnormalities in type 2 diabetes. Diabetes Metab 2005;31:429–39.

19. Cholesterol Treatment Trialists' (CTT) Collaborators, Kearney PM, Blackwell L, Collins R, et al. Efficacy of cholesterol-lowering therapy in 18,686 people

with diabetes in 14 randomised trials of statins: a meta-analysis. Lancet 2008;371:117–25.

20. Scherer DJ, Nelson A, Psaltis PJ, et al. Targeting low-density lipoprotein cholesterol with PCSK9 inhibitors. Intern Med J 2017;47(8):856–65.

21. Cannon CP, Braunwald E, McCabe CH, et al. Intensive versus moderate lipid lowering with statins after acute coronary syndromes. N Engl J Med 2004;350: 1495–504.

22. Hsia J, MacFadyen JG, Monyak J, et al. Cardiovascular event reduction and adverse events among subjects attaining low-density lipoprotein cholesterol <50 mg/dl with rosuvastatin. The JUPITER trial (Justification for the Use of Statins in Prevention: an Intervention Trial Evaluating Rosuvastatin). J Am Coll Cardiol 2011;57:1666–75.

23. LaRosa JC, Grundy SM, Waters DD, et al. Intensive lipid lowering with atorvastatin in patients with stable coronary disease. N Engl J Med 2005;352:1425–35.

24. Nicholls SJ, Ballantyne CM, Barter PJ, et al. Effect of two intensive statin regimens on progression of coronary disease. N Engl J Med 2011;365:2078–87.

25. Pedersen TR, Faergeman O, Kastelein JJ, et al. High-dose atorvastatin vs usual-dose simvastatin for secondary prevention after myocardial infarction: the IDEAL study: a randomized controlled trial. JAMA 2005;294:2437–45.

26. Colhoun HM, Betteridge DJ, Durrington PN, et al. Primary prevention of cardiovascular disease with atorvastatin in type 2 diabetes in the Collaborative Atorvastatin Diabetes Study (CARDS): multicentre randomised placebo-controlled trial. Lancet 2004; 364:685–96.

27. Swerdlow DI, Preiss D, Kuchenbaecker KB, et al. HMG-coenzyme A reductase inhibition, type 2 diabetes, and bodyweight: evidence from genetic analysis and randomised trials. Lancet 2015;385: 351–61.

28. Schmidt AF, Swerdlow DI, Holmes MV, et al. PCSK9 genetic variants and risk of type 2 diabetes: a mendelian randomisation study. Lancet Diabetes Endocrinol 2017;5:97–105.

29. Besseling J, Kastelein JJ, Defesche JC, et al. Association between familial hypercholesterolemia and prevalence of type 2 diabetes mellitus. JAMA 2015;313:1029–36.

30. Cai R, Yuan Y, Zhou Y, et al. Lower intensified target LDL-c level of statin therapy results in a higher risk of incident diabetes: a meta-analysis. PLoS One 2014; 9:e104922.

31. Wang S, Cai R, Yuan Y, et al. Association between reductions in low-density lipoprotein cholesterol with statin therapy and the risk of new-onset diabetes: a meta-analysis. Sci Rep 2017;7:39982.

32. Morrone D, Weintraub WS, Toth PP, et al. Lipid-altering efficacy of ezetimibe plus statin and statin monotherapy and identification of factors associated

with treatment response: a pooled analysis of over 21,000 subjects from 27 clinical trials. Atherosclerosis 2012;223:251–61.

33. Bohula EA, Giugliano RP, Cannon CP, et al. Achievement of dual low-density lipoprotein cholesterol and high-sensitivity C-reactive protein targets more frequent with the addition of ezetimibe to simvastatin and associated with better outcomes in IMPROVE-IT. Circulation 2015;132:1224–33.

34. Cannon CP, Blazing MA, Giugliano RP, et al. Ezetimibe added to statin therapy after acute coronary syndromes. N Engl J Med 2015;372:2387–97.

35. Sattar N, Preiss D, Robinson JG, et al. Lipid-lowering efficacy of the PCSK9 inhibitor evolocumab (AMG 145) in patients with type 2 diabetes: a meta-analysis of individual patient data. Lancet Diabetes Endocrinol 2016;4:403–10.

36. Nicholls SJ, Puri R, Anderson T, et al. Effect of evolocumab on progression of coronary disease in statin-treated patients: the GLAGOV randomized clinical trial. JAMA 2016;316:2373–84.

37. Sabatine MS, Giugliano RP, Keech AC, et al. Evolocumab and clinical outcomes in patients with cardiovascular disease. N Engl J Med 2017;376: 1713–22.

38. Sabatine MS, Leiter LA, Wiviott SD, et al. Cardiovascular safety and efficacy of the PCSK9 inhibitor evolocumab in patients with and without diabetes and the effect of evolocumab on glycaemia and risk of new-onset diabetes: a prespecified analysis of the FOURIER randomised controlled trial. Lancet Diabetes Endocrinol 2017;5(12):941–50.

39. Gutierrez MJ, Rosenberg NL, Macdougall DE, et al. Efficacy and safety of ETC-1002, a novel investigational low-density lipoprotein-cholesterol-lowering therapy for the treatment of patients with hypercholesterolemia and type 2 diabetes mellitus. Arterioscler Thromb Vasc Biol 2014;34:676–83.

40. Staels B, Dallongeville J, Auwerx J, et al. Mechanism of action of fibrates on lipid and lipoprotein metabolism. Circulation 1998;98:2088–93.

41. Ikewaki K, Tohyama J, Nakata Y, et al. Fenofibrate effectively reduces remnants, and small dense LDL, and increases HDL particle number in hypertriglyceridemic men - a nuclear magnetic resonance study. J Atheroscler Thromb 2004;11:278–85.

42. Bloomfield Rubins H, Davenport J, Babikian V, et al. Reduction in stroke with gemfibrozil in men with coronary heart disease and low HDL cholesterol: the Veterans Affairs HDL Intervention Trial (VA-HIT). Circulation 2001;103:2828–33.

43. Rubins HB, Robins SJ, Collins D, et al. Gemfibrozil for the secondary prevention of coronary heart disease in men with low levels of high-density lipoprotein cholesterol. Veterans Affairs High-Density Lipoprotein Cholesterol Intervention Trial Study Group. N Engl J Med 1999;341:410–8.

44. Guo J, Meng F, Ma N, et al. Meta-analysis of safety of the coadministration of statin with fenofibrate in patients with combined hyperlipidemia. Am J Cardiol 2012;110:1296–301.

45. Effect of fenofibrate on progression of coronary-artery disease in type 2 diabetes: the Diabetes Atherosclerosis Intervention Study, a randomised study. Lancet 2001;357:905–10.

46. Keech A, Simes RJ, Barter P, et al. Effects of long-term fenofibrate therapy on cardiovascular events in 9795 people with type 2 diabetes mellitus (the FIELD study): randomised controlled trial. Lancet 2005;366:1849–61.

47. ACCORD Study Group, Ginsberg HN, Elam MB, Lovato LC, et al. Effects of combination lipid therapy in type 2 diabetes mellitus. N Engl J Med 2010;362: 1563–74.

48. Lee M, Saver JL, Towfighi A, et al. Efficacy of fibrates for cardiovascular risk reduction in persons with atherogenic dyslipidemia: a meta-analysis. Atherosclerosis 2011;217:492–8.

49. Nissen SE, Nicholls SJ, Wolski K, et al. Comparison of pioglitazone vs glimepiride on progression of coronary atherosclerosis in patients with type 2 diabetes: the PERISCOPE randomized controlled trial. JAMA 2008;299:1561–73.

50. Dormandy JA, Charbonnel B, Eckland DJ, et al. Secondary prevention of macrovascular events in patients with type 2 diabetes in the PROactive Study (PROspective pioglitAzone Clinical Trial in macroVascular Events): a randomised controlled trial. Lancet 2005;366:1279–89.

51. Nicholls SJ, Tuzcu EM, Wolski K, et al. Lowering the triglyceride/high-density lipoprotein cholesterol ratio is associated with the beneficial impact of pioglitazone on progression of coronary atherosclerosis in diabetic patients: insights from the PERISCOPE (Pioglitazone Effect on Regression of Intravascular Sonographic Coronary Obstruction Prospective Evaluation) study. J Am Coll Cardiol 2011;57:153–9.

52. Nissen SE, Wolski K. Effect of rosiglitazone on the risk of myocardial infarction and death from cardiovascular causes. N Engl J Med 2007;356:2457–71.

53. Hennuyer N, Duplan I, Paquet C, et al. The novel selective PPARalpha modulator (SPPARMalpha) pemafibrate improves dyslipidemia, enhances reverse cholesterol transport and decreases inflammation and atherosclerosis. Atherosclerosis 2016;249: 200–8.

54. Fruchart JC. Pemafibrate (K-877), a novel selective peroxisome proliferator-activated receptor alpha modulator for management of atherogenic dyslipidaemia. Cardiovasc Diabetol 2017;16:124.

55. Ballantyne CM, Bays HE, Kastelein JJ, et al. Efficacy and safety of eicosapentaenoic acid ethyl ester (AMR101) therapy in statin-treated patients with

persistent high triglycerides (from the ANCHOR study). Am J Cardiol 2012;110:984–92.

56. Yokoyama M, Origasa H, Matsuzaki M, et al. Effects of eicosapentaenoic acid on major coronary events in hypercholesterolaemic patients (JELIS): a randomised open-label, blinded endpoint analysis. Lancet 2007;369:1090–8.

57. Dewey FE, Gusarova V, Dunbar RL, et al. Genetic and Pharmacologic inactivation of ANGPTL3 and cardiovascular disease. N Engl J Med 2017;377:211–21.

58. Pollin TI, Damcott CM, Shen H, et al. A null mutation in human APOC3 confers a favorable plasma lipid profile and apparent cardioprotection. Science 2008;322:1702–5.

59. Stitziel NO, Khera AV, Wang X, et al. ANGPTL3 deficiency and protection against coronary artery disease. J Am Coll Cardiol 2017;69:2054–63.

60. Stitziel NO, the Myocardial Infarction Genetics and CARDIoGRAM Exome Consortia Investigators. Variants in ANGPTL4 and the risk of coronary artery disease. N Engl J Med 2016;375:2306.

61. Do R, Willer CJ, Schmidt EM, et al. Common variants associated with plasma triglycerides and risk for coronary artery disease. Nat Genet 2013;45:1345–52.

62. Graham MJ, Lee RG, Brandt TA, et al. Cardiovascular and metabolic effects of ANGPTL3 antisense oligonucleotides. N Engl J Med 2017;377:222–32.

63. Gordon DJ, Probstfield JL, Garrison RJ, et al. High-density lipoprotein cholesterol and cardiovascular disease. Four prospective American studies. Circulation 1989;79:8–15.

64. Barter PJ, Nicholls S, Rye KA, et al. Antiinflammatory properties of HDL. Circ Res 2004;95:764–72.

65. Brewer HB Jr. HDL metabolism and the role of HDL in the treatment of high-risk patients with cardiovascular disease. Curr Cardiol Rep 2007;9:486–92.

66. Canner PL, Berge KG, Wenger NK, et al. Fifteen year mortality in Coronary Drug Project patients: long-term benefit with niacin. J Am Coll Cardiol 1986;8:1245–55.

67. Brown BG, Zhao XQ, Chait A, et al. Simvastatin and niacin, antioxidant vitamins, or the combination for the prevention of coronary disease. N Engl J Med 2001;345:1583–92.

68. AIM-HIGH Investigators, Boden WE, Probstfield JL, Anderson T, et al. Niacin in patients with low HDL cholesterol levels receiving intensive statin therapy. N Engl J Med 2011;365:2255–67.

69. HPS2-THRIVE Collaborative Group, Landray MJ, Haynes R, Hopewell JC, et al. Effects of extended-release niacin with laropiprant in high-risk patients. N Engl J Med 2014;371:203–12.

70. Waksman R, Torguson R, Kent KM, et al. A first-in-man, randomized, placebo-controlled study to evaluate the safety and feasibility of autologous delipidated high-density lipoprotein plasma infusions in patients with acute coronary syndrome. J Am Coll Cardiol 2010;55:2727–35.

71. Tardif JC, Ballantyne CM, Barter P, et al. Effects of the high-density lipoprotein mimetic agent CER-001 on coronary atherosclerosis in patients with acute coronary syndromes: a randomized trial. Eur Heart J 2014;35:3277–86.

72. Barter PJ, Caulfield M, Eriksson M, et al. Effects of torcetrapib in patients at high risk for coronary events. N Engl J Med 2007;357:2109–22.

73. Lincoff AM, Nicholls SJ, Riesmeyer JS, et al. Evacetrapib and cardiovascular outcomes in high-risk vascular disease. N Engl J Med 2017;376:1933–42.

74. Schwartz GG, Olsson AG, Abt M, et al. Effects of dalcetrapib in patients with a recent acute coronary syndrome. N Engl J Med 2012;367:2089–99.

75. HPS3/TIMI55–REVEAL Collaborative Group, Bowman L, Hopewell JC, Chen F, et al. Effects of anacetrapib in patients with atherosclerotic vascular disease. N Engl J Med 2017;377:1217–27.

76. Tall AR, Rader DJ. The trials and tribulations of CETP inhibitors. Circ Res 2017;122(1):106–12.

Proprotein Convertase Subtilisin Kexin 9 Inhibitors

Angela Pirillo, PhD[a,b], Alberico Luigi Catapano, PhD[b,c],*

KEYWORDS

- PCSK9 • Monoclonal antibodies • Evolocumab • Alirocumab • LDL-C • Hypercholesterolemia
- Cardiovascular disease • Proprotein convertase subtilisin kexin 9

KEY POINTS

- Low-density lipoprotein (LDL) is a major risk factor for cardiovascular disease.
- Patients at high or very high cardiovascular risk may benefit from large LDL-C reduction.
- Many patients often cannot achieve their LDL-C goals with the starting therapy.

INTRODUCTION

Low-density lipoprotein (LDL) is a major risk factor for cardiovascular disease (CVD), and a large number of epidemiologic studies have established the strong and direct relationship between high LDL-cholesterol (LDL-C) levels and coronary heart disease (CHD), and a wealth of clinical trials have shown that reducing LDL-C levels results in a reduced incidence of cardiovascular (CV) events. In fact, 12% reduction in all-cause mortality, 19% reduction in coronary mortality, and 17% reduction in any vascular cause of mortality per millimole per liter reduction in LDL-C have been observed,[1] and the higher the degree of reduction of LDL-C levels, the greater the benefit in terms of reduction of CV risk, as suggested by the comparison between more intensive and less intensive lipid-lowering therapies.[2] Thus, patients at high or very high CV risk may benefit from achieving the largest LDL-C reduction, as suggested by current guidelines,[3] which need to be maintained over

time to gain a clinical benefit. However, many patients often cannot achieve their LDL-C goals with the starting therapy, which thus require adjustment based on the individual response to the lipid-lowering approach. Statins represent the first-line choice, and their efficacy in reducing CV morbidity and mortality in both primary and secondary prevention has been established in several clinical trials and meta-analyses.[1,2,4–9]

However, despite the efficacy of statins, many patients do not reach their LDL-C level goals due to several reasons, including the occurrence of statin-related adverse events (mainly muscle-related disorders) leading to therapy discontinuation.[10] In addition, a large proportion of patients with high or very high CV risk, including those with genetically determined forms of familial hypercholesterolemia (FH), does not achieve the recommended LDL-C level target even with maximally tolerated doses of drugs. Thus, there is the need of additional interventions that can efficiently reduce

Disclosure: A.L. Catapano has received research funding and/or honoraria from Aegerion, Amgen, AstraZeneca, Eli Lilly, Genzyme, Mediolanum, Merck or MSD, Pfizer, Recordati, Rottapharm, Sanofi-Regeneron, Sigma-Tau. A. Pirillo has nothing to disclose.
[a] Center for the Study of Atherosclerosis, E. Bassini Hospital, Via M. Gorki, 50, Cinisello Balsamo, Milan 20092, Italy; [b] IRCCS MultiMedica, Via Milanese, 300, Sesto S. Giovanni, Milan 20099, Italy; [c] Department of Pharmacological and Biomolecular Sciences, University of Milan, Via Balzaretti, 9, Milan 20133, Italy
* Corresponding author. Department of Pharmacological and Biomolecular Sciences, University of Milan, Via Balzaretti 9, Milan 20133, Italy.
E-mail address: alberico.catapano@unimi.it

Cardiol Clin 36 (2018) 241–256
https://doi.org/10.1016/j.ccl.2017.12.006
0733-8651/18/© 2017 Elsevier Inc. All rights reserved.

LDL-C levels below those achievable with the common cholesterol-lowering drugs.

PROPROTEIN CONVERTASE SUBTILISIN KEXIN 9

Proprotein convertase subtilisin kexin 9 (PCSK9) is a serine protease that plays a key role in the regulation of hepatic low-density lipoprotein receptor (LDLR) function, which represents the key regulator of cellular LDL uptake and plasma cholesterol levels (**Fig. 1**). Following the binding to LDL particles, the complex LDLR/LDL particle is internalized within the cell where it dissociates allowing receptor recycling and lysosomal degradation of LDL particle. When circulating PCSK9 binds to the epidermal growth factor-like repeat domain of LDLR, a conformational change of LDLR occurs, making it more vulnerable to degradation within lysosomes.[11] The binding PCSK9/LDLR thus results in a reduced LDLR surface expression, reduced LDL uptake, and increased plasma levels of LDL-C.

The relevance of PCSK9 as main regulator of plasmatic cholesterol levels derives from the observations that genetic variants of PCSK9 associated with loss or gain of function of this protein resulted in lower or higher levels of LDL-C, respectively.[12,13] More importantly, an association with protection against cardiovascular disease (CVD) was observed in subjects carrying loss-of-function mutations in PCSK9 gene,[13–17] whereas gain-of-function mutations are associated with an increased risk of premature CVD.[18–20] These findings suggested that PCSK9 may be a useful pharmacologic target for the control of hypercholesterolemia (**Fig. 2**) and led to the development

of 2 fully human monoclonal antibodies (mAbs) against circulating PCSK9, evolocumab and alirocumab, which are now approved for the treatment of hypercholesterolemia. The development of a third mAb against PCSK9 (bococizumab) was recently halted because of a high titer of antidrug antibodies, which may significantly attenuate the LDL-C-lowering effect.[21] Another mAb to PCSK9, named LY3015014, the safety and efficacy of which have been so far tested in a phase 2 study, is still in development.[22] Recently, other approaches are being developed, such as RNA interfering drugs; inclisiran is a long-acting RNA interference drug that produces a specific and sustained inhibition of hepatic PCSK9 synthesis. Finally, an approach for long-term LDL-C management through PCSK9-specific active vaccines has been evaluated in preclinical models.[23–25]

It is worth noting that although PCSK9 targets mainly the LDLR in the liver, the protein is expressed also in extrahepatic tissues, including kidney, pancreas, and brain,[26] suggesting that pharmacologic inhibition of PCSK9 may lead to extrahepatic effects of PCSK9, which may raise concerns about this approach. To date, there is no evidence indicating a direct association between lipid-lowering therapy (LLT) with PCSK9 inhibitors with or without statins and the risk of cognitive disorders,[27] but specifically designed long-term clinical trials are awaited to clarify this aspect.

CLINICAL STUDIES ON EVOLOCUMAB AND ALIROCUMAB

Several clinical studies have evaluated the efficacy and safety of evolocumab and alirocumab in

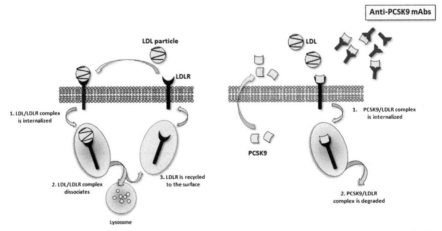

Fig. 1. Mechanism of action of PCSK9 and mAbs to PCSK9. In the absence of PCSK9, following the binding with LDL, LDLR is internalized and then recycled to the cell surface to restart the cycle. PCSK9 binds to LDLR and targets it to the degradation. MAbs to PCSK9 neutralize the circulating protein and block its binding to LDLR. (*Modified from* Pirillo A, Norata GD, Catapano AL. Advances in hypercholesterolemia. In: Chackalamannil S, editor. Comp Med Chem III. 3rd edition. Cambridge (MA): Elsevier; 2017. p. 669; with permission.)

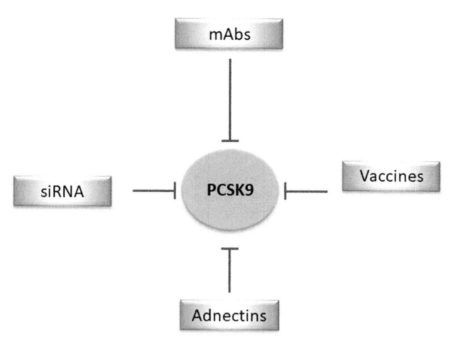

Fig. 2. Different approaches available or under current evaluation for the inhibition of PCSK9.

different groups of hypercholesterolemic patients with high CV risk; 2 meta-analyses have shown their safety and efficacy in reducing persistently LDL-C levels,[28–30] which translates into a lower incidence of CV events.

Evolocumab

A large number of clinical trials have assessed the efficacy and safety of evolocumab in different groups of patients. Most of them were 12-week phase 2 and phase 3 trials in which participants showed significant reductions of LDL-C levels in the group treated with evolocumab compared with either placebo or ezetimibe[31,32] (**Table 1**). Evolocumab was tested as monotherapy in the MENDEL studies, showing that in hypercholesterolemic patients (LDL-C ≥100 mg/dL [≥2.6 mmol/L], <190 mg/dL [<4.9 mmol/L]) the administration of evolocumab every 2 weeks or every 4 weeks for 3 months produced a significant reduction of LDL-C levels compared with either ezetimibe or placebo (see **Table 1**); other lipids and lipoproteins, including very low density lipoprotein cholesterol (VLDL-C) and lipoprotein(a) (Lp[a]), were also significantly reduced; adverse events were comparable among treatment groups.[33,34]

Since then, evolocumab has been evaluated as add-on to background lipid-lowering therapies, mainly statins, in patients who did not reach their recommended LDL-C goal. The LAPLACE-TIMI 57 trial showed that in hypercholesterolemic patients taking a statin with or without ezetimibe

the administration of evolocumab at different doses for 12 weeks reduced LDL-C levels by up to 66% compared with placebo[35] (see **Table 1**). All doses of evolocumab were more likely than placebo to reduce LDL-C levels less than 70 mg/dL (1.8 mmol/L).[35] In the phase 3 LAPLACE-2 study, patients taking moderate- or high-intensity statin therapy were administered with evolocumab (140 mg every 2 weeks or 420 mg every 4 weeks), placebo, or ezetimibe for 12 weeks: a significant additional reduction of LDL-C was observed (see **Table 1**), and most patients (86%–94%) achieved LDL-C levels less than 70 mg/dL, compared with the group receiving ezetimibe (17%–62%).[36] Similar results were obtained when hyperlipidemic patients were treated with evolocumab added to a background LLT for 52 weeks (DESCARTES study): LDL-C levels were significantly reduced by 57% (see **Table 1**); no decrement in the efficacy of evolocumab was observed from week 12 to week 52 and was similar across all the background lipid-lowering therapies.[37] More patients in the evolocumab group experienced serious adverse events or events leading to drug discontinuation; however, the analysis of such events did not reveal a clear association with evolocumab use.[38] Recently, the GLAGOV study evaluated the effect of evolocumab in addition to statins in patients with angiographic coronary disease after 78 weeks.[39] Very low levels of LDL-C were observed in evolocumab-treated patients (mean value: 36.6 mg/dL), which associated with a decrease in percent atheroma volume (PAV) not

Table 1
Effect of evolocumab on low-density lipoprotein cholesterol levels and cardiovascular outcomes in randomized clinical trials

Clinical Trial (Duration)	Characteristics of Selected Patients	Background LLT	Evolocumab Dosing	LDL-C (% Change From Baseline)	Clinical Outcomes
MENDEL (12 wk)[33]	LDL-C ≥100, <190 mg/dL	None	1. 70 mg, 105 mg, 140 mg q2w 280 mg, 350 mg, 420 mg q4w 2. 280 mg, 350 mg, 420 mg q4w 3. Eze 4. Placebo	1. −26.7% to −36.7% vs Eze; −37.3% to −47.2% vs placebo 2. −25.2% to −34.1% vs Eze; −43.6% to −52.5% vs placebo	
MENDEL-2 (12 wk)[34]	LDL-C ≥100 and <190 mg/dL	None	1. 140 mg q2w 2. 420 mg q4w 3. Eze 4. Placebo	1. −39.3% vs Eze; −57.4% vs placebo 2. −37.6% vs Eze; −54.8% vs placebo	
LAPLACE-TIMI 57 (12 wk)[35]	Fasting LDL-C ≥85 mg/dL	Statin ± Eze	1. 70, 105, or 140 mg q2w 2. 280, 350, or 420 mg q4w 3. Placebo	1. −41.8% to −66.1% vs placebo 2. −41.8% to −50.3% vs placebo	
LAPLACE-2 (12 wk)[36]	Primary hypercholesterolemia and mixed dyslipidemia	Atorva 10/80 mg ± Eze 10 mg; rosuva 5/40 mg; simva 40 mg	1. 140 mg q2w 2. 420 mg q4w 3. Eze 4. Placebo	1. −66% to −75% vs placebo; −39.6% to −47.2% vs Eze 2. −63% to −75% vs placebo; −38.9% to −41.1% vs Eze	
DESCARTES (52 wk)[37]	Fasting LDL-C ≥75 mg/dL	Diet; Diet + Atorva 10/80 mg; Diet + Atorva 80 mg + eze 10 mg	1. 420 mg q4w 2. Placebo	−57.0% vs placebo	
GLAGOV (78 wk)[39]	Fasting LDL-C ≥80 mg/dL	Statin	1. 420 mg q4w 2. Placebo	−61% vs placebo	Nominal change in PAV: −1.0%, P<.001
FOURIER (5 y)[41]	CVD at high risk for a recurrent event LDL-C ≥70 mg/dL	Atorva 20 mg or equivalent	1. 140 mg q2w + statin 2. 420 mg q4w + statin 3. Placebo	−59% vs placebo	Time to CV death, MI, hospitalization for unstable angina, stroke, or coronary revascularization: HR 0.85 (0.79–0.92) P<.001

Trial	Population		Treatment	LDL-C reduction	Outcome
GAUSS (12 wk)[42]	Statin intolerant	Stable LLT therapy	1. 280, 350, or 420 mg q4w 2. 420 mg q4w + Eze 10 mg 3. Eze 10 mg	1. −26% to −35.9 vs Eze 2. −47.3% vs Eze	
GAUSS-2 (12 wk)[43]	Statin intolerant; subjects not at LDL-C goal	Not on statin or on low-dose statin	1. 140 mg q2w 2. 420 mg q4w 3. Eze 10	1. −38.1% vs Eze 2. −37.6% vs Eze	
GAUSS-3 (Part B: 24 wk; Part C: 2 y)[44]	Statin intolerant; subjects not at LDL-C goal	Stable LLT	Part A: atorva rechallenge Part B: evo q4w vs Eze Part C: evo q2w	Part B −37.8% vs Eze Part C ONGOING	
RUTHERFORD (12 wk)[45]	HeFH Fasting LDL-C ≥100 mg/dL	Statin ± ezetimibe	1. 350 mg q4w 2. 420 mg q4w 3. Placebo	1. −43.8% vs placebo 2. −56.4% vs placebo	
RUTHERFORD-2 (12 wk)[46]	HeFH Fasting LDL-C ≥100 mg/dL	Statin ± ezetimibe	1. 140 mg q2w 2. 420 mg q4w 3. Placebo	1. −59.2% vs placebo 2. −61.3% vs placebo	
TESLA part A (36 wk)[47]	HoFH; LDL-C ≥130 mg/dL	Stable LLT	1. 420 mg q4w for 24 we 2. +420 mg q2w for 12 we	1. −16.5% from baseline 2. −13.9% from baseline	
TESLA part B (12 wk)[48]	HoFH; LDL-C ≥130 mg/dL	Stable LLT	1. 420 mg q4w 2. Placebo	−30.9% vs placebo	
TAUSSIG (5 y)[49]	Severe FH	Stable LLT	q2w or q4w	ONGOING (2020) Interim analysis: −20.6% at week 12	
OSLER-1 and OSLER-2 (1 y)[50]	Subjects from phase 2 and 3 evolocumab trials		1. 420 mg q4w + standard therapy 2. Placebo	−61% vs placebo	HR: 0.47 (0.28–0.78), $P = .003$

Abbreviation: Eze, ezetimibe.

observed in patients receiving placebo (−0.95% with evolocumab vs +0.05% with placebo)[39] (see **Table 1**); a greater percentage of patients showed plaque regression with evolocumab than with placebo (64.3% and 47.3%, respectively).[39] This study showed for the first time that lowering LDL-C levels aggressively with a PCSK9 inhibitor as add-on to a background statin therapy may result in a reduction of atherosclerosis. The FOUR-IER trial confirmed and extended this finding, showing that adding evolocumab to a background lipid therapy (mainly statin) resulted in a reduction of CV events after a median follow-up of 2.2 years, with a hazard ratio (HR) of 0.85 (95% confidence interval [CI], 0.79–0.92) for the primary endpoint (including CV death, myocardial infarction [MI], stroke, hospitalization for unstable angina, or coronary revascularization) and 0.80 (95% CI, 0.73–0.88) for secondary endpoint (CV death, MI, or stroke)[40] (see **Table 1**). A prespecified analysis of this trial showed that evolocumab significantly reduced the incidence of CV events with similar efficacy in patients with and without diabetes, but the absolute risk reduction was higher in patients with diabetes[41]; evolocumab did not increase the risk of new-onset diabetes and did not worsen glycemia.[41] A median of 30 mg/dL was reached following evolocumab treatment (median LDL-C at baseline: 92 mg/dL), and the reduction of LDL-C levels was maintained over time.[40] Interestingly, a 22% reduction of CV events was observed in the lowest quartile for baseline LDL-C level, in which patients reached an LDL-C level of 22 mg/dL[40]; this finding, together with the observations from the GLAGOV, suggests that a CV benefit may be accrued even when LDL-C levels are reduced at levels well below those recommended by the current guidelines.[3]

Statin intolerance represents a major issue during the treatment of patients at high or very high CV risk; it is characterized by the occurrence of adverse events, mainly muscle-related events following therapy, which may lead to the discontinuation of the statin therapy and the increase of CV risk. The most effective drug used in alternative is ezetimibe, but given the relatively modest reduction achieved, it does not allow to reach the recommended LDL-C levels. Thus statin-intolerant patients, who need a very effective therapy to reduce their cholesterol levels, may significantly benefit from the therapy with anti-PCSK9. To address this question, evolocumab has been specifically tested in statin-intolerant patients in the GAUSS studies[42–44] (see **Table 1**). As monotherapy, evolocumab dose dependently reduced LDL-C levels by 41% up to 63% compared with a 14.8% reduction achieved

with ezetimibe[42]; more importantly, no signs of muscle-related adverse events were observed in evolocumab-treated patients.[42] The association with ezetimibe further reduced LDL-C levels.[42] A higher proportion of patients in the evolocumab group reached the LDL-C target less than 100 mg/dL; patients receiving the combination evolocumab + ezetimibe were more likely to reach the recommended LDL-C (90% for LDL-C <100 mg/dL and 62% for LDL-C <70 mg/dL).[42] In the GAUSS-2 study, statin-intolerant patients were treated with evolocumab or ezetimibe for 12 weeks: evolocumab induced a significant reduction of LDL-C levels compared with ezetimibe (see **Table 1**), and more than 75% of patients reached an LDL-C level less than 100 mg/dL, whereas most of the patients treated with ezetimibe were unable to achieve LDL-C target levels.[43] The incidence of myalgia among these patients was low.[43] These findings have been confirmed by the GAUSS-3 clinical trial (see **Table 1**), which aimed at identifying patients with muscle symptoms confirmed by statin rechallenge and comparing the effect of evolocumab and ezetimibe.[44]

Despite that commonly used cholesterol-lowering drugs have significantly improved the management of FH patients, particularly when used in combination, a large proportion of FH patients still does not achieve the recommended LDL-C level target even with maximally tolerated doses of drugs. These considerations directed the attention on the need of a new pharmacologic approach for the treatment of these high CV risk patients. Some drugs have been developed for these needs, including mipomersen and lomitapide, which reduce LDL-C levels by mechanisms that are independent of LDLR and thus are indicated specifically for homozygous FH (HoFH) patients who do not respond well to conventional lipid-lowering therapies. Two specific studies aimed at evaluating the effect of evolocumab in heterozygous FH (HeFH) patients[45,46] (see **Table 1**). Evolocumab significantly reduced LDL-C levels in these patients at week 12 (43%-55%) when added to intensive statin therapy with or without ezetimibe.[45] A high percentage of patients treated with evolocumab reached either LDL-C less than 100 mg/dL (70% and 89%) or LDL-C less than 70 mg/dL (44% and 65%).[45] The lipid profile was generally improved, and a significant reduction of Lp(a), a CV risk factor whose levels are particularly elevated in FH patients, was observed.[45] The phase 3 RUTHERFORD-2 study, performed in HeFH patients on stable LLT, confirmed the high ability of evolocumab to reduce significantly LDL-C levels (∼60%) independently of the type of background LLT.[46] Interestingly, some patients recruited as HeFH were then reclassified as homozyogotes; in these patients, the reduction of LDL-C induced by evolocumab treatment was comparable to those observed in heterozygotes, and much greater than those reported in other studies on HoFH, probably because of a residual receptor activity.[46] The pilot study TESLA part A, which recruited 8 HoFH patients (6 receptor-defective and 2 receptor negative) with a mean baseline LDL-C level of 440 mg/dL (11.4 mmol/L), showed that patients with defective LDLR activity had a significant reduction in their LDL-C levels following the treatment with evolocumab (~23%), whereas receptor-negative patients did not respond to this therapy.[47] This finding suggests that the mechanism by which evolocumab reduces LDL-C levels is through the upregulation of residual LDLR activity, but the large variation in the response of patients carrying the same mutation merits investigation, because it assumes that other factors may contribute to this observation. It is worth noting that the baseline PCSK9 levels of these patients was much higher than those reported in other cohorts of FH patients, which requires higher dose and more frequent administration of evolocumab to reduce PCSK9 levels at the same levels observed in other trials.[47] Another relevant finding of this study, that however needs to be verified in a larger population, is the similar reduction of Lp(a) levels observed in both receptor-defective and receptor-negative HoFH patients.[47] The TESLA part B trial reported similar results, with an overall 30.9% reduction of LDL-C levels compared with placebo (see **Table 1**); the intensity of the response was significantly correlated with the type of genetic defects, with receptor-negative patients not responding to the therapy and a maximal response (~40% reduction) in patients carrying 1 or 2 defective LDLR mutations.[48] The ongoing TAUSSIG clinical trial will evaluate the long-term efficacy and safety of evolocumab in HoFH patients (completion date March, 2020). An interim subset analysis showed a 20.6% reduction of LDL-C levels, which is persistent at week 48 (see **Table 1**), and no differences were observed between patients with or without apheresis.[49]

Patients who completed one of the described phase 2 or 3 studies were then enrolled in 2 open-label, randomized trials (OSLER-1 and OSLER-2); combined data from these 2 studies showed that evolocumab significantly reduced LDL-C levels by 61% compared with the standard LLT, and that patients on evolocumab had a significantly lower rate of CV events compared with patients on standard therapy (HR0.47; 95% CI, 0.28–0.78, P = .003)[50]

(see **Table 1**), a finding that has been confirmed by the above discussed FOURIER trial.[40]

Alirocumab

Alirocumab is a fully human mAb against PCSK9. Hypercholesterolemic patients on stable atorvastatin therapy administered with alirocumab showed a further reduction of LDL-C (40% up to 72%); the reductions were dose dependent and dose regimen dependent, with the highest efficacy observed when alirocumab was given every 2 weeks[51] (**Table 2**). Almost all patients reached the LDL-C level less than 100 mg/dL, and a great proportion reached the level less than 70 mg/dL.[51] Lp(a) levels significantly decreased in all tested conditions[51]; total cholesterol, non–high-density lipoprotein cholesterol (non–HDL-C), and apolipoprotein B (apoB) were also significantly reduced.[51] Similar observations were reported in other 2 studies. A significant decrease of LDL-C levels was observed when alirocumab was added to atorvastatin 10 mg or 80 mg compared with atorvastatin 80 mg alone (−66.2%, −73.2%, and −17.3%, respectively)[52] (see **Table 2**); all patients on alirocumab reached the LDL-C level target less than 100 mg/dL, and more than 90% had an LDL-C level less than 70 mg/dL.[52] Alirocumab was effective in reducing LDL-C levels also in a population of young HeFH patients with a background treatment of low to moderate dose of atorvastatin: reductions ranged from 28.9% with alirocumab 150 mg every 4 weeks up to 67.90% with 150 mg every 2 weeks, compared with a reduction of 10.65% with placebo[53] (see **Table 2**). The patients who completed this study and were receiving stable statin + ezetimibe therapy entered the open-label extension during which they received alirocumab 150 mg every 2 weeks; after 3 years, sustained LDL-C reductions were observed (~60%), without specific safety signals, including in those patients who achieved very low levels of LDL-C (<25 mg/dL).[54]

The *ODYSSEY* program, which included 14 phase 3 trials on alirocumab, aimed at evaluating the efficacy and safety of alirocumab alone or in combination with other lipid-lowering therapies in different groups of hypercholesterolemic patients (see **Table 2**). Most of these trials used a dosage of 75 mg every 2 weeks uptitrated to 150 every 2 weeks if LDL-C target is not reached after 8 weeks. The *ODYSSEY COMBO* studies (I and II) have evaluated the efficacy and safety of alirocumab in high CV risk patients with suboptimal levels of LDL-C at baseline despite on maximal tolerated dose of statin, with or without other lipid-lowering drugs (see **Table 2**). The

Table 2
Effect of alirocumab on low-density lipoprotein cholesterol levels and cardiovascular outcomes in randomized clinical trials

Clinical Trial (Duration)	Characteristics of Selected Patients	Background LLT	Alirocumab Dosing	LDL-C Change	CV Outcomes
DFI11565 (12 wk)[51]	LDL-C ≥100 mg/dL	Atorva 10, 20, or 40 mg	1. 50, 100, 150 mg q2w 2. 200, 300 mg q4w 3. Placebo	1. −39.6% to −72.4% 2. −43.2%, −47.7% 3. −5.1%	
DFI11566 (8 wk)[52]	LDL-C ≥100 mg/dL	Atorva 10 mg	1. 150 mg q2w + atorva 10 mg 2. 150 mg q2w + atorva 80 mg 3. Atorva 80 mg	1. −66.2% 2. −73.2% 3. −17.3%	
R727-CL-1003 (12 wk)[53]	HeFH; LDL-C ≥100 mg/dL	Diet + statin	1. 150 mg q2w 2. 150 mg, 200 mg, 300 mg q4w 3. Placebo	1. −57.2% vs placebo 2. −18.2% to −31.9% vs placebo	
ODYSSEY COMBO I (52 wk)[55]	Established CHD or CHD equivalent, LDL-C ≥70 mg/dL	Maximum tolerated statin ± other LLT	75 mg q2w (increased at 150 mg q2w if LDL-C ≥70 mg/dL at week 8) 2. Placebo	−45.9% vs placebo	
ODYSSEY COMBO II (52 wk)[56]	Established CHD or CHD equivalent, LDL-C ≥70 mg/dL with maximally tolerate dose of statin	High-intensity statins	1. 75 mg q2w (increased at 150 mg q2w if LDL-C ≥70 mg/dL at week 8) 2. Eze 10 mg	−29.8% vs Eze	
ODYSSEY OPTIONS I (24 wk)[58]	Very high CVD risk, LDL-C ≥70 mg/dL; high CVD risk and LDL-C ≥100 mg/dL	Atorva 20/40 mg	1. 75 mg q2w 2. Eze 10 mg 3. Doubling atorva dose 4. Atorva 40 mg → Rosuva 40 mg	Entry statin: Atorva 20 Atorva 40 1. −44.1% −54% 2. −20.5% −22.6% 3. −5% −4.8% 4. — −21.4%	
ODYSSEY OPTIONS II (24 wk)[59]	Very high CVD risk, LDL-C ≥70 mg/dL; high CVD risk and LDL-C ≥100 mg/dL	Rosuva 10/20 mg	1. 75 mg q2w 2. Eze 10 mg 3. Doubling rosuva dose	Entry statin: Rosuva 10 Rosuva 20 1. −50.6% −36.3% 2. −14.4% −11.0% 3. −16.3% −15.9%	

Study	Population	Background LLT	Treatment arms	Results	Endpoint
ODYSSEY ALTERNATIVE (24 wk)[60]	Moderate or high CV risk with statin intolerance, LDL-C ≥100 or ≥70 mg/dL	Non-statin LLT	1. 75 mg q2w 2. Eze 10 mg	−30.4% vs Eze	
ODYSSEY MONO (24 wk)[61]	LDL-C ≥100 mg/dL and <190 mg/dL	None	1. 75 mg q2w 2. Eze 10 mg	−31.6% vs Eze	
ODYSSEY LONG TERM (78 wk)[62]	HeFH or established CHD or CHD equivalent LDL-C ≥70 mg/dL	Maximum tolerated statin ± other LLT	1. 150 mg q2w 2. Placebo	−61.9% vs placebo	
ODYSSEY OUTCOMES (64 mo)[63]	Recent acute coronary syndrome, LDL-C ≥70 mg/dL	Atorva 40/80 mg or Rosuva 20/40 mg or the maximum tolerated dose	1. 75 mg q2w 2. 150 mg q2w 3. Placebo	ONGOING (2017)	Time from randomization to first occurrence of CHD death, nonfatal MI, stroke, or UA requiring hospitalization
ODYSSEY FH I and FH II (78 wk)[64]	HeFH; LDL-C ≥100 mg/dL (for primary prevention) or LDL-C ≥70 mg/dL (for secondary prevention)	Maximum tolerated statin ± other LLT	1. 75 mg q2w (increased at 150 mg q2w if LDL-C ≥70 mg/dL at week 8) 2. Placebo	FH I: −57.9% vs placebo FH II: −51.4% vs placebo	
ODYSSEY JAPAN (52 wk)[65]	HeFH or non-FH at high CV risk not at target	Stable statin therapy	1. 75 mg q2w (increased at 150 mg q2w if LDL-C ≥70 mg/dL at week 8) 2. Placebo	−58.9% vs placebo	
ODYSSEY HIGH FH (78 wk)[66]	HeFH LDL-C ≥160	Stable LLT	1. 150 mg q2w 2. Placebo	−39.1% vs placebo	
ODYSSEY ESCAPE (18 wk)[67]	HeFH undergoing apheresis	Stable LLT	1. 150 mg q2w 2. Placebo	−46.4% vs placebo	
ODYSSEY OLE (176 wk)[68]	HeFH who have completed one of the 4 parent studies			ONGOING (2017) Preliminary data at week 48: −46.9%	
CHOICE I (48 wk)[69]	Hypercholesterolemic at moderate to very high CV risk	± Statin ± other LLT	1. 300 mg q4w 2. 75 mg q2w 3. Placebo	1. −52.4% vs placebo (no statin); −58.7 vs placebo (statin) 2. −49.8% vs placebo (no statin); −51.4% vs placebo (statin)	
CHOICE II (24 wk)[71]	Inadequately controlled hypercholesterolemia	No statin Fenofibrate, ezetimibe, or diet	1. 150 mg q4w 2. 75 mg q2w 3. Placebo	1. −56.4% vs placebo 2. −58.2% vs placebo	

COMBO I study showed that alirocumab treatment induced a greater reduction of LDL-C levels (−48.2% at week 24, compared with −2.3% with placebo); in addition, a greater proportion of patients (77.5% on-treatment) reached the recommended LDL-C level less than 70 mg/dL.[55] The COMBO II study showed a greater efficacy of alirocumab in reducing LDL-C levels compared with ezetimibe in the 104-week treatment period, and many more patients achieved LDL-C goals.[56]

The ODYSSEY OPTIONS studies were designed to evaluate the efficacy and safety of alirocumab in patients at high CV risk with LDL-C levels not adequately controlled[57] (see **Table 2**). The ODYSSEY OPTIONS I trial recruited patients with very high CVD risk and LDL-C ≥70 mg/dL (≥1.8 mmol/L) or high CVD risk and LDL-C ≥100 mg/dL (≥2.6 mmol/L); these patients were randomized to one of the following treatments: (1) alirocumab 75 mg every 2 weeks (switched to 150 mg every 2 weeks if LDL-C target was not achieved after 12 weeks) added to atorvastatin 20 or 40 mg; (2) ezetimibe 10 mg added to atorvastatin; (3) double atorvastatin dose; (4) switch from atorvastatin 40 mg to rosuvastatin 40 mg.[58] The greatest reductions of LDL-C levels were observed in patients treated with alirocumab as add-on (−44.1% and −54.0% with atorvastatin 20 or 40 mg), whereas the addition of ezetimibe reduced LDL-C levels by 20.5% and 22.6%, respectively, similarly to the reduction observed following the switch from atorvastatin to rosuvastatin; doubling the atorvastatin dose resulted in additional reduction of 5.0% and 4.8% compared with the baseline[58] (see **Table 2**). Patients treated with alirocumab were more likely to achieve the recommended LDL-C target; alirocumab also induced a higher reduction of apoB, non-HDL-C, and Lp(a) levels compared with all other treatments.[58] Similarly, the ODYSSEY OPTIONS II showed the higher efficacy of adding alirocumab to a background of rosuvastatin 10 or 20 mg in the same type of patients[59]: LDL-C levels were reduced by −50.6% and −36.3%, respectively, whereas adding ezetimibe or doubling rosuvastatin dose was less effective (−14.4% and −11.0% with ezetimibe; −16.3% and −15.9% doubling rosuvastatin)[59] (see **Table 2**). Altogether, these results suggest that high CV risk patients with not controlled LDL-C levels despite on maximal tolerated LLT may significantly benefit from the addition of alirocumab to their therapy.

As for evolocumab, a specific trial has addressed the efficacy and safety of alirocumab in statin-intolerant patients, with a statin rechallenge arm. The ODYSSEY ALTERNATIVE trial showed that alirocumab was superior to ezetimibe in reducing LDL-C levels in patients intolerant to statins, with reduction of −45% and −14.6% from baseline, respectively, at week 24 (P<.0001) (see **Table 2**); following the treatment with alirocumab, patients were more likely to achieve the recommended LDL-C levels (41.9% vs 4.4% with ezetimibe).[60] Myalgia was the most common adverse event reported in all groups, but alirocumab treatment was associated with the lowest rate of muscle-related adverse events.[60] The higher efficacy of alirocumab compared with ezetimibe has been reported also by the ODYSSEY MONO trial, conducted in patients on no LLT[61] (see **Table 2**).

To evaluate the long-term efficacy and safety of alirocumab, 2 studies have been designed to specifically address these questions. The ODYSSEY LONG TERM, conducted in a population of high CV risk patients with LDL-C levels ≥70 mg/dL while receiving the maximal tolerated dose of statin, showed that addition of alirocumab produced a further −62% reduction of LDL-C levels after 24 weeks[62] (see **Table 2**); these reductions, which were maintained during the course of the study, did not differ between HeFH and non-HeFH patients.[62] Interestingly, a high percentage of patients (37.1%) reached very low levels of LDL-C (<25 mg/dL), but the rate of adverse events in these patients was not increased.[62] A post hoc analysis reported a lower rate of major adverse CV events in the alirocumab group than in the placebo group (1.7% vs 3.3%, HR 0.52, nominal P = .02), with cumulative probability of event curves tending to diverge over time.[62] The ongoing ODYSSEY OUTCOMES is evaluating the effect of adding alirocumab or placebo to the current LLT in patients with a recent acute coronary syndrome; the primary outcome is the time from randomization to first occurrence of a clinical CV event, including CHD death, MI, fatal and nonfatal ischemic stroke, and unstable angina requiring hospitalization.[63] It is expected to be completed at the end of 2017.

The ODYSSEY program also included clinical trials evaluating the effect of alirocumab in HeFH patients with inadequate LDL-C level control despite maximal tolerated dose of LLT (see **Table 2**). In the ODYSSEY FH I and FH II studies, patients (mean LDL-C levels 144.7 mg/dL) received alirocumab 75 mg every 2 weeks uptitrated to 150 mg if LDL-C was ≥70 mg/dL (≥1.8 mmol/L) at week 8; LDL-C levels significantly decreased by 57.9% (FH I) and 51.4% (FH II) versus placebo. These reductions were maintained up to week 78, and most alirocumab-receiving patients reached LDL-C levels less than 70 mg/dL.[64] Alirocumab also reduced apoB, non–HDL-C, and Lp(a).[64] The ODYSSEY JAPAN trial, which included 41 HeFH patients, reported similar results.[65] In the ODYSSEY HIGH FH trial, HeFH patients with LDL-C $\geq$160 mg/dL ($\geq$4.1 mmol/L) despite maximally tolerated dose of statin with or without other lipid-lowering drugs were treated with alirocumab 150 mg every 2 weeks or placebo for 78 weeks.[66] At week 24, in patients treated with alirocumab, LDL-C levels were reduced by −45.7% compared with −6.6% with placebo.[66] This reduction was comparable with that observed in a subgroup of patients with HeFH with high baseline LDL-C levels in the ODYSSEY LONG TERM trial, which reported a −52.2% with alirocumab and −8.1% with placebo.[62] The ODYSSEY ESCAPE trial showed that, in HeFH patients undergoing regular lipoprotein apheresis, the addition of alirocumab to their LLT led to the discontinuation of apheresis in 63.4% of patients, whereas in 29.3% of patients the standardized rate was reduced by at least 50%,[67] which suggests that these specific subgroups of HeFH patients may significantly benefit from an anti-PCSK9 therapy. The ODYSSEY OLE is an open-label extension study of 4 phase 3 studies (FH I, FH II, LONG TERM, HIGH FH) that is evaluating the long-term (176 weeks) efficacy and safety of alirocumab in patients with HeFH. Preliminary data show a mean reduction in LDL-C levels of 46.9% at week 48 compared with baseline; significant reductions are observed also in other parameters, including non-HDL-C, Lp(a), and apoB.[68]

Recently, alirocumab has been approved as a once-monthly dosing option, based on the results of the ODYSSEY CHOICE I clinical trial, which compared the well-established 75 mg every 2 weeks alirocumab dosing with 300 mg every 4 weeks as a monotherapy or add-on to statin therapy in patients with moderate to very high CV risk, with a 48-week follow-up[69] (see Table 2). The monthly dosing was as effective in reducing LDL-C levels as the every 2 weeks dosing; the reductions were significant both in patients on statin therapy and in patients not receiving statins.[69] The analysis of a subgroup of patients with atherosclerotic CVD showed a significant reduction of LDL-C levels with alirocumab 300 mg every 4 weeks both in patients on statin (−64.2%) and in the group not receiving statin (−56.8%)[70]; the reductions were similar to that observed in the whole population of the study.[69] The most relevant finding of this study is that the variations of LDL-C week by week are small, and at week 48, a large proportion of patients achieved the recommended LDL-C levels following the treatment with alirocumab. Alirocumab has been tested also as a 150-mg dose every 4 weeks in the ODYSSEY CHOICE II clinical

trial, conducted in patients with inadequately controlled hypercholesterolemia and not on statin therapy because of muscle-related adverse events[71] (see Table 2). The LDL-C level reductions obtained with this dosing regimen did not differ from that observed with the reference dose (−51.7% vs −53.5% vs baseline with 75 mg every 2 weeks); some patients required a dose adjustment at week 12, which was associated with higher LDL-C levels at baseline.[71] About 90% of the patients included in this trial had muscle-related adverse events with statins, leading to therapy discontinuation, but during the treatment with alirocumab, the rate of these events was low.[71] All these observations represent a relevant step in the development of these drugs; in fact, reducing the timing of injection maintaining the effect on LDL-C levels may result in an increased adherence of the patients to the therapy, but can also have a positive effect on the costs of the therapy.

OTHER MONOCLONAL ANTIBODIES TO PROPROTEIN CONVERTASE SUBTILISIN KEXIN 9
Bococizumab

Bococizumab is a humanized mAb targeting PCSK9; because it contains a 3% murine sequence, the development of anti-drug antibodies may occur. Two randomized clinical trials have recently shown that bococizumab treatment did not reduce major adverse CV events in low-risk patients, whereas a benefit was reported for higher risk patients, despite similar LDL-C level reductions; the combined analysis of these 2 trials did not report benefit with respect to the primary end point.[72] In the SPIRE lipid-lowering program, which included several trials on bococizumab, high-titer anti-drug antibodies developed in a high percentage of patients receiving bococizumab after week 12, which markedly reduced the magnitude and durability of LDL-C lowering ($\sim$50%).[21] In addition, a high variability in the LDL-C lowering was observed among patients with no anti-drug antibodies, a variation that was present as early as 12 weeks, and thus before the detection of anti-drug antibodies.[21] Bococizumab immunogenicity seems also to increase the rate of adverse events, such as injection-site reactions, that were higher than those previously reported with the other anti-PCSK9 mAbs.[21] Following these observations, the development of bococizumab has been discontinued.

LY3015014

PCSK9 secreted from cells is formed by a 14-kDa prodomain associated noncovalently with a

60-kDa mature domain; in addition to this form, serum contains also a truncated form of PCSK9 (representing up to 40% of total circulating PCSK9) in which the N terminus of the catalytic domain is truncated by 7 to 8 kDa following the activity of furin. This truncated form seems to be inactive at LDLR degradation.[73,74] This observation can have a specific relevance when using mAbs, because if the antibody binds to both intact and truncated forms, it may be consumed unproductively. LY3015014 antibody binds to intact but not to truncated form of PCSK9, thus blocking its interaction with LDLR but allowing the normal proteolytic cleavage of PCSK9 and limiting its accumulation.[75] LY3015014 has been tested in hypercholesterolemic patients as add-on to their background lipid-lowering therapy in a phase 2 randomized clinical trial.[22] A dose-dependent significant and durable reduction of LDL-C levels was reported (-14.9% up to -50.5% for every 4 weeks and -14.9% to -37.1% for every 8 weeks dosing).[22] LY3015014 also reduced significantly other lipid parameters, including non–HDL-C, apoB, and Lp(a).[22] The development of LY3015014 has been discontinued because of lower reductions of LDL-C induced compared with approved PCSK9 mAbs.

NEW APPROACHES FOR THE INHIBITION OF PROPROTEIN CONVERTASE SUBTILISIN KEXIN 9
Adnectins

Adnectins are a new family of therapeutic proteins based on the 10th fibronectin type III domain, designed to bind with high affinity and specificity to therapeutic targets, which may translate into a higher pharmacologic activity and increased therapeutic efficacy.[76] BMS-962476 targets circulating PCSK9; in hypercholesterolemic mice overexpressing human PCSK9, it rapidly reduces cholesterol and free PCSK9 levels, and the treatment of cynomolgus monkeys suppressed PCSK9 by more than 99% and LDL-C levels by $\sim55\%$.[77] BMS-962476 was well tolerated in healthy subjects on diet and LDL-C greater than 130 mg/dL or statins and LDL-C greater than 100 mg/dL; in these subjects, it produced reductions of 48% in LDL-C and greater than 90% in PCSK9 levels at maximal dose.[78] Also, the development of this molecule has been discontinued.[79]

Inclisiran

A more recent approach for the inhibition of PCSK9 is through a biological process referred to as RNA interference; this approach uses a small interfering RNA (siRNA), which induces the degradation of specific mRNA, resulting in the suppression of the corresponding protein synthesis. Thus, preclinical studies have shown that the treatment with PCSK9-specific siRNA results in the reduction of PCSK9 and LDL-C plasma levels.[80] In healthy volunteers with serum LDL-C levels ≥116 mg/dL (≥3.00 mmol/L), a single intravenous dose of ALN-PCS, a siRNA that inhibits PCSK9 synthesis in a lipid nanoparticle formulation, resulted in a mean 70% reduction in circulating PCSK9 plasma levels and a 40% reduction of LDL-C.[81]

Inclisiran (ALN-PCSsc) is a long-acting synthetic siRNA against PCSK9 that is conjugated to triantennary N-acetylgalactosamine carbohydrates, which bind to the asialoglycoprotein receptors abundantly expressed in the liver, thus resulting in a specific uptake of inclisiran into hepatocytes. In a phase 1 trial, inclisiran has been tested in healthy volunteers with LDL-C ≥100 mg/dL (2.6 mmol/L) in either a single ascending dose (25–800 mg) or multiple dose[82]; at day 84, in the single-dose phase, a dose of 300 mg or higher significantly reduced PCSK9 levels (up to a least-squares mean reduction of 74.5%), which corresponded to a reduction of LDL-C levels by $\sim50\%$.[82] All multiple dose regimens massively reduced PCSK9 levels (up to 83.8%) and LDL-C levels (up to 59.7%).[82] No serious adverse events were reported.[82]

Inclisiran has been tested in a phase 2 trial (ORION-1) in patients at high CV risk with high LDL-C levels.[83] Patients were randomly assigned to receive a single dose of placebo or 200, 300, or 500 mg of inclisiran or 2 doses (at days 1 and 90) of placebo or 100, 200, or 300 mg of inclisiran; the greatest reduction in LDL-C levels (52.6%) was observed in patients who received the 2-dose 300-mg regimen of inclisiran (first injection at day 1, second injection at day 90).[83] LDL-C levels were reduced in every patient enrolled in the trial.[83] In terms of safety, during the 210 days of exposure to inclisiran, the rate of adverse events was similar in inclisiran and placebo group, and also injection-site reactions were uncommon and similar to those reported with mAbs.[83] So far, symptoms of immune activation after exposure to inclisiran were rare, but longer trials are warranted to evaluate the safety of a long-term exposure to this drug as well as to establish a long-term duration of the effect.

Anti–Proprotein Convertase Subtilisin Kexin 9 Vaccines

Active vaccination represents one of the recent approaches that are currently under investigation for cholesterol management and prevention of CVD. The goal of this approach is to induce a therapeutic response similar to that induced by the administration of mAbs, but with reduced interventions and avoiding the possibility of the formation of anti-drug antibodies, which may limit the pharmacologic effect. To this end, a peptide-based anti-PCSK9 active vaccination has been evaluated in preclinical models[23]: vaccines induced the generation of high-affine antibodies specific for PCSK9, resulting in the reduction of LDL-C up to 50% in treated animals.[23] The humoral immune response induced by vaccine persisted for 1 year, and LDL-C level reduction persisted for the entire period of the study.[23] Similar results were reported in another study that evaluated the effect of vaccination with various PCSK9 peptides in mice, and reported a consistent effect on LDL-C levels, that were even lower in vaccinated animals treated with statins.[24] The vaccine against PCSK9, besides the effect on LDL-C levels, also reduced plasma inflammatory markers and decreased significantly the atherosclerotic lesion area (−64%) and aortic inflammation in mice.[25] One main problem of this type of approach might be the high variability in the antibody response, thus suggesting the need of vaccine protocols able to induce a high-titer response; on the other hand, to be effective, it requires the maintenance of high levels of antibodies.

SUMMARY

In summary, PCSK9 is a viable target for hypolipidemic therapy. The current available drugs target the circulating protein, and clinical results are in line with the reduction of LDL-C induced by the drugs. Other therapies targeting PCSK9 albeit with different mechanisms are being developed and will certainly help to widen the range of possible choices for treatment. Whether PCSK9 inhibition will become directly second-line therapy is still pending, but data are accumulating especially from clinical trials, which will provide the wealth of evidence needed.

REFERENCES

1. Baigent C, Keech A, Kearney PM, et al, Cholesterol Treatment Trialists' (CTT) Collaborators. Efficacy and safety of cholesterol-lowering treatment: prospective meta-analysis of data from 90,056 participants in 14 randomised trials of statins. Lancet 2005;366(9493): 1267–78.
2. Baigent C, Blackwell L, Emberson J, et al. Efficacy and safety of more intensive lowering of LDL cholesterol: a meta-analysis of data from 170,000 participants in 26 randomised trials. Lancet 2010; 376(9753):1670–81.
3. Catapano AL, Graham I, De Backer G, et al. 2016 ESC/EAS guidelines for the management of dyslipidaemias: the task force for the management of dyslipidaemias of the European Society of Cardiology (ESC) and European Atherosclerosis Society (EAS) developed with the special contribution of the European Assocciation for Cardiovascular Prevention & Rehabilitation (EACPR). Atherosclerosis 2016;253: 281–344.
4. Naci H, Brugts JJ, Fleurence R, et al. Comparative benefits of statins in the primary and secondary prevention of major coronary events and all-cause mortality: a network meta-analysis of placebo-controlled and active-comparator trials. Eur J Prev Cardiol 2013;20(4):641–57.
5. Mills EJ, Wu P, Chong G, et al. Efficacy and safety of statin treatment for cardiovascular disease: a network meta-analysis of 170,255 patients from 76 randomized trials. QJM 2011;104(2):109–24.
6. Tonelli M, Lloyd A, Clement F, et al. Efficacy of statins for primary prevention in people at low cardiovascular risk: a meta-analysis. CMAJ 2011;183(16): E1189–202.
7. Mills EJ, O'Regan C, Eyawo O, et al. Intensive statin therapy compared with moderate dosing for prevention of cardiovascular events: a meta-analysis of >40 000 patients. Eur Heart J 2011; 32(11):1409–15.
8. Chan DK, O'Rourke F, Shen Q, et al. Meta-analysis of the cardiovascular benefits of intensive lipid lowering with statins. Acta Neurol Scand 2011; 124(3):188–95.
9. Taylor F, Huffman MD, Macedo AF, et al. Statins for the primary prevention of cardiovascular disease. Cochrane Database Syst Rev 2013;(1): CD004816.
10. Corrao G, Conti V, Merlino L, et al. Results of a retrospective database analysis of adherence to statin therapy and risk of nonfatal ischemic heart disease in daily clinical practice in Italy. Clin Ther 2010; 32(2):300–10.
11. Leren TP. Sorting an LDL receptor with bound PCSK9 to intracellular degradation. Atherosclerosis 2014;237(1):76–81.
12. Abifadel M, Varret M, Rabes JP, et al. Mutations in PCSK9 cause autosomal dominant hypercholesterolemia. Nat Genet 2003;34(2):154–6.
13. Cohen JC, Boerwinkle E, Mosley TH Jr, et al. Sequence variations in PCSK9, low LDL, and protection against coronary heart disease. N Engl J Med 2006;354(12):1264–72.
14. Cohen J, Pertsemlidis A, Kotowski IK, et al. Low LDL cholesterol in individuals of African descent resulting from frequent nonsense mutations in PCSK9. Nat Genet 2005;37(2):161–5.

15. Kathiresan S. A PCSK9 missense variant associated with a reduced risk of early-onset myocardial infarction. N Engl J Med 2008;358(21):2299–300.

16. Kent ST, Rosenson RS, Avery CL, et al. PCSK9 loss-of-function variants, low-density lipoprotein cholesterol, and risk of coronary heart disease and stroke: data from 9 studies of blacks and whites. Circ Cardiovasc Genet 2017;10(4):e001632.

17. Benn M, Nordestgaard BG, Grande P, et al. PCSK9 R46L, low-density lipoprotein cholesterol levels, and risk of ischemic heart disease: 3 independent studies and meta-analyses. J Am Coll Cardiol 2010;55(25):2833–42.

18. Hopkins PN, Defesche J, Fouchier SW, et al. Characterization of autosomal dominant hypercholesterolemia caused by PCSK9 gain of function mutations and its specific treatment with alirocumab, a PCSK9 monoclonal antibody. Circ Cardiovasc Genet 2015;8(6):823–31.

19. Qiu C, Zeng P, Li X, et al. What is the impact of PCSK9 rs505151 and rs11591147 polymorphisms on serum lipids level and cardiovascular risk: a meta-analysis. Lipids Health Dis 2017;16(1):111.

20. Naoumova RP, Tosi I, Patel D, et al. Severe hypercholesterolemia in four British families with the D374Y mutation in the PCSK9 gene: long-term follow-up and treatment response. Arterioscler Thromb Vasc Biol 2005;25(12):2654–60.

21. Ridker PM, Tardif JC, Amarenco P, et al, SPIRE Investigators. Lipid-reduction variability and antidrug-antibody formation with bococizumab. N Engl J Med 2017;376(16):1517–26.

22. Kastelein JJ, Nissen SE, Rader DJ, et al. Safety and efficacy of LY3015014, a monoclonal antibody to proprotein convertase subtilisin/kexin type 9 (PCSK9): a randomized, placebo-controlled Phase 2 study. Eur Heart J 2016;37(17):1360–9.

23. Galabova G, Brunner S, Winsauer G, et al. Peptide-based anti-PCSK9 vaccines - an approach for long-term LDLc management. PLoS One 2014;9(12): e114469.

24. Crossey E, Amar MJ, Sampson M, et al. A cholesterol-lowering VLP vaccine that targets PCSK9. Vaccine 2015;33(43):5747–55.

25. Landlinger C, Pouwer MG, Juno C, et al. The AT04A vaccine against proprotein convertase subtilisin/kexin type 9 reduces total cholesterol, vascular inflammation, and atherosclerosis in APOE*3Leiden.CETP mice. Eur Heart J 2017; 38(32):2499–507.

26. Norata GD, Tavori H, Pirillo A, et al. Biology of proprotein convertase subtilisin kexin 9: beyond low-density lipoprotein cholesterol lowering. Cardiovasc Res 2016;112(1):429–42.

27. Banach M, Rizzo M, Nikolic D, et al. Intensive LDL-cholesterol lowering therapy and neurocognitive function. Pharmacol Ther 2017;170:181–91.

28. Navarese EP, Kolodziejczak M, Schulze V, et al. Effects of proprotein convertase subtilisin/kexin type 9 antibodies in adults with hypercholesterolemia: a systematic review and meta-analysis. Ann Intern Med 2015;163(1):40–51.

29. Li C, Lin L, Zhang W, et al. Efficiency and safety of proprotein convertase subtilisin/kexin 9 monoclonal antibody on hypercholesterolemia: a meta-analysis of 20 randomized controlled trials. J Am Heart Assoc 2015;4(6):e001937.

30. Qian LJ, Gao Y, Zhang YM, et al. Therapeutic efficacy and safety of PCSK9-monoclonal antibodies on familial hypercholesterolemia and statin-intolerant patients: a meta-analysis of 15 randomized controlled trials. Sci Rep 2017;7(1):238.

31. Zhang XL, Zhu QQ, Zhu L, et al. Safety and efficacy of anti-PCSK9 antibodies: a meta-analysis of 25 randomized, controlled trials. BMC Med 2015;13:123.

32. Langslet G, Emery M, Wasserman SM. Evolocumab (AMG 145) for primary hypercholesterolemia. Expert Rev Cardiovasc Ther 2015;13(5):477–88.

33. Koren MJ, Scott R, Kim JB, et al. Efficacy, safety, and tolerability of a monoclonal antibody to proprotein convertase subtilisin/kexin type 9 as monotherapy in patients with hypercholesterolaemia (MENDEL): a randomised, double-blind, placebo-controlled, phase 2 study. Lancet 2012;380(9858): 1995–2006.

34. Koren MJ, Lundqvist P, Bolognese M, et al. Anti-PCSK9 monotherapy for hypercholesterolemia: the MENDEL-2 randomized, controlled phase III clinical trial of evolocumab. J Am Coll Cardiol 2014;63(23): 2531–40.

35. Giugliano RP, Desai NR, Kohli P, et al. Efficacy, safety, and tolerability of a monoclonal antibody to proprotein convertase subtilisin/kexin type 9 in combination with a statin in patients with hypercholesterolaemia (LAPLACE-TIMI 57): a randomised, placebo-controlled, dose-ranging, phase 2 study. Lancet 2012;380(9858):2007–17.

36. Robinson JG, Nedergaard BS, Rogers WJ, et al. Effect of evolocumab or ezetimibe added to moderate- or high-intensity statin therapy on LDL-C lowering in patients with hypercholesterolemia: the LAPLACE-2 randomized clinical trial. JAMA 2014; 311(18):1870–82.

37. Blom DJ, Hala T, Bolognese M, et al. A 52-week placebo-controlled trial of evolocumab in hyperlipidemia. N Engl J Med 2014;370(19):1809–19.

38. Blom T, Back N, Mutka AL, et al. FTY720 stimulates 27-hydroxycholesterol production and confers atheroprotective effects in human primary macrophages. Circ Res 2010;106(4):720–9.

39. Nicholls SJ, Puri R, Anderson T, et al. Effect of evolocumab on progression of coronary disease in statin-treated patients: the GLAGOV randomized clinical trial. JAMA 2016;316(22):2373–84.

40. Sabatine MS, Giugliano RP, Keech AC, et al. Evolocumab and clinical outcomes in patients with cardiovascular disease. N Engl J Med 2017. https://doi.org/10.1056/NEJMoa1615664.

41. Sabatine MS, Leiter LA, Wiviott SD, et al. Cardiovascular safety and efficacy of the PCSK9 inhibitor evolocumab in patients with and without diabetes and the effect of evolocumab on glycaemia and risk of new-onset diabetes: a prespecified analysis of the FOURIER randomised controlled trial. Lancet Diabetes Endocrinol 2017;5(12):941–50.

42. Sullivan D, Olsson AG, Scott R, et al. Effect of a monoclonal antibody to PCSK9 on low-density lipoprotein cholesterol levels in statin-intolerant patients: the GAUSS randomized trial. JAMA 2012;308(23):2497–506.

43. Stroes E, Colquhoun D, Sullivan D, et al. Anti-PCSK9 antibody effectively lowers cholesterol in patients with statin intolerance: the GAUSS-2 randomized, placebo-controlled phase 3 clinical trial of evolocumab. J Am Coll Cardiol 2014;63(23):2541–8.

44. Nissen SE, Stroes E, Dent-Acosta RE, et al, GAUSS-3 Investigators. Efficacy and tolerability of evolocumab vs ezetimibe in patients with muscle-related statin intolerance: the GAUSS-3 randomized clinical trial. JAMA 2016;315(15):1580–90.

45. Raal F, Scott R, Somaratne R, et al. Low-density lipoprotein cholesterol-lowering effects of AMG 145, a monoclonal antibody to proprotein convertase subtilisin/kexin type 9 serine protease in patients with heterozygous familial hypercholesterolemia: the reduction of LDL-C with PCSK9 inhibition in heterozygous familial hypercholesterolemia disorder (RUTHERFORD) randomized trial. Circulation 2012;126(20):2408–17.

46. Raal FJ, Stein EA, Dufour R, et al. PCSK9 inhibition with evolocumab (AMG 145) in heterozygous familial hypercholesterolaemia (RUTHERFORD-2): a randomised, double-blind, placebo-controlled trial. Lancet 2015;385(9965):331–40.

47. Stein EA, Honarpour N, Wasserman SM, et al. Effect of the proprotein subtilisin/kexin 9 monoclonal antibody, AMG 145, in homozygous familial hypercholesterolemia. Circulation 2013;128(19):2113–20.

48. Raal FJ, Honarpour N, Blom DJ, et al. Inhibition of PCSK9 with evolocumab in homozygous familial hypercholesterolaemia (TESLA Part B): a randomised, double-blind, placebo-controlled trial. Lancet 2015;385(9965):341–50.

49. Raal FJ, Hovingh GK, Blom D, et al. Long-term treatment with evolocumab added to conventional drug therapy, with or without apheresis, in patients with homozygous familial hypercholesterolaemia: an interim subset analysis of the open-label TAUSSIG study. Lancet Diabetes Endocrinol 2017;5(4):280–90.

50. Sabatine MS, Giugliano RP, Wiviott SD, et al. Efficacy and safety of evolocumab in reducing lipids and cardiovascular events. N Engl J Med 2015;372(16):1500–9.

51. McKenney JM, Koren MJ, Kereiakes DJ, et al. Safety and efficacy of a monoclonal antibody to proprotein convertase subtilisin/kexin type 9 serine protease, SAR236553/REGN727, in patients with primary hypercholesterolemia receiving ongoing stable atorvastatin therapy. J Am Coll Cardiol 2012;59(25):2344–53.

52. Roth EM, McKenney JM, Hanotin C, et al. Atorvastatin with or without an antibody to PCSK9 in primary hypercholesterolemia. N Engl J Med 2012;367(20):1891–900.

53. Stein EA, Gipe D, Bergeron J, et al. Effect of a monoclonal antibody to PCSK9, REGN727/SAR236553, to reduce low-density lipoprotein cholesterol in patients with heterozygous familial hypercholesterolaemia on stable statin dose with or without ezetimibe therapy: a phase 2 randomised controlled trial. Lancet 2012;380(9836):29–36.

54. Dufour R, Bergeron J, Gaudet D, et al. Open-label therapy with alirocumab in patients with heterozygous familial hypercholesterolemia: results from three years of treatment. Int J Cardiol 2017;228:754–60.

55. Kereiakes DJ, Robinson JG, Cannon CP, et al. Efficacy and safety of the proprotein convertase subtilisin/kexin type 9 inhibitor alirocumab among high cardiovascular risk patients on maximally tolerated statin therapy: the ODYSSEY COMBO I study. Am Heart J 2015;169(6):906–15.e13.

56. Cannon CP, Cariou B, Blom D, et al. Efficacy and safety of alirocumab in high cardiovascular risk patients with inadequately controlled hypercholesterolaemia on maximally tolerated doses of statins: the ODYSSEY COMBO II randomized controlled trial. Eur Heart J 2015;36(19):1186–94.

57. Robinson JG, Colhoun HM, Bays HE, et al. Efficacy and safety of alirocumab as add-on therapy in high-cardiovascular-risk patients with hypercholesterolemia not adequately controlled with atorvastatin (20 or 40 mg) or rosuvastatin (10 or 20 mg): design and rationale of the ODYSSEY OPTIONS Studies. Clin Cardiol 2014;37(10):597–604.

58. Bays H, Gaudet D, Weiss R, et al. Alirocumab as add-on to atorvastatin versus other lipid treatment strategies: ODYSSEY OPTIONS I randomized trial. J Clin Endocrinol Metab 2015;100(8):3140–8.

59. Farnier M, Jones P, Severance R, et al. Efficacy and safety of adding alirocumab to rosuvastatin versus adding ezetimibe or doubling the rosuvastatin dose in high cardiovascular-risk patients: the ODYSSEY OPTIONS II randomized trial. Atherosclerosis 2016;244:138–46.

60. Moriarty PM, Thompson PD, Cannon CP, et al. Efficacy and safety of alirocumab vs ezetimibe in statin-intolerant patients, with a statin rechallenge arm: the ODYSSEY ALTERNATIVE randomized trial. J Clin Lipidol 2015;9(6):758–69.

61. Roth EM, McKenney JM. ODYSSEY MONO: effect of alirocumab 75 mg subcutaneously every 2 weeks as monotherapy versus ezetimibe over 24 weeks. Future Cardiol 2015;11(1):27–37.

62. Robinson JG, Farnier M, Krempf M, et al. Efficacy and safety of alirocumab in reducing lipids and cardiovascular events. N Engl J Med 2015;372(16): 1489–99.

63. Schwartz GG, Bessac L, Berdan LG, et al. Effect of alirocumab, a monoclonal antibody to PCSK9, on long-term cardiovascular outcomes following acute coronary syndromes: rationale and design of the ODYSSEY outcomes trial. Am Heart J 2014;168(5): 682–9.

64. Kastelein JJ, Ginsberg HN, Langslet G, et al. ODYSSEY FH I and FH II: 78 week results with alirocumab treatment in 735 patients with heterozygous familial hypercholesterolaemia. Eur Heart J 2015;36(43): 2996–3003.

65. Teramoto T, Kobayashi M, Tasaki H, et al. Efficacy and safety of alirocumab in Japanese patients with heterozygous familial hypercholesterolemia or at high cardiovascular risk with hypercholesterolemia not adequately controlled with statins- ODYSSEY Japan randomized controlled trial. Circ J 2016; 80(9):1980–7.

66. Kastelein JJ, Robinson JG, Farnier M, et al. Efficacy and safety of alirocumab in patients with heterozygous familial hypercholesterolemia not adequately controlled with current lipid-lowering therapy: design and rationale of the ODYSSEY FH studies. Cardiovasc Drugs Ther 2014;28(3): 281–9.

67. Moriarty PM, Parhofer KG, Babirak SP, et al. Alirocumab in patients with heterozygous familial hypercholesterolaemia undergoing lipoprotein apheresis: the ODYSSEY ESCAPE trial. Eur Heart J 2016;37(48): 3588–95.

68. Farnier M, Hovingh GK, Langslet G, et al. Durability of alirocumab effect: data from an open-label extension to the ODYSSEY program for patients with heterozygous familial hypercholesterolemia. J Clin Lipidol 2017;11(3):840.

69. Roth EM, Moriarty PM, Bergeron J, et al, ODYSSEY CHOICE I investigators. A phase III randomized trial evaluating alirocumab 300 mg every 4 weeks as monotherapy or add-on to statin: ODYSSEY CHOICE I. Atherosclerosis 2016;254:254–62.

70. Roth E, Moriarty PM, Bergeron J, et al. Efficacy and safety of the PCSK9 inhibitor alirocumab 300 mg every 4 weeks in patients with ASCVD. Atherosclerosis 2017;263:e102–3.

71. Stroes E, Guyton JR, Lepor N, et al, ODYSSEY CHOICE II Investigators. Efficacy and safety of alirocumab 150 mg every 4 weeks in patients with hypercholesterolemia not on statin therapy: the ODYSSEY CHOICE II study. J Am Heart Assoc 2016;5(9) [pii:e003421].

72. Ridker PM, Revkin J, Amarenco P, et al. Cardiovascular efficacy and safety of bococizumab in high-risk patients. N Engl J Med 2017; 376(16):1527–39.

73. Essalmani R, Susan-Resiga D, Chamberland A, et al. In vivo evidence that furin from hepatocytes inactivates PCSK9. J Biol Chem 2011;286(6):4257–63.

74. Han B, Eacho PI, Knierman MD, et al. Isolation and characterization of the circulating truncated form of PCSK9. J Lipid Res 2014;55(7):1505–14.

75. Schroeder KM, Beyer TP, Hansen RJ, et al. Proteolytic cleavage of antigen extends the durability of an anti-PCSK9 monoclonal antibody. J Lipid Res 2015;56(11):2124–32.

76. Lipovsek D. Adnectins: engineered target-binding protein therapeutics. Protein Eng Des Sel 2011; 24(1–2):3–9.

77. Mitchell T, Chao G, Sitkoff D, et al. Pharmacologic profile of the adnectin BMS-962476, a small protein biologic alternative to PCSK9 antibodies for low-density lipoprotein lowering. J Pharmacol Exp Ther 2014;350(2):412–24.

78. Stein EA, Kasichayanula S, Turner T, et al. LDL cholesterol reduction with BMS-962476, an adnectin inhibitor of Pcsk9: results of a single ascending dose study. J Am Coll Cardiol 2014;63(12):A1372.

79. Mullard A. Nine paths to PCSK9 inhibition. Nat Rev Drug Discov 2017;16(5):299–301.

80. Frank-Kamenetsky M, Grefhorst A, Anderson NN, et al. Therapeutic RNAi targeting PCSK9 acutely lowers plasma cholesterol in rodents and LDL cholesterol in nonhuman primates. Proc Natl Acad Sci U S A 2008;105(33):11915–20.

81. Fitzgerald K, Frank-Kamenetsky M, Shulga-Morskaya S, et al. Effect of an RNA interference drug on the synthesis of proprotein convertase subtilisin/kexin type 9 (PCSK9) and the concentration of serum LDL cholesterol in healthy volunteers: a randomised, single-blind, placebo-controlled, phase 1 trial. Lancet 2014;383(9911):60–8.

82. Fitzgerald K, White S, Borodovsky A, et al. A highly durable RNAi therapeutic inhibitor of PCSK9. N Engl J Med 2017;376(1):41–51.

83. Ray KK, Landmesser U, Leiter LA, et al. Inclisiran in patients at high cardiovascular risk with elevated LDL cholesterol. N Engl J Med 2017; 376(15):1430–40.

Bempedoic Acid (ETC-1002)
A Current Review

Anum Saeed, MD[a,b,1], Christie M. Ballantyne, MD[a,b,c],*

KEYWORDS

- Bempedoic acid • Cholesterol • Cardiovascular disease • Lipids • Lipid-lowering agents
- Statin intolerance • Nonstatin therapy

KEY POINTS

- ETC-1002 (bempedoic acid) is a novel, once-daily oral lipid-lowering agent that inhibits adenosine triphosphate citrate lyase, an enzyme in the cholesterol synthesis pathway, and leads to upregulation of LDL receptors.
- ETC-1002 has shown efficacious low-density lipoprotein–cholesterol (LDL-C) lowering in early-phase clinical studies.
- Once-daily dosing of ETC-1002 at various doses has excellent tolerability in patients with or without statin intolerance.
- This novel drug is a potential nonstatin therapeutic option for high-risk patients who require additional LDL-C reduction and/or are statin intolerant.
- Currently, phase 3 clinical studies are investigating the cardiovascular outcomes, long-term safety, and tolerability of ETC-1002 use in individuals with high cardiovascular risk.

INTRODUCTION

Cardiovascular disease (CVD) is one of the leading causes of mortality and morbidity worldwide.[1] Approximately 92.1 million American adults are living with some form of CVD. In the *Heart Disease and Stroke Statistics—2017 Update* by the American Heart Association, the direct and indirect costs of CVD, including health expenditures and lost productivity, are estimated to total more than $316 billion.[1]

The pathogenesis of CVD is largely driven by the atherosclerotic disease process. One of the most important causes of atherosclerotic CVD is dyslipidemia. Epidemiologic data confirm an independent positive association between low-density lipoprotein cholesterol (LDL-C) and CVD.[2–4] In genetic studies, persistent exposure to lower LDL-C beginning early in life has been shown to have a three-times greater reduction in the risk of coronary heart disease for each unit lower LDL-C level than treatment with a statin started later in life.[2] Based on evidence from large observational studies and randomized clinical trials, reduction in LDL-C levels leads to reduced CVD mortality and morbidity.[5,6]

Statins, which inhibit 3-hydroxy-3-methylglutaryl–coenzyme A reductase, the rate-limiting enzyme of cholesterol synthesis, are the standard of therapy for dyslipidemia management and

Disclosure Statement: C.M. Ballantyne receives institutional grants and research support from Amarin, Amgen, Esperion, Ionis, Novartis, Pfizer, Regeneron, and Sanofi-Synthelabo; and is a consultant for Amarin, Amgen, Astra Zeneca, Boehringer Ingelheim, Eli Lilly, Esperion, Ionis, Matinas BioPharma Inc, Merck, Novartis, Pfizer, Regeneron, and Sanofi-Synthelabo. A. Saeed has nothing to disclose.
[a] Section of Cardiovascular Research, Department of Medicine, Baylor College of Medicine, One Baylor Plaza, M.S. BCM285, Suite 524D, Houston, TX 77030, USA; [b] Center for Cardiometabolic Disease Prevention, 6655 Travis Street, Suite 320, Houston, TX 77030, USA; [c] Section of Cardiology, Department of Medicine, Baylor College of Medicine, One Baylor Plaza, M.S. BCM285, Suite 524D, Houston, TX 77030, USA
[1] 6655 Travis Street, Suite 320, Houston, TX 77030.
* Corresponding author. One Baylor Plaza, M.S. BCM285, Suite 524D, Houston, TX 77030.
E-mail address: cmb@bcm.edu

Cardiol Clin 36 (2018) 257–264
https://doi.org/10.1016/j.ccl.2017.12.007
0733-8651/18/© 2017 Elsevier Inc. All rights reserved.

first-line agents for reduction of LDL-C levels. The efficacy of statins in reducing LDL-C levels and decreasing CVD-associated morbidity and mortality has been well established. High levels of adherence with statins have proven to have beneficial outcomes in primary and secondary prevention populations.[7]

Although high-intensity statins are recommended for high-risk patients, such as those with clinical CVD, diabetes, and very high levels of LDL-C greater than or equal 190 mg/dL, numerous surveys show that most patients are not on guideline-recommended doses.[8–10] Statin therapy can yield a range of muscle complaints, which vary between simple myalgia or myositis to the rare but life-threatening rhabdomyolysis.[11] A large observational survey reported that approximately 29% of statin users suffered from statin-associated side effects, which led 15% of these individuals to discontinue their therapy.[12] Furthermore, a significant proportion of patients do not have sufficient therapeutic response despite complying with statin therapy. Therefore, additional lipid-lowering medications are needed in this large group of individuals, who are either intolerant to statin therapy or continue to have elevated LDL-C levels on maximally tolerated statin therapy.

Several nonstatin therapies, when added to background statin therapy, have improved CVD outcomes as shown in large clinical trials. The Improved Reduction of Outcomes: Vytorin Efficacy International Trial (IMPROVE-IT; n = 18,144) evaluated the effect of ezetimibe combined with simvastatin, compared with that of simvastatin alone, in stable patients who had had an acute coronary syndrome and whose LDL-C values were within guideline recommendations.[5] IMPROVE-IT showed a 6% relative reduction in CVD events when ezetimibe was added to background statin therapy, with a mean achieved LDL-C of 54 mg/dL compared with a mean of 70 mg/dL in the statin monotherapy group.

More recently, the proprotein convertase subtilisin/kexin type 9 (PCSK9) inhibitors have emerged as a promising nonstatin therapy for LDL-C reduction. PCSK9 inhibitors are effective LDL-C–lowering agents[13,14] and have also shown favorable cardiovascular outcomes.[6] The Further Cardiovascular Outcomes Research with PCSK9 Inhibition in Subjects with Elevated Risk (FOURIER) trial (n = 27,564) showed a 15% reduction in cardiovascular events with the addition of the PCSK9 inhibitor evolocumab to statin therapy.[6] Another PCSK9 inhibitor, bococizumab, a humanized monoclonal antibody, was assessed in Studies of PCSK9 Inhibition and the Reduction of Vascular Events (SPIRE),

multicenter randomized clinical trials in high-risk patients (n = 27,438) and also was associated with a reduction in cardiovascular events but had an increased incidence of neutralizing antibodies, which attenuated the LDL-C lowering by bococizumab over time.[15] Another novel nonstatin agent, anacetrapib, a potent cholesterol ester transfer protein inhibitor, was studied in the Randomized Evaluation of the Effects of Anacetrapib through Lipid Modification (REVEAL) trial (n = 30,449), in which LDL-C level was reduced by 17% relative to placebo and major coronary event risk was reduced by 9%.[16] Collectively, these outcomes trials of nonstatin therapy include more than 100,000 participants.

Bempedoic acid (ETC-1002) is a novel first-in-class, oral small molecule that inhibits cholesterol synthesis by inhibiting action of ATP citrate lyase (ACL), a cystolic enzyme upstream of 3-hydroxy-3-methylglutaryl–coenzyme A reductase. In this article, we discuss the mechanism of action of ETC-1002, its lipid-lowering effect on atherosclerosis, and genetic data currently available. We also discuss the efficacy and safety profile of ETC-1002 in patients with or without statin intolerance based on recent clinical studies.

MECHANISM OF ACTION

ETC-1002 acts in the same biosynthetic pathway as the statins. ACL plays an integral part in linking energy metabolism from carbohydrates to the production of fatty acids through catalyzing acetyl-CoA synthesis, the fundamental substrate for the biosynthesis of fatty acids and cholesterol.[17] ACL has been a potential target of therapeutic intervention given its centralized role in cholesterol synthesis. However, prior efforts in inhibition of ACL in vitro have been hampered by the compound's poor ability to cross cell membranes, reduced affinity for ACL, and nonspecific inhibition of other essential enzymes in vivo.

ETC-1002, with its improved bioavailability and specificity, is the most clinically advanced ACL inhibitor. In preclinical models, ETC-1002 inhibited sterol and fatty acid synthesis by ACL inhibition and adenosine monophosphate–activated protein kinase activation.[18] This small molecule is an oral, once-daily ingested compound that is absorbed rapidly through the small intestine. Once taken up by the liver, its half-life varies between 15 and 24 hours.

ETC-1002 is a prodrug, and in the liver it is converted to ETC-1002-CoA, its active metabolite, by endogenous liver acyl-CoA synthetase. It is ETC-1002-CoA, the active metabolite of ETC-1002, that is responsible for the inhibition of ACL and thereby the upregulation of the LDL receptor.[19] Upregulation of the LDL receptor results in an increased uptake and removal of LDL particles by the liver and reduction in blood LDL-C levels.[20] Initial studies have reported up to a 27% decrease in LDL-C with ETC-1002 used as monotherapy,[21] up to 24% additional decrease in LDL-C when added to stable background statin therapy,[22] and up to 48% total reduction in combination with ezetimibe.[23]

POTENTIAL MECHANISM OF LOWERING MYOTOXICITY AND ATHEROSCLEROSIS

Recently, the basic mechanism for LDL-C lowering by ETC-1002 and the efficacy of ETC-1002 for attenuating atherosclerosis were examined by Pinkosky and colleagues[24] by using genetic, pharmacologic, and mouse models. ETC-1002 was shown to moderate ACL and adenosine monophosphate–activated protein kinase activities only in cells capable of activation of this prodrug into its active forms. The activation of the prodrug is achieved by action of very-long-chain acyl-CoA synthetase-1 (ACSVL1), an enzyme expressed in the liver but not in adipose tissue or the skeletal muscles.[24] In humans, ACSVL1 was shown to be present in the liver extensively but only nominally expressed in the kidneys and undetectable in the skeletal muscles.[24] In vitro, ETC-1002 did not inhibit cholesterol synthesis nor did it induce muscle apoptosis or myotoxicity as compared with myotubes containing simvastatin and atorvastatin.[24] Reduced cholesterol synthesis and LDL receptor upregulation via ACL inhibition by ETC-1002 results in lower LDL-C levels. In mice, these reductions in LDL-C levels were associated with equivalent decreases in whole aortic cholesterol and lesion size within the aortic sinus in vivo.[24]

GENETIC DATA ON ATP CITRATE LYASE INHIBITION

Recently, Ference and colleagues[25] carried out a Mendelian randomization study to evaluate the effect of lowering LDL-C by genetic variants in the gene encoding ACL (ACLY). A genetic score, which included independently inherited variants in the gene encoding ACL that were associated with lower LDL-C, was used as a simulator for the effect of ACL inhibition. The primary outcome was major cardiovascular events (MCE), a composite of coronary death, myocardial infarction, stroke, and coronary revascularization, and 101,236 participants from 14 prospective cohort or case-control studies were included in the analysis.

Individuals with ACL scores lower than the median had 2.0 mg/dL lower LDL-C, 1.8 mg/dL lower apolipoprotein B (apoB), and 3.5% lower risk of MCE (odds ratio [OR], 0.965; 95% confidence interval [CI], 0.942–0.988; $P = .003$). Variants that mimic the effect of an ACL inhibitor had comparable effects on MCE risk (OR, 0.832; 95% CI, 0.736–0.940) as variants that mimic the effects of statins (OR, 0.844; 95% CI, 0.806–0.885), ezetimibe (OR, 0.833; 95% CI, 0.755–0.920), and PCSK9 inhibitors (OR, 0.843; 95% CI, 0.805–0.882), all of which lower LDL-C through the LDL receptor pathway.

The results of this study suggest that bempedoic acid–associated LDL-C reduction may reduce cardiovascular event risk favorably and that this risk reduction may be comparable with that achieved with the statins per unit decrease in LDL-C.

PHASE 1 AND 2 STUDIES

In phase 1 studies of ETC-1002, the safety, tolerability, and pharmacokinetics of the compound were evaluated in a small number of healthy subjects compared with placebo. ETC-1002-001 demonstrated the drug's safety in 18 healthy subjects,[26] whereas ETC-1002-002 was a staged 2-week and 4-week phase Ib trial that evaluated multiple dosing tolerance in 53 subjects.[27] The doses in ETC-1002-002 were divided into 20, 60, 100, or 120 mg of ETC-1002 or placebo. The tolerability and safety of doses greater than 120 mg/d were demonstrated in ETC-1002-004, a 2-week phase Ib, multiple-dose tolerance clinical trial in 24 subjects of whom 18 subjects received ETC-1002 in different doses of 140, 180, or 220 mg for a total of 14 days.[28] Subjects taking ETC-1002 showed an average LDL-C reduction of 36% (220 mg/d dose) compared with a 4% increase in the placebo arm. ETC-1002 was observed to be safe and well tolerated in this trial, without any adverse events.

A total of nine phase 2 clinical studies of ETC-1002 have been completed (**Table 1**), evaluating ETC-1002 as monotherapy,[21,23,29–31] added onto statin background therapy,[32–34] and as combination therapy with ezetimibe[23] and triple therapy with ezetimibe + statin.[35] ETC-1002-007, a phase 2a clinical study spanning an 8-week period, primarily evaluated adverse events, laboratory derangements, and other safety data findings when using ETC-1002 as an add-on therapy to atorvastatin, 10 mg. This study showed that ETC-1002 was safely tolerated without any serious adverse events. Furthermore, the addition of ETC-1002 to a background therapy of atorvastatin, 20 mg reduced LDL-C levels by an average of

Table 1
Phase 2 studies of ETC-1002

Study Number	Patient Population (Other Therapy) (n = Total/ Assigned Bempedoic Acid)	LDL-C Lowering (Placebo Corrected)	Dose (mg)	Treatment Duration (wk)
003[21]	Hypercholesterolemia (n = 177/133)	≤27% (25%)	40, 80, 120	12
005[29]	Hypercholesterolemia and type 2 diabetes (n = 60/30)	43% (39%)	80, 120	4
006[30]	Hypercholesterolemia and history of statin intolerance (n = 56/37)	32% (29%)	60, 120, 180, 240	8
007[32]	Hypercholesterolemia (added on to atorvastatin, 10 mg) (n = 58/42)	22% (22%)	60, 120, 180, 240	8
008[23]	Hypercholesterolemia with or without statin intolerance (± ezetimibe, 10 mg) (n = 349/249)	≤30% (monotherapy); ≤48% (+ ezetimibe)	120, 180	12
009[33]	Hypercholesterolemia (on stable statin therapy) (n = 134/88)	24% (20%)	120, 180	12
014[31]	Hypercholesterolemia and hypertension (n = 143/72)	21% (24%)	180	6
035[34]	Hypercholesterolemia (added on to high-dose statin) (n = 68/45)	13% (22%)	180	4
038[35]	Hypercholesterolemia (+ ezetimibe + atorvastatin, 20 mg) (n = 63/43)	64% (61%)	180	6

22% versus 0% reduction in the placebo arm (P<.0001).[32]

ETC-1002-006 and ETC-1002-008 were phase 2a and 2b clinical studies that evaluated LDL-C–lowering efficacy, tolerability, and safety, including muscle-associated adverse events, in individuals with intolerance to at least one statin (defined as new myalgia, muscle cramps, muscle aches, or weakness that developed during statin treatment and resolved/reduced markedly on discontinuation of the statin). In ETC-1002-006,[30] eligible subjects were given increasing doses of ETC-1002 (60, 120, 180, and 240 mg) for 2 weeks each or placebo for 8 weeks. After 8 weeks of therapy, the ETC-1002 treatment arm had an average 32% LDL-C reduction, whereas the placebo group had only approximately 3% reduction in LDL-C (P<.0001). Furthermore, ETC-1002 also reduced high-sensitivity C-reactive protein (hs-CRP) levels by 42%, versus 0% in the placebo arm of the study.

In ETC-1002-008, a phase 2b study, 348 patients with (n = 177) or without (n = 171) statin intolerance were enrolled to assess the LDL-C-lowering efficacy of ETC-1002 versus ezetimibe and to assess the safety and tolerability of ETC-1002 in statin-intolerant individuals.[23] During the 12-week duration of the study, two doses of ETC-1002 (120 mg and 180 mg) were assessed for comparison with ezetimibe. The combination of ETC-1002 and ezetimibe was also assessed for LDL-C–lowering efficacy. ETC-1002 lowered LDL-C significantly both as monotherapy (30% reduction) and in combination with ezetimibe (48% reduction) in statin-intolerant individuals.[23] Furthermore, ETC-1002 treatment also lowered hs-CRP by up to 40% compared with ezetimibe. Reported muscle complaints were comparable across both ETC-1002 arms and placebo.

Overall, in phase 2 studies, the LDL-C–lowering effect of ETC-1002 was robust as a monotherapy (LDL-C reduction of 28.7% compared with placebo[30]) and when added with ezetimibe as a combination therapy (LDL-C reduction up to 48% compared with ezetimibe monotherapy).[22] The incremental LDL-C reduction was somewhat reduced (~20%–25% change from baseline) when ETC-1002 was added onto stable background statin therapy. Moreover, ETC-1002 was a safe, well tolerated, and efficacious drug in subjects with statin intolerance.

PHASE 3 STUDIES

Currently, four phase 3 clinical studies evaluating the long-term safety and LDL-C–lowering efficacy are ongoing in patients who have high risk for CVD, established atherosclerotic CVD, heterozygous familial hypercholesterolemia (HeFH), or statin intolerance (Table 2). The phase 3 program has now fully enrolled approximately 3500 patients. CLEAR Harmony is a 52-week global pivotal phase 3 randomized, double-blind, placebo-controlled study evaluating the long-term safety of 180 mg of ETC-1002 versus placebo in subjects with hypercholesterolemia and established atherosclerotic CVD or HeFH who are at high CVD risk and whose LDL-C is not adequately controlled with current lipid-modifying therapies.[36] CLEAR Harmony Open-Label Extension provides 78-week follow-up in CLEAR Harmony participants.[37] CLEAR Serenity is also a 52-week randomized, multicenter,

Table 2
Ongoing phase 3 clinical studies of ETC-1002

Study	Patient Population	Background Therapy	Study Duration	End Points
CLEAR Harmony[36]; CLEAR Harmony OLE[37]	ASCVD and/or HeFH; on maximally tolerated statin therapy (LDL-C ≥70 mg/dL)	Maximally tolerated statin therapy	52 wk; OLE: 78 wk	Primary: long-term safety Secondary: efficacy
CLEAR Wisdom[39]	ASCVD and/or HeFH; on maximally tolerated statin therapy (LDL-C ≥100 mg/dL)	Maximally tolerated statin therapy	52 wk	Primary: 12-wk LDL-C–lowering efficacy Secondary: 24-wk LDL-C–lowering efficacy; 52-wk safety and tolerability; effects on risk markers, including non-HDL-C, total cholesterol, apoB, and hs-CRP
CLEAR Serenity[38]	Statin intolerance and elevated LDL-C not adequately controlled with current lipid-modifying therapy	< Low-dose statin	24 wk	Primary: 24-wk LDL-C–lowering efficacy Secondary: safety and tolerability; effect on risk markers, including hs-CRP, apoB, and total cholesterol
CLEAR Tranquility[40]	Elevated LDL-C with statin intolerance not adequately controlled with current lipid-modifying therapy	Ezetimibe ± low-dose statin	12 wk	Primary: 12-wk LDL-C–lowering efficacy Secondary: safety and tolerability; effect on other biomarkers including hs-CRP
CLEAR Outcomes[41]	Patients with ASCVD, or at high risk, and statin intolerance	Maximally tolerated statin	~3.5 y	Primary: effect on major cardiovascular event occurrence vs placebo

Abbreviations: ASCVD, atherosclerotic cardiovascular disease; HDL, high-density lipoprotein; OLE, open-label extension.

double-blind, placebo-controlled study evaluating the safety and efficacy of 180 mg of bempedoic acid versus placebo in 750 patients with hypercholesterolemia, atherosclerotic CVD, and/or HeFH, and high CVD risk whose LDL-C is not adequately controlled with current maximally tolerated lipid-modifying therapies, including high-intensity statins.[38] The primary end point of this clinical study is the 12-week LDL-C–lowering efficacy of ETC-1002 versus placebo. Secondary end points include the 24-week LDL-C–lowering efficacy, and 52-week safety and tolerability of ETC-1002 versus placebo. Effects on other risk markers, including hs-CRP, will also be evaluated. CLEAR Wisdom[39] and CLEAR Tranquility[40] are randomized, multicenter, double-blind, placebo-controlled trials evaluating the safety and efficacy of ETC-1002 added onto background lipid-lowering therapy in patients with elevated LDL-C on their current therapy.

CLEAR Outcomes, an event-driven, global, randomized, double-blind, placebo-controlled study, is currently in the recruitment stage.[41] This study is evaluating the effects of bempedoic acid in statin-intolerant patients with atherosclerotic CVD or at high risk for CVD. The primary end point is time to first occurrence of cardiovascular death, nonfatal myocardial infarction, nonfatal stroke, or coronary revascularization over an estimated time period of approximately 3.5 years.

SUMMARY

ETC-1002 is an oral, once-daily compound that has shown beneficial lowering of LDL-C by inhibiting ACL, which upregulates LDL receptors in the liver. ETC-1002 achieves significant LDL-C reductions as monotherapy or as add-on therapy to background statin or ezetimibe without any serious adverse events. Based on currently available clinical studies data, ETC-1002 may be a promising addition to lipid-lowering agents as a nonstatin, once-daily oral therapy for high-risk patients who are intolerant to statins and/or unable to achieve recommended LDL-C levels. Furthermore, evolving genetic and basic research data suggest a favorable effect on atherosclerosis by ETC-1002–associated LDL-C lowering. The long-term safety and efficacy of ETC-1002, including effects on cardiometabolic risk parameters and cardiovascular outcomes, are currently being evaluated in phase 3 clinical trials.

REFERENCES

1. Benjamin EJ, Blaha MJ, Chiuve SE, et al. Heart disease and stroke statistics-2017 update: a report from the American Heart Association. Circulation 2017;135:e146–603.
2. Ference BA, Yoo W, Alesh I, et al. Effect of long-term exposure to lower low-density lipoprotein cholesterol beginning early in life on the risk of coronary heart disease: a Mendelian randomization analysis. J Am Coll Cardiol 2012;60:2631–9.
3. Mihaylova B, Emberson J, Blackwell L, et al. The effects of lowering LDL cholesterol with statin therapy in people at low risk of vascular disease: meta-analysis of individual data from 27 randomised trials. Lancet 2012;380:581–90.
4. Collins R, Reith C, Emberson J, et al. Interpretation of the evidence for the efficacy and safety of statin therapy. Lancet 2016;388:2532–61.
5. Cannon CP, Blazing MA, Giugliano RP, et al. Ezetimibe added to statin therapy after acute coronary syndromes. N Engl J Med 2015;372:2387–97.
6. Sabatine MS, Giugliano RP, Keech AC, et al. Evolocumab and clinical outcomes in patients with cardiovascular disease. N Engl J Med 2017;376: 1713–22.
7. Simpson RJ Jr, Mendys P. The effects of adherence and persistence on clinical outcomes in patients treated with statins: a systematic review. J Clin Lipidol 2010;4:462–71.
8. Pokharel Y, Gosch K, Nambi V, et al. Practice-level variation in statin use among patients with diabetes: insights from the PINNACLE registry. J Am Coll Cardiol 2016;68:1368–9.
9. Pokharel Y, Tang F, Jones PG, et al. Adoption of the 2013 American College of Cardiology/American Heart Association cholesterol management guideline in cardiology practices nationwide. JAMA Cardiol 2017;2:361–9.
10. Salami JA, Warraich H, Valero-Elizondo J, et al. National trends in statin use and expenditures in the US adult population from 2002 to 2013: insights from the medical expenditure panel survey. JAMA Cardiol 2017;2:56–65.
11. Jacobson TA, Ito MK, Maki KC, et al. National lipid association recommendations for patient-centered management of dyslipidemia: part 1–full report. J Clin Lipidol 2015;9:129–69.
12. Ito MK, Maki KC, Brinton EA, et al. Muscle symptoms in statin users, associations with cytochrome P450, and membrane transporter inhibitor use: a subanalysis of the USAGE study. J Clin Lipidol 2014;8:69–76.
13. Sabatine MS, Giugliano RP, Wiviott SD, et al. Efficacy and safety of evolocumab in reducing lipids and cardiovascular events. N Engl J Med 2015; 372:1500–9.
14. Robinson JG, Farnier M, Krempf M, et al. Efficacy and safety of alirocumab in reducing lipids and cardiovascular events. N Engl J Med 2015;372: 1489–99.

15. Ridker PM, Revkin J, Amarenco P, et al. Cardiovascular efficacy and safety of bococizumab in high-risk patients. N Engl J Med 2017;376:1527–39.

16. HPS3/TIMI55–REVEAL Collaborative Group. Effects of anacetrapib in patients with atherosclerotic vascular disease. N Engl J Med 2017;377:1217–27.

17. Pearce NJ, Yates JW, Berkhout TA, et al. The role of ATP citrate-lyase in the metabolic regulation of plasma lipids. Hypolipidaemic effects of SB-204990, a lactone prodrug of the potent ATP citrate-lyase inhibitor SB-201076. Biochem J 1998; 334(Pt 1):113–9.

18. Pinkosky SL, Filippov S, Srivastava RA, et al. AMP-activated protein kinase and ATP-citrate lyase are two distinct molecular targets for ETC-1002, a novel small molecule regulator of lipid and carbohydrate metabolism. J Lipid Res 2013; 54:134–51.

19. Berkhout TA, Havekes LM, Pearce NJ, et al. The effect of (−)-hydroxycitrate on the activity of the low-density-lipoprotein receptor and 3-hydroxy-3-methylglutaryl-CoA reductase levels in the human hepatoma cell line Hep G2. Biochem J 1990;272: 181–6.

20. Hamilton JG, Sullivan AC, Kritchevsky D. Hupolipidemic activity of (−)-hydroxycitrate. Lipids 1977;12: 1–9.

21. Ballantyne CM, Davidson MH, Macdougall DE, et al. Efficacy and safety of a novel dual modulator of adenosine triphosphate-citrate lyase and adenosine monophosphate-activated protein kinase in patients with hypercholesterolemia: results of a multicenter, randomized, double-blind, placebo-controlled, parallel-group trial. J Am Coll Cardiol 2013;62: 1154–62.

22. Ballantyne CM, McKenney JM, MacDougall DE, et al. Effect of ETC-1002 on serum low-density lipoprotein cholesterol in hypercholesterolemic patients receiving statin therapy. Am J Cardiol 2016;117: 1928–33.

23. Thompson PD, MacDougall DE, Newton RS, et al. Treatment with ETC-1002 alone and in combination with ezetimibe lowers LDL cholesterol in hypercholesterolemic patients with or without statin intolerance. J Clin Lipidol 2016;10:556–67.

24. Pinkosky SL, Newton RS, Day EA, et al. Liver-specific ATP-citrate lyase inhibition by bempedoic acid decreases LDL-C and attenuates atherosclerosis. Nat Commun 2016;7:13457.

25. Ference BA, Neff D, Cabot M, et al. Genetic target validation for ATP-citrate lyase inhibition [abstract]. J Am Coll Cardiol 2017;69:1655.

26. Nikolic D, Mikhailidis DP, Davidson MH, et al. ETC-1002: a future option for lipid disorders? Atherosclerosis 2014;237:705–10.

27. ClinicalTrials.gov. A multiple ascending dose study of ETC-1002 in subjects with mild dyslipidemia. Available at: https://clinicaltrials.gov/ct2/show/NCT01105598. Accessed January 20, 2016.

28. ClinicalTrials.gov. A multiple ascending dose study of ETC-1002 in healthy subjects. Available at: https://clinicaltrials.gov/ct2/show/NCT01485146. Accessed January 20, 2016.

29. Gutierrez MJ, Rosenberg NL, Macdougall DE, et al. Efficacy and safety of ETC-1002, a novel investigational low-density lipoprotein-cholesterol-lowering therapy for the treatment of patients with hypercholesterolemia and type 2 diabetes mellitus. Arterioscler Thromb Vasc Biol 2014;34: 676–83.

30. Thompson PD, Rubino J, Janik MJ, et al. Use of ETC-1002 to treat hypercholesterolemia in patients with statin intolerance. J Clin Lipidol 2015;9: 295–304.

31. ClinicalTrials.gov. Evaluation of ETC-1002 in patients with hypercholesterolemia and hypertension. Available at: https://clinicaltrials.gov/ct2/show/NCT02178098. Accessed January 20, 2016.

32. ClinicalTrials.gov. A study of the safety, pharmacokinetic drug interaction and efficacy of ETC-1002 and atorvastatin in subjects with hypercholesterolemia. Available at: https://clinicaltrials.gov/ct2/show/study/NCT01779453. Accessed January 20, 2016.

33. ClinicalTrials.gov. Evaluation of ETC-1002 vs placebo in patients receiving ongoing statin therapy. Available at: https://clinicaltrials.gov/ct2/show/NCT02072161. Accessed 19 October 2017.

34. ClinicalTrials.gov. A study of pharmacokinetics, pharmacodynamics and safety of adding ETC-1002 To atorvastatin 80 mg. Available at: https://clinicaltrials.gov/ct2/show/NCT02659397. Accessed October 19, 2017.

35. ClinicalTrials.gov. Evaluation of the efficacy and safety of bempedoic acid (ETC-1002) 180 mg, ezetimibe 10 mg, and atorvastatin 20 mg triplet therapy in patients with elevated LDL-C. Available at: https://clinicaltrials.gov/ct2/show/NCT03051100. Accessed October 19, 2017.

36. ClinicalTrials.gov. Evaluation of long-term safety and tolerability of ETC-1002 in high-risk patients with hyperlipidemia and high CV risk (CLEAR Harmony). Available at: https://clinicaltrials.gov/ct2/show/NCT02666664. Accessed October 19, 2017.

37. ClinicalTrials.gov. Assessment of the long-term safety and efficacy of bempedoic acid (CLEAR Harmony OLE). Available at: https://clinicaltrials.gov/ct2/show/NCT03067441. Accessed October 19, 2017.

38. ClinicalTrials.gov. Evaluation of the efficacy and safety of bempedoic acid (ETC-1002) in patients with hyperlipidemia and statin intolerant (CLEAR Serenity). Available at: https://clinicaltrials.gov/ct2/show/NCT02988115. Accessed October 19, 2017.

39. ClinicalTrials.gov. Evaluation of long-term efficacy of bempedoic acid (ETC-1002) in patients with hyperlipidemia at high cardiovascular risk (CLEAR Wisdom). Available at: https://clinicaltrials.gov/ct2/show/NCT02991118. Accessed October 19, 2016.

40. ClinicalTrials.gov. Evaluation of the efficacy and safety of bempedoic acid (ETC-1002) as add-on to ezetimibe therapy in patients with elevated LDL-C (CLEAR Tranquility). Available at: https://clinicaltrials.gov/ct2/show/NCT03001076. Accessed October 19, 2017.

41. ClinicalTrials.gov. Evaluation of major cardiovascular events in patients with, or at high risk for, cardiovascular disease who are statin intolerant treated with bempedoic acid (ETC-1002) or placebo (CLEAR Outcomes). Available at: https://clinicaltrials.gov/ct2/show/NCT02993406. Accessed October 19, 2017.

Triglyceride-Rich Lipoproteins

Maaike Kockx, PhD[a], Leonard Kritharides, MBBS, PhD, FRACP, FCSANZ, FESC[b],*

KEYWORDS

- Triglycerides • Triglyceride-rich lipoproteins • Cardiovascular risk • Triglyceride-lowering therapy
- Lipoprotein lipase • Apolipoprotein CIII • Angiopoietin-like proteins

KEY POINTS

- A substantial residual cardiovascular risk remains after effective lowering of plasma low-density lipoprotein cholesterol.
- A causal relationship between plasma triglyceride (TG) levels and risk of cardiovascular disease has been indicated by Mendelian randomization studies and epidemiologic studies.
- TG metabolism is complex: genetic association studies have identified LPL, apoCIII, apoAV, ANGPTL3/4, LMF1, GPIHBP1, and TRIB1 as important regulators of TG levels.
- There are numerous emerging pharmacologic and biological therapies for elevated TG.

INTRODUCTION

Elevated levels of triglyceride-rich lipoproteins (TRLs), the main carriers of triglycerides (TG) in the blood, have been associated with an increased risk of cardiovascular disease (CVD) for decades. It has been debated whether increased plasma TG are causally linked to CVD. The difficulty in establishing causality between plasma TG levels and an increased risk of CVD is due to the postprandial variability of TG levels, which makes associations difficult, the confounding association with decreased high-density lipoprotein (HDL) levels, and the fact that subjects with extremely high TG levels do not typically develop CVD.[1] Recent genetic association and Mendelian randomization studies have identified many loci linked with TG, of which 7 are causally associated with CVD independently of plasma high-density lipoprotein cholesterol (HDL-C) or low-density lipoprotein cholesterol levels (LDL-C).[2] Because a substantial risk for CVD remains even after effective lowering of LDL-C, this and other studies relating to genetic deficiencies

of apolipoproteinCIII (apoCIII) and angiopoietin-like proteins (ANGPTLs)[3,4] have sparked renewed interest in elevated TG levels as valid independent targets in the prevention of CVD. Here, the authors summarize their understanding of TG-rich lipoproteins and their relevance as candidate targets for therapeutic intervention.

TRIGLYCERIDE METABOLISM

Although classifications of severity vary between guidelines, plasma TG levels are generally considered elevated greater than 150 mg/dL (1.7 mmol/L). Severely elevated levels are greater than 885 mg/dL (10 mmol/L).[5] The standard measurement of plasma TG is performed under fasting conditions. However nonfasting levels have become accepted and are suggested to represent a more true reflection of average TG concentrations. Importantly, both elevated fasting and nonfasting concentrations of TG are associated with increased risk of CVD.[6]

Disclosure: The authors have nothing to disclose.
a Atherosclerosis Laboratory, ANZAC Research Institute, University of Sydney, Concord Repatriation General Hospital, Gate 3 Hospital Road, Concord, New South Wales 2139, Australia; b Department of Cardiology, Concord Hospital, Atherosclerosis laboratory, ANZAC Research Institute, University of Sydney, 3rd Floor, Hospital Road, Concord, NSW 2139, Australia
* Corresponding author.
E-mail address: leonard.kritharides@sydney.edu.au

Cardiol Clin 36 (2018) 265–275
https://doi.org/10.1016/j.ccl.2017.12.008
0733-8651/18/© 2017 Elsevier Inc. All rights reserved

In the circulation, TG are carried within a variety of lipoproteins, transporting TG to and from tissues depending on demand. TG are most abundant in intestine-derived chylomicrons and in liver-derived very low-density lipoproteins (VLDL). Remnant lipoproteins such as intermediate-density lipoprotein (IDL) and chylomicron remnants, as well as HDL, also contain TG. It is important to note that the cholesterol content of TG-containing lipoproteins may link them causally to increased atherosclerotic plaque development.[7] Unlike VLDL and chylomicrons, remnant particles are small and have been demonstrated to enter the arterial wall.[8] It has been estimated that remnants contain 40 times more cholesterol compared with LDL and could therefore contribute substantially to cholesterol accumulation in the arterial wall.[9] Particle size may also explain why subjects with severe hypertriglyceridemia do not develop CVD because large chylomicrons do not enter the arterial wall.[9]

Postprandially, diet-derived fatty acids are used to synthesize TG, which are subsequently packed into chylomicrons containing apolipoproteinB48 by intestinal microsomal triglyceride transfer protein (MTTP). The chylomicrons are released from the intestine into the lymph before entering the blood, where hydrolysis of TG quickly converts these large chylomicrons into smaller chylomicron remnants, which are cleared by the liver.

In the liver, TG are assembled from fatty acids that are either synthesized locally or derived from the circulation. TG are packed into VLDL in a stepwise process lipidating apolipoproteinB100 (apoB) during translation in the rough endoplasmic reticulum (ER). Further addition of lipids by MTTP generates triglyceride-poor VLDL2. Subsequent fusion with TG-rich particles in the smooth ER leads to the formation of larger TG-rich VLDL1.[10] VLDL formation is highly dependent on the availability of both lipids and apoB, and a proportion of newly synthesized apoB is degraded intracellularly.[11] Although both VLDL1 and VLDL2 are secreted from the liver, it is VLDL1 that primarily contributes to plasma TG levels. Lipolysis on the capillary endothelium via lipoprotein lipase (LPL) converts VLDL into IDL, and further, lipolysis via hepatic triglyceride lipase (HTGL) on the luminal surface of endothelial cells in liver sinusoids generates LDL. LPL activity is promoted by apolipoproteinCII (apoCII) and apolipoproteinAV (apoAV) and inhibited by apolipoproteinCIII (apoCIII) and ANGPTLs.[9] As a consequence, genetic increases in apoCIII and loss of function (LOF) in apoAV increase TG levels and the risk of coronary disease, and decreased or LOF of apoCIII or ANGPTL3/4 decreases plasma TG and the risk of CVD.[3,4]

HDL acquires TG through the action of cholesteryl ester transfer protein, which mediates the exchange of cholesteryl esters and TG between HDL and apoB-containing lipoproteins. ApolipoproteinAIV (apoAIV) is added to chylomicrons during their formation in the intestine, whereas apoAV is added to VLDL during synthesis in the liver. In the circulation, exchange of apolipoproteins between TRLs and other lipoproteins occurs leading to an increase in apoCII, apoCIII, and apoE content and a decrease in apoAIV or apoAV.

Clearance of TRLs is mediated by LPL. Bound to heparin sulfate proteoglycans (HPSGs) on the surface of endothelial cells, LPL releases fatty acids for uptake by tissues, thereby generating triglyceride-containing remnants. During this process, lipids and proteins are transferred to HDL, explaining the tight link between TRLs and HDL levels. TRLs and remnants are taken up by the liver via interaction with HSPGs, the low-density lipoprotein receptor (LDLr), the low-density lipoprotein receptor related protein-1 (LRP1), and possibly the scavenger receptor type-1.[12] Small remnants bind the LDLr via apoE or apoB, while larger remnants are cleared via binding of apoE to HSPGs, LPL, HTGL, and other undefined receptors.[12] TG that are taken up in the liver are either resecreted or catabolized via β-oxidation. Although VLDL catabolism is much slower than that of chylomicrons, the clearance of chylomicrons and VLDL is understood to be mediated through the same pathways. Therefore, conditions leading to increased chylomicron levels will affect plasma VLDL levels and vice versa. Several factors that regulate LPL activity and TRL clearance are discussed later.

CAUSES OF HYPERTRIGLYCERIDEMIA

There are many factors that can contribute to elevated TG levels, which include genetic and nongenetic factors.[5,13] Severe hypertriglyceridemia can be caused by monogenic LOF mutations in *LPL*, *APOCII*, *APOAV*, lipase maturation factor-1 (*LMF1*), glycosylphosphatidylinositol-anchored high-density lipoprotein binding protein-1 (*GPIHBP1*), and glycerol-3-phosphate dehydrogenase. Most of these are linked to inhibited clearance of TRLs. Monogenic LOF mutations are particularly rare. Polygenetic hypertriglyceridemia is more common, leads in general to moderate hypertriglyceridemia, and can be linked to the presence of multiple predisposing genetic variants. More than 40 common single-nucleotide polymorphisms (SNP) have been identified, many linked to pathways not previously known to affect plasma triglyceride levels. Each SNP has a small effect on TG levels explaining the wide populational variation in TG. High TG are commonly observed after the interaction of genetic predisposition with lifestyle factors such as metabolic syndrome, obesity, overnutrition, insulin resistance/type 2 diabetes mellitus (T2DM), kidney disease, hypothyroidism, alcohol excess, or the use of certain medications such as cyclosporine, or oral contraceptives (see Ref.[14] or Ref.[5] for comprehensive review). The degree of hypertriglyceridemia will depend on the severity of genetic and environmental factors present.

ApoE plays a quantitative as well as a qualitative role in regulating plasma TG levels. Mutations in *APOE* resulting in complete apoE deficiency or the apoε2 isoform lead to type III hyperlipoproteinemia, which is characterized by increased TG, LDL-C, and deceased HDL levels. Apoε2 is unable to bind lipoprotein receptors, thereby preventing TRL clearance. The apoε2 isoform is however not sufficient because a secondary factor needs to be present for hyperlipidemia to occur.[15] It has been estimated that 20% to 40% of variability in plasma TG levels can be explained by plasma apoE concentrations. Interestingly, the apoε2 isoform itself is associated with higher plasma levels of apoE protein.[16] Both complete deficiency as well as increased levels of apoE leads to hypertriglyceridemia.[17,18] Lack of apoE on TRL reduces clearance, while accumulation stimulates VLDL production and impairs LPL-mediated clearance, indicating that for optimal TG metabolism, physiologic levels of apoE are required.

Of lifestyle factors, poor diet and excess alcohol intake are the best known to affect plasma TG levels. Plasma TG levels are dose dependently linked to amounts of dietary fat ingested.[19] Diets high in carbohydrates increase the secretion of apoE-poor VLDL, which is cleared at a slower rate.[20] Excessive chronic alcohol intake leads to increased lipolysis in adipose tissue, thereby providing free fatty acid as a substrate to the liver for more VLDL production.[21]

Hypertriglyceridemia is prevalent in patients with insulin resistance and related diseases, such as T2DM and obesity. Insulin resistance is associated with elevated fasting and nonfasting TG levels and is attributed to an overproduction and secretion of VLDL1 and chylomicron secretion.[22,23] Under normal physiologic conditions, postprandial insulin release increases apoB degradation, thereby limiting VLDL formation. However, under conditions of insulin resistance, apoB degradation is not suppressed, and an increased influx of fatty acids from adipose tissue leads to increased hepatic VLDL assembly and secretion of VLDL1.[22] The increased influx of fatty acids into the circulation also drives increased intestinal chylomicron secretion.[23] Increased VLDL1 production contributes to elevated plasma TG levels in abdominal obesity but to a lesser extent. Kinetic studies have indicated that in obesity hypertriglyceridemia is predominantly the result of impaired remnant clearance due to elevated apoCIII levels.[24]

High TG levels are observed in more than 50% of patients with chronic kidney disease (CKD).[25] Adults frequently show multiple other comorbidities, such as insulin resistance, metabolic syndrome, or obesity. However, the fact that elevated TG levels are found in young patients without any comorbidities suggests a direct effect of renal dysfunction. Elevated TG levels result from decreased clearance of TRLs[26,27] with that the degree of clearance impairment directly correlating to the severity of CKD.[27] Decreased clearance in CKD has been linked to decreased LPL and HTGL activity, increased apoCIII, and decreased apoCII levels.[26]

APPROACH TO THE CONVENTIONAL TREATMENT OF ELEVATED TRIGLYCERIDES

Several excellent reviews have addressed therapeutic options currently available for the treatment of elevated TRLs.[5,28] The authors summarize important issues in the approach to these patients based on their understanding of the nature of TRLs as described above. First, lifestyle factors should be carefully explored. They include reduction of carbohydrate and fat intake, increased exercise, avoidance of obesity and alcohol, and the treatment of underlying medical conditions, such as diabetes and hypothyroidism. In the acute setting, fasting and the regulation of diabetes with insulin can immediately reduce chylomicron and VLDL production.

The first issue to identify is the treatment objective- reduction of CVD risk or prevention of pancreatitis. The former requires an initial focus on lower levels of non-HDL cholesterol and apoB-containing particles. The latter requires a focus on the reduction of plasma TG. The considerations prioritize the use of cholesterol-lowering (statin) and TG-lowering therapies as first-line treatment.

In patients in whom TG are moderately or mildly elevated, and in whom non-HDL cholesterol is decreased, and there is increased risk for CVD, the first treatment target is reduction of non-HDL cholesterol in apoB-containing lipoproteins.[29] A meta-regression has recently concluded that lowering of TG in at-risk populations reduces risk in proportion to the degree that TG are lowered.[6]

Lowering of non-HDL cholesterol is pharmacologically achieved by use of a high-potency statin, and where required, ezetimibe (**Table 1**). In patients with diabetes already on a statin who have residual TG >2.0 mmol/L in conjunction with low HDL, subgroup analyses indicate that the addition of fibrates lowers the risk of future cardiovascular events.[6] Because the population with high TG and low HDL was not specifically targeted in the ACCORD and FIELD studies, or in other studies lowering TG with omega-3 fish oil or nicotinic acid, forthcoming studies targeting this group will be very important to prove benefit for drug combinations.[5] In addition, newer more specific fibrates may have improved outcomes (**Table 2**). For patients with markedly elevated TG where the primary focus of treatment is prevention of pancreatitis, treatment should commence with fibrates and fish oil and consider other agents such as nicotinic acid derivatives (see **Table 1**).

OTHER AND NOVEL THERAPIES TARGETING ELEVATED TRIGLYCERIDES
Triglycerides Production

Inhibition of either MTTP or apoB synthesis in the liver is expected to affect the production of all apoB-containing lipoproteins and could therefore be a strategy to target both elevated plasma TG and LDL-C levels (see **Table 2**). That inhibition of MTTP or apoB synthesis leads to lowering of all apoB-containing lipoproteins is corroborated in subjects with *MTTP* deficiency who have low levels of circulating TG and subjects carrying apoB truncation mutations who show reduced

hepatic secretion of VLDL, low plasma apoB levels, and low incidence of CVD.[30,31]

Mipomersen is an antisense oligonucleotide inhibiting apoB synthesis.[32] Mouse studies indicate a robust decrease in plasma apoB and apoB-containing lipoproteins leading to reduced atherosclerosis.[32] However, studies including high-fat diets show accumulation of liver fat most likely due to induction of compensatory lipid synthesis pathways.[33] Similar effects are observed in humans. Mipomersen dose dependently decreases circulating apoB levels with decreases of all apoB-containing lipoproteins.[32] Mild hepatic steatosis is observed, which stabilizes or declines after long-term treatment.[34] Investigation of fractional catabolic and production rates of apoB-containing lipoproteins in healthy volunteers indicated unexpected complex effects of mipomersen whereby VLDL production may only be affected when apoB degradation is limiting.[33]

Lopitamide is an antisense oligonucleotide targeting MTTP. Lopitamide effectively lowers plasma TG and cholesterol in animal models by inhibiting hepatic and intestinal TG secretion and markedly reduces TG and cholesterol levels in healthy human subjects.[35] Unfortunately, lopitamide treatment is associated with increased liver fat accumulation in healthy and diseased subjects.[36] Because of their lipotoxic effects, both mipomersen and lopitamide are currently only used to treat markedly elevated TG levels associated with life-threatening pancreatitis.

Table 1
Conventional treatments

Compound	Effect on TRL	Molecular Mechanism for TRL Effect	Other Effects
Fibrates (PPARα agonist)	Increased ß-oxidation Reduced TRL secretion Increased lipolysis/clearance	↑ ACSL1, ACO ↓ FAS ↑ LPL, apoAV, ANGPTL4 ↓ apoCIII	Increases HDL Decreases LDL Decreases CRP
Ezetimibe	Decreases postprandial lipemia	Blocks NPC1L1	Decreases LDL
Niacin/nicotinic acid	Reduced VLDL formation/secretion Increased adipose fatty acid uptake	↓ DGAT2 ↑ adipose LPL	Decreases LDL Shift to larger LDL Increases HDL
n-3 PUFA (PPARα agonist)	Increased ß-oxidation Decreased lipogenesis Reduced TRL secretion Increased lipolysis/clearance	PPARα agonist ↓ SREBP1c ↓ DGAT2 ↑ LPL ↓ apoCIII	Antioxidant Antithrombotic
Statins	Increased remnant clearance	Block HMGCoAr, ↑ LDLr	Decreases LDL

Abbreviations: ACO, acyl-CoA oxidase; ACSL1, acyl-CoA synthase; HMGCoAr, 3-hydroxy-3-methyl-glutaryl-coenzyme A reductase; NPC1L1, Niemann-pick C1-like 1.

Table 2
Novel therapies

Compound	Target	Mechanisms of TRL Lowering	Other Effects	Ref.
New PPARα agonist				
Pemafibrate (K-877)	PPARα	Decreased TRL production/secretion Increased clearance	Increased HDL Shift to larger LDL and small HDL Decreases CRP	78
BMS-711939	PPARα	Decreased TRL production/secretion Increased clearance	Increases HDL Lowers LDL	79
Hepatic TG synthesis inhibitors				
ACC	ACC	Decreased ACC activity	Increased TG levels and liver fat	39
FAS	FAS	Decreased VLDL production/secretion	Increased liver fat accumulation	40
SCAP antisense	SCAP	Decreased VLDL production/secretion	Decreased LDL	41
DGAT2 antisense	DGAT2	Decreased VLDL production/secretion	Suppressed liver fat accumulation	37,38
LCQ908, AZD7687; pradigastat	DGAT1	Decreases intestinal TRL production	Improved glucose and insulin response	13
Lopitamide	MTTP	Decreased TRL production/secretion	Increased liver fat accumulation	35,36
Mipomersen	APOB	Decreased VLDL production/secretion	Increased liver fat accumulation	32
APOCIII inhibitors				
Volanersorsen	APOCIII	Increased TRL lipolysis and clearance/decreased VLDL production secretion	Increased HDL Increased LDL	61
APOV gene therapy	APOAV	Increased TRL lipolysis/decreased VLDL production-secretion	Decreased LDL Increased HDL	58
ANGTPL3 inhibitors				
REGN1500; evinacumab/ ISIS 703802	ANGPTL3	Increased TRL lipolysis	Decreased HDL Decreased LDL	3,66
ANGTPL4 inhibitors	ANGPTL4	Increased TRL lipolysis	Lipid accumulation in abdominal lymph nodes	71
ANGTPL8 inhibitors	ANGPTL8	Increased TRL lipolysis	Affects body weight	73
LPL gene therapy				
Glybera	LPL	Increased TRL lipolysis	Transient	48
LPL activating compounds				
NO1886;ibrolipim/ C10d/50F10	LPL	Increased TRL lipolysis	Decreased LDL and liver fat accumulation	50

Other approaches include inhibition of enzymes involved in the TG synthesis pathway. Acyl-CoA:diacylglycerol acyltransferase (DGAT) mediates the last reaction in triglyceride synthesis. Two isoforms exist, DGAT1, which is most highly expressed in the small intestine, and DGAT2, which is primarily expressed in liver. Several DGAT1 inhibitors are under investigation (see **Table 2**). So far, marked reductions in postprandial TG secretion and beneficial effects on insulin and glucose metabolism are observed; however, treatment is associated with severe gastrointestinal side effects and requires dietary fat restriction.[13] DGAT2 antisense therapy targets TG synthesis in the liver. Animal studies show effective reduction of VLDL secretion.[37] In parallel, DGAT2 inhibition decreases sterol regulatory binding protein 1 (SREBP1) levels, thereby reducing liver fat content.[38] Inhibition of acetyl-CoA carboxylase (ACC), the first enzyme in the TG synthesis cascade, unexpectedly raised plasma TG levels.[39] Others show that inhibition of fatty acid synthase (FAS) increased liver TG content by activating SREBP1.[40] More promising are therapies targeting SREBP cleavage-activating protein (SCAP). Antisense-mediated inhibition of SCAP lowers TG as well as LDL-C levels in dyslipidemic rhesus monkeys.[41]

A novel target affecting VLDL production is the tribbles homolog-1 (TRIB1). *TRIB1* was identified in Mendelian randomization studies casually linking plasma TG levels and CVD.[2] Studies in mice show that hepatic overexpression of TRIB1 lowers plasma TG and cholesterol levels, while mice with liver-specific deletion of TRIB1 show increased TG and cholesterol levels.[42,43] The mechanisms by which TRIB1 affects TG metabolism are complex. In liver, TRIB1 mediates hepatic lipogenesis and glycogenesis. Although increased lipogenesis and glycogenesis explains increased hepatic fatty accumulation, it appears unrelated to changes in plasma lipids.[43] TRIB1 may also affect MTTP levels and hepatic VLDL secretion through binding to SAP18.[44] Differentiating the pathways by which TRIB1 regulates liver fat and plasma TG levels will be necessary before TRIB1 can be considered a therapeutic target.

TARGETING CLEARANCE OF TRIGLYCERIDE-RICH LIPOPROTEINS

More successful in decreasing plasma TG levels have been strategies targeting lipolysis. Interestingly, most loci identified in Mendelian randomization are those mediating LPL levels or LPL activity. Loci identified by Mendelian Randomization studies include *LPL, APOA5, APOC3,* and *ANGPTL4.*[45] In addition, genetic association studies have identified several other proteins linked to LPL that have a regulatory role in determining plasma TG including apoCII, apoAV, GPIHBP1, ANGPTL3, and LMF-1.[46] Many of these are currently pursued as treatment targets to lower plasma TG levels.

Lipoprotein Lipase

LPL is the most common gene linked to plasma TG, and clear association between plasma LPL levels, plasma TG, and risk of CVD has

been established.[2,47] The link between plasma TG and the LPL gene relates to LOF mutations that lead to partial LPL deficiency.[47] Mutations resulting in complete lack of LPL activity are typically not associated with CVD but are associated with severe hypertriglyceridemia.

Gene replacement therapy was developed for patients with severe hypertriglyceridemia and recurrent pancreatitis because of complete loss of LPL activity and involves delivery of a gain of function variant into muscle using an adeno-associated viral vector (AAV1-LPL^{S447X}; Alipogene tiparvovec).[48] Although fasting TG levels decreased initially by up to 40% in some patients, levels returned to baseline after 26 weeks of treatment. This transient reduction was ascribed to development of antibodies to viral proteins. Phase 2 and 3 studies therefore included immunosuppression using cyclosporine A and mycophenolate mofetil; however, this did not suppress antibody formation.[48] Immunosuppressant agents, especially cyclosporine A, are known to cause dyslipidemia and increase plasma TG.[49] Although the effect on TG was transient, a long-lasting reduction in postprandial chylomicron TG content leading to fewer pancreatitis-related hospitalizations was observed.[48]

A second approach targeting LPL activity is the use of small organic LPL activating compounds. So far 3 LPL activators called NO-1886 (ibrolipim), C10d, and 50F10 have been identified.[50] All compounds increase LPL activity but by different mechanisms. NO-1886 primarily increases adipose LPL messenger RNA levels, whereas C10d directly affects the hydrolytic activity and 50F10 stabilizes the active homodimer structure of LPL.[50] All have been tested in rodent models and decrease elevated TG; however, clinical development of NO-1886 was terminated because of side effects. Besides reducing TG, C10d also lowered plasma cholesterol, total body fat, and reduced fatty liver formation.[50] Interestingly, C10d and 50F10 reverse the inhibition of LPL by ANGPTL4 (see later discussion), while this was not observed with NO-1886.[51]

ApolipoproteinCII

ApoCII is a potent activator of LPL necessary for the interaction between lipoproteins and LPL and for efficient hydrolysis of TRLs. However, excess apoCII may inhibit LPL activity through as yet unknown mechanisms.[52] Complete LOF of apoCII leads to severe hypertriglyceridemia.[46] An apoCII mimetic peptide (C-II-a) reduces elevated TG in many animal models and stimulates LPL activity in plasma from different types of dyslipidemia.[53] To the best of the authors' knowledge, these peptides have not been tested in humans.

ApolipoproteinAV

Genetic association studies established a clear link between *APOA5* variants and TG levels.[9] The discovery of apoAV as a major regulator of plasma TG levels raises some intriguing questions. Plasma apoAV levels are very low. It has been estimated that only 4% of circulating VLDL particles contain apoAV.[9] Thus, although present on only a small proportion of TRLs, apoAV seems to be an important regulator of plasma triglyceride levels. In mice, deficiency of apoAV leads to hypertriglyceridemia, whereas overexpression of human apoAV diminishes plasma TG.[54] It should be mentioned that in humans a positive correlation between plasma apoAV and TG is often observed.[9] The mechanisms by which apoAV affects triglyceride levels remain unclear. It is generally considered that apoAV enhances LPL-mediated hydrolysis through its interaction with GPIHBP because the TG-lowering effect of apoAV is lost in $Gpihbp1^{-/-}$ mice.[55] ApoAV may also affect remnant uptake through its ability to bind to HSPG, LDLr, and LRP1,[56] and others have indicated an intracellular role mediating lipidation of VLDL.[57] So far, effective lowering of plasma TG and cholesterol levels has been shown in mice using adenoviral delivery of human apoAV.[58]

ApolipoproteinCIII

Plasma levels of apoCIII show a clear association with plasma TG levels. Polymorphism analysis and Mendelian randomization studies suggest a causal relationship between the *APOC3* gene and risk of CVD.[59] LOF mutations decrease plasma TG and are associated with a 40% lower risk of CVD.[4] It is not clear which metabolic pathway is the most important in mediating these effects. ApoCIII promotes secretion of TRLs from the liver and inhibits clearance by interfering with the binding of remnants to lipoprotein receptors and HSPGs as well as by displacing apoE from TRLs.[59] Although well known for its capacity to inhibit LPL-mediated lipolysis in vitro, this does not seem to occur in vivo.[60] It can stimulate hepatic lipase, resulting in enhanced conversion of VLDL to LDL and LDL to small dense LDL particles.

Current apoCIII therapies focus on antisense oligonucleotides, which markedly decrease plasma TG levels in rodents, primates, and humans.[59,61] Interestingly, apoCIII antisense therapy decreased TG levels in LPL-deficient patients, supporting the notion that apoCIII-mediated regulation of TG can occur by LPL-independent mechanisms. A recent study has indicated a role of hepatic clearance through LDLr and LRP1, but not HPSGs in TG lowering by apoCIII-antisense therapy.[62]

HDL-C as well as LDL-C levels are concomitantly increased.

Angiopoietin-Like Proteins

Several members of the ANGPTL proteins (ANGPTL3, 4, and 8) regulate tissue-specific activation of LPL under conditions such as feeding, exercise, and cold exposure.[63,64]

ANGPTL3 inhibits LPL by unknown mechanisms. Produced and secreted by the liver, ANGPTL3 mediates VLDL hydrolysis and uptake of fatty acids in heart, muscle, and adipose tissue in an endocrine manner. Several studies suggest a reciprocal requirement between ANGPTL3 and ANGPTL8 for inhibition of LPL.[64] LOF variants in *ANGPTL3* are associated with lower TG, LDL-C, and HDL-C, reduced risk of CVD,[3] and increased insulin sensitivity.[65] Targeting of ANGPTL3 using either monoclonal antibodies or antisense therapy decreases TG effectively and to a lesser extent lowers LDL cholesterol and HDL cholesterol.[3,66] The HDL-C-lowering effect is mediated by interference with endothelial lipase activity.[67] The mechanism behind the LDL-C lowering by ANGPTL3 most likely relates to increased clearance but seems independent of the LDLr, indicating that ANGPTL3 may be a good target for therapy for hypertriglyceridemia in patients with homozygous FH. That ANGPTL3 may be a good target for TG-lowering therapy is corroborated by a recent study in which ANGPTL3 monoclonal antibodies showed a marked decrease in plasma TG and LDL-C in FH patients already receiving LDL-lowering therapy.[68]

ANGPTL4 is predominantly expressed in adipose tissue, where it inhibits LPL under fasting conditions.[63] Its been suggested to inhibit LPL activity by acting as a reversible, noncompetitive inhibitor and/or by converting active LPL dimer to inactive monomers. Besides directly affecting LPL activity, ANGPTL4 may regulate LPL degradation intracellularly.[69] A rare mutational variant leading to nonfunctional ANGPTL4 was associated with low TG, high HDL-C levels, and protection against CVD. In mice, ANGPTL4 upregulates cholesterol synthesis secondary to inhibition of LPL- and HTGL-dependent cholesterol uptake in fasting conditions.[70] In humans, ANGPTL4 genetic variants do not affect plasma LDL-C levels.[71] *Angtpl4* knockout mice have low plasma TG but decreased survival and lymphogranulomatous inflammation.[72] Monoclonal antibody therapy inhibiting ANGPTL4 decreased plasma TG in mice and nonhuman primates. Effects on LDL-C were not reported. In both mouse and primate studies, accumulation of lipid in abdominal lymph nodes was observed, raising doubt about the safety of ANGPTL4 therapy.[71]

ANGPTL8, also known as lipasin/betatrophin, regulates LPL activity in heart and skeletal muscle.[64] It is expressed in liver and adipose tissue and released into the circulation. ANGPTL8 appears to interact with ANGPTL3 and is highly upregulated after feeding. LPL-independent functions of ANGPTL8 in adipose tissue such as mediating adipocyte differentiation have also been suggested.[64] Recently, a human monoclonal antibody against ANGPTL8 increased plasma LPL activity and decreased plasma TG in mice, and lowered TG in nonhuman primates. No effects on plasma LDL-C levels were observed, whereas HDL-C levels were increased.[73]

Glycosylphosphatidylinositol-Anchored High-Density Lipoprotein Binding Protein-1

GPIHBP1 binds LPL and mediates its transfer to the luminal surface of capillary endothelial cells.[74] Deficiency of GPIHBP1 in mice leads to impaired LPL activity and severe hypertriglyceridemia. In humans, several *GPIHBP1* mutations have been identified that lead to chylomicronemia.[74] Recently, it was shown that patients with GPIHBP1 autoantibodies have impaired lipase-mediated processing of TRLs causing severe hypertriglyceridemia, supporting a role of GPIHBP1 in determining plasma triglyceride levels.[75] To date, no therapies targeting GPIHBP1 have been reported.

Lipase Maturation Factor-1

LMF1 is an ER chaperone membrane protein that interacts with LPL and mediates posttranslational processing of LPL and HTGL. In humans, an association between *LMF1* gene variants and post–heparin LPL activity exists. If completely defective, no lipase activity is observed.[76] LMF1 knockout mice show extreme hypertriglyceridemia and die within the first 4 days of life.[77] Currently, no treatments targeting LMF1 have been reported.

SUMMARY

There are numerous emerging therapies for the treatment of elevated TRLs. Their application will require a sound understanding of the basic biochemistry and physiology of these lipoproteins and their treatment targets.

REFERENCES

1. Brunzell JD. Clinical practice. Hypertriglyceridemia. N Engl J Med 2007;357(10):1009–17.
2. Do R, Willer CJ, Schmidt EM, et al. Common variants associated with plasma triglycerides and risk for coronary artery disease. Nat Genet 2013;45(11): 1345–52.
3. Dewey FE, Gusarova V, Dunbar RL, et al. Genetic and pharmacologic inactivation of ANGPTL3 and cardiovascular disease. N Engl J Med 2017; 377(3):211–21.
4. TG and HDL Working Group of the Exome Sequencing Project, National Heart, Lung, and Blood Institute, Crosby J, Peloso GM, Auer PL, et al. Loss-of-function mutations in APOC3, triglycerides, and coronary disease. N Engl J Med 2014;371(1):22–31.
5. Watts GF, Ooi EMM, Chan DC. Demystifying the management of hypertriglyceridaemia. Nat Rev Cardiol 2013;10(11):648–61.
6. Nordestgaard BG, Varbo A. Triglycerides and cardiovascular disease. Lancet 2014;384(9943):626–35.
7. Borén J, Williams KJ. The central role of arterial retention of cholesterol-rich apolipoprotein-B-containing lipoproteins in the pathogenesis of atherosclerosis: a triumph of simplicity. Curr Opin Lipidol 2016;27(5):473–83.
8. Rapp JH, Lespine A, Hamilton RL, et al. Triglyceride-rich lipoproteins isolated by selected-affinity anti-apolipoprotein B immunosorption from human atherosclerotic plaque. Arterioscler Thromb 1994; 14(11):1767–74.
9. Dallinga-Thie GM, Kroon J, Borén J, et al. Triglyceride-rich lipoproteins and remnants: targets for therapy? Curr Cardiol Rep 2016;18(7):67.
10. Shelness GS, Sellers JA. Very-low-density lipoprotein assembly and secretion. Curr Opin Lipidol 2001;12(2):151–7.
11. Ginsberg HN, Fisher EA. The ever-expanding role of degradation in the regulation of apolipoprotein B metabolism. J Lipid Res 2009;50(Suppl):S162–6.
12. Williams KJ, Chen K. Recent insights into factors affecting remnant lipoprotein uptake. Curr Opin Lipidol 2010;21(3):218–28.
13. Brahm AJ, Hegele RA. Chylomicronaemia–current diagnosis and future therapies. Nat Rev Endocrinol 2015;11(6):352–62.
14. Miller M, Stone NJ, Ballantyne C, et al. Triglycerides and cardiovascular disease: a scientific statement from the American Heart Association. Circulation 2011;123(20):2292–333.
15. Utermann G. Apolipoprotein E polymorphism in health and disease. Am Heart J 1987;113(2 Pt 2):433–40.
16. Kritharides L, Nordestgaard BG, Tybjærg-Hansen A, et al. Effect of APOE ε genotype on lipoprotein(a) and the associated risk of myocardial infarction and aortic valve stenosis. J Clin Endocrinol Metab 2017;102(9):3390–9.
17. Schaefer EJ, Gregg RE, Ghiselli G, et al. Familial apolipoprotein E deficiency. J Clin Invest 1986; 78(5):1206–19.
18. Huang Y, Liu XQ, Rall SC, et al. Overexpression and accumulation of apolipoprotein E as a cause of

hypertriglyceridemia. J Biol Chem 1998;273(41): 26388–93.

19. Lairon D. Macronutrient intake and modulation on chylomicron production and clearance. Atheroscler Suppl 2008;9(2):45–8.

20. Sacks FM. The crucial roles of apolipoproteins E and C-III in apoB lipoprotein metabolism in normolipidemia and hypertriglyceridemia. Curr Opin Lipidol 2015;26(1):56–63.

21. Klop B, do Rego AT, Cabezas MC. Alcohol and plasma triglycerides. Curr Opin Lipidol 2013;24(4): 321–6.

22. Borén J, Taskinen M-R, Olofsson S-O, et al. Ectopic lipid storage and insulin resistance: a harmful relationship. J Intern Med 2013;274(1):25–40.

23. Adeli K, Lewis GF. Intestinal lipoprotein overproduction in insulin-resistant states. Curr Opin Lipidol 2008;19(3):221–8.

24. Björnson E, Adiels M, Taskinen M-R, et al. Kinetics of plasma triglycerides in abdominal obesity. Curr Opin Lipidol 2017;28(1):11–8.

25. Nestel PJ, Fidge NH, Tan MH. Increased lipoprotein-remnant formation in chronic renal failure. N Engl J Med 1982;307(6):329–33.

26. Vaziri ND. Causes of dysregulation of lipid metabolism in chronic renal failure. Semin Dial 2009; 22(6):644–51.

27. Saland JM, Satlin LM, Zalsos-Johnson J, et al. Impaired postprandial lipemic response in chronic kidney disease. Kidney Int 2016;90(1):172–80.

28. Chapman MJ, Ginsberg HN, Amarenco P, et al. Triglyceride-rich lipoproteins and high-density lipoprotein cholesterol in patients at high risk of cardiovascular disease: evidence and guidance for management. Eur Heart J 2011;32(11):1345–61.

29. Reith C, Armitage J. Management of residual risk after statin therapy. Atherosclerosis 2016;245: 161–70.

30. Wetterau JR, Aggerbeck LP, Bouma ME, et al. Absence of microsomal triglyceride transfer protein in individuals with abetalipoproteinemia. Science 1992;258(5084):999–1001.

31. Schonfeld G, Lin X, Yue P. Familial hypobetalipoproteinemia: genetics and metabolism. Cell Mol Life Sci 2005;62(12):1372–8.

32. Visser ME, Witztum JL, Stroes ESG, et al. Antisense oligonucleotides for the treatment of dyslipidaemia. Eur Heart J 2012;33(12):1451–8.

33. Reyes-Soffer G, Moon B, Hernandez-Ono A, et al. Complex effects of inhibiting hepatic apolipoprotein B100 synthesis in humans. Sci Transl Med 2016; 8(323):323ra12.

34. Akdim F, Stroes ESG, Sijbrands EJG, et al. Efficacy and safety of mipomersen, an antisense inhibitor of apolipoprotein B, in hypercholesterolemic subjects receiving stable statin therapy. J Am Coll Cardiol 2010;55(15):1611–8.

35. Chandler CE, Wilder DE, Pettini JL, et al. CP-346086: an MTP inhibitor that lowers plasma cholesterol and triglycerides in experimental animals and in humans. J Lipid Res 2003;44(10): 1887–901.

36. Cuchel M, Bloedon LT, Szapary PO, et al. Inhibition of microsomal triglyceride transfer protein in familial hypercholesterolemia. N Engl J Med 2007;356(2): 148–56.

37. Liu Y, Millar JS, Cromley DA, et al. Knockdown of acyl-CoA:diacylglycerol acyltransferase 2 with antisense oligonucleotide reduces VLDL TG and ApoB secretion in mice. Biochim Biophys Acta 2008; 1781(3):97–104.

38. Choi CS, Savage DB, Kulkarni A, et al. Suppression of diacylglycerol acyltransferase-2 (DGAT2), but not DGAT1, with antisense oligonucleotides reverses diet-induced hepatic steatosis and insulin resistance. J Biol Chem 2007;282(31): 22678–88.

39. Kim C-W, Addy C, Kusunoki J, et al. Acetyl CoA carboxylase inhibition reduces hepatic steatosis but elevates plasma triglycerides in mice and humans: a bedside to bench investigation. Cell Metab 2017;26(2):394–406.e6.

40. Chakravarthy MV, Pan Z, Zhu Y, et al. "New" hepatic fat activates PPARalpha to maintain glucose, lipid, and cholesterol homeostasis. Cell Metab 2005; 1(5):309–22.

41. Murphy BA, Tadin-Strapps M, Jensen K, et al. siRNA-mediated inhibition of SREBP cleavage-activating protein reduces dyslipidemia in spontaneously dysmetabolic rhesus monkeys. Metabolism 2017;71:202–12.

42. Ishizuka Y, Nakayama K, Ogawa A, et al. TRIB1 downregulates hepatic lipogenesis and glycogenesis via multiple molecular interactions. J Mol Endocrinol 2014;52(2):145–58.

43. Bauer RC, Sasaki M, Cohen DM, et al. Tribbles-1 regulates hepatic lipogenesis through posttranscriptional regulation of C/EBPα. J Clin Invest 2015; 125(10):3809–18.

44. Makishima S, Boonvisut S, Ishizuka Y, et al. Sin3A-associated protein, 18 kDa, a novel binding partner of TRIB1, regulates MTTP expression. J Lipid Res 2015;56(6):1145–52.

45. Musunuru K, Kathiresan S. Surprises from genetic analyses of lipid risk factors for atherosclerosis. Circ Res 2016;118(4):579–85.

46. Surendran RP, Visser ME, Heemelaar S, et al. Mutations in LPL, APOC2, APOA5, GPIHBP1 and LMF1 in patients with severe hypertriglyceridaemia. J Intern Med 2012;272(2):185–96.

47. Khera AV, Won H-H, Peloso GM, et al. Association of rare and common variation in the lipoprotein lipase gene with coronary artery disease. JAMA 2017; 317(9):937–46.

48. Gaudet D, Méthot J, Kastelein J. Gene therapy for lipoprotein lipase deficiency. Curr Opin Lipidol 2012; 23(4):310–20.

49. Kockx M, Kritharides L. Cyclosporin a-induced hyperlipidemia. In: Sasa Frank, Gerhard Kostner, editors. Lipoproteins- Role in Health and Diseases. Rijeka (Croatia): InTech Publishers; 2012. p. 337–54.

50. Geldenhuys WJ, Caporoso J, Leeper TC, et al. Structure-activity and in vivo evaluation of a novel lipoprotein lipase (LPL) activator. Bioorg Med Chem Lett 2017;27(2):303–8.

51. Geldenhuys WJ, Aring D, Sadana P. A novel lipoprotein lipase (LPL) agonist rescues the enzyme from inhibition by angiopoietin-like 4 (ANGPTL4). Bioorg Med Chem Lett 2014;24(9):2163–7.

52. Shachter NS, Hayek T, Leff T, et al. Overexpression of apolipoprotein CII causes hypertriglyceridemia in transgenic mice. J Clin Invest 1994;93(4):1683–90.

53. Amar MJA, Sakurai T, Sakurai-Ikuta A, et al. A novel apolipoprotein C-II mimetic peptide that activates lipoprotein lipase and decreases serum triglycerides in apolipoprotein E-knockout mice. J Pharmacol Exp Ther 2015;352(2):227–35.

54. Pennacchio LA, Olivier M, Hubacek JA, et al. An apolipoprotein influencing triglycerides in humans and mice revealed by comparative sequencing. Science 2001;294(5540):169–73.

55. Gin P, Beigneux AP, Voss C, et al. Binding preferences for GPIHBP1, a glycosylphosphatidylinositol-anchored protein of capillary endothelial cells. Arterioscler Thromb Vasc Biol 2011;31(1):176–82.

56. Mendoza-Barberá E, Julve J, Nilsson SK, et al. Structural and functional analysis of APOA5 mutations identified in patients with severe hypertriglyceridemia. J Lipid Res 2013;54(3):649–61.

57. Schaap FG, Rensen PCN, Voshol PJ, et al. ApoAV reduces plasma triglycerides by inhibiting very low density lipoprotein-triglyceride (VLDL-TG) production and stimulating lipoprotein lipase-mediated VLDL-TG hydrolysis. J Biol Chem 2004;279(27): 27941–7.

58. van der Vliet HN, Schaap FG, Levels JHM, et al. Adenoviral overexpression of apolipoprotein A-V reduces serum levels of triglycerides and cholesterol in mice. Biochem Biophys Res Commun 2002; 295(5):1156–9.

59. Taskinen M-R, Borén J. Why is apolipoprotein CIII emerging as a novel therapeutic target to reduce the burden of cardiovascular disease? Curr Atheroscler Rep 2016;18(10):59.

60. Mendivil CO, Zheng C, Furtado J, et al. Metabolism of very-low-density lipoprotein and low-density lipoprotein containing apolipoprotein C-III and not other small apolipoproteins. Arterioscler Thromb Vasc Biol 2010;30(2):239–45.

61. Gaudet D, Alexander VJ, Baker BF, et al. Antisense inhibition of apolipoprotein C-III in patients with hypertriglyceridemia. N Engl J Med 2015;373(5): 438–47.

62. Gordts PLSM, Nock R, Son N-H, et al. ApoC-III inhibits clearance of triglyceride-rich lipoproteins through LDL family receptors. J Clin Invest 2016; 126(8):2855–66.

63. Dijk W, Kersten S. Regulation of lipid metabolism by angiopoietin-like proteins. Curr Opin Lipidol 2016; 27(3):249–56.

64. Zhang R. The ANGPTL3-4-8 model, a molecular mechanism for triglyceride trafficking. Open Biol 2016;6(4):150272.

65. Wang Y, McNutt MC, Banfi S, et al. Hepatic ANGPTL3 regulates adipose tissue energy homeostasis. Proc Natl Acad Sci U S A 2015;112(37): 11630–5.

66. Graham MJ, Lee RG, Brandt TA, et al. Cardiovascular and metabolic effects of ANGPTL3 antisense oligonucleotides. N Engl J Med 2017;377(3):222–32.

67. Gusarova V, Alexa CA, Wang Y, et al. ANGPTL3 blockade with a human monoclonal antibody reduces plasma lipids in dyslipidemic mice and monkeys. J Lipid Res 2015;56(7):1308–17.

68. Gaudet D, Gipe DA, Pordy R, et al. ANGPTL3 inhibition in homozygous familial hypercholesterolemia. N Engl J Med 2017;377(3):296–7.

69. Dijk W, Beigneux AP, Larsson M, et al. Angiopoietin-like 4 promotes intracellular degradation of lipoprotein lipase in adipocytes. J Lipid Res 2016;57(9): 1670–83.

70. Lichtenstein L, Berbée JFP, van Dijk SJ, et al. Angptl4 upregulates cholesterol synthesis in liver via inhibition of LPL- and HL-dependent hepatic cholesterol uptake. Arterioscler Thromb Vasc Biol 2007;27(11):2420–7.

71. Dewey FE, Gusarova V, O'Dushlaine C, et al. Inactivating variants in ANGPTL4 and risk of coronary artery disease. N Engl J Med 2016;374(12):1123–33.

72. Desai U, Lee E-C, Chung K, et al. Lipid-lowering effects of anti-angiopoietin-like 4 antibody recapitulate the lipid phenotype found in angiopoietin-like 4 knockout mice. Proc Natl Acad Sci U S A 2007; 104(28):11766–71.

73. Gusarova V, Banfi S, Alexa-Braun CA, et al. ANGPTL8 blockade with a monoclonal antibody promotes triglyceride clearance, energy expenditure, and weight loss in mice. Endocrinology 2017; 158(5):1252–9.

74. Fong LG, Young SG, Beigneux AP, et al. GPIHBP1 and plasma triglyceride metabolism. Trends Endocrinol Metab 2016;27(7):455–69.

75. Beigneux AP, Miyashita K, Ploug M, et al. Autoantibodies against GPIHBP1 as a cause of hypertriglyceridemia. N Engl J Med 2017;376(17): 1647–58.

76. Hosseini M, Ehrhardt N, Weissglas-Volkov D, et al. Transgenic expression and genetic variation of

Lmf1 affect LPL activity in mice and humans. Arterioscler Thromb Vasc Biol 2012;32(5):1204–10.

77. Ehrhardt N, Bedoya C, Péterfy M. Embryonic viability, lipase deficiency, hypertriglyceridemia and neonatal lethality in a novel LMF1-deficient mouse model. Nutr Metab (Lond) 2014;11:37.

78. Arai H, Yamashita S, Yokote K, et al. Efficacy and safety of K-877, a novel selective peroxisome proliferator-activated receptor α modulator (SPPARMα), in combination with statin treatment: two randomised, double-blind, placebo-controlled clinical trials in patients with dyslipidaemia. Atherosclerosis 2017;261:144–52.

79. Shi Y, Li J, Kennedy LJ, et al. Discovery and preclinical evaluation of BMS-711939, an oxybenzylglycine based PPARα selective agonist. ACS Med Chem Lett 2016;7(6):590–4.

Evolution of Omega-3 Fatty Acid Therapy and Current and Future Role in the Management of Dyslipidemia

Lane B. Benes, MD[a], Nikhil S. Bassi, MD[b],
Mohamad A. Kalot, MD[c], Michael H. Davidson, MD[a],*

KEYWORDS

- Omega-3 fatty acids • Omega-3 icosapent ethyl • Omega-3 carboxylic acids • Hypertriglyceridemia
- Residual risk • Dyslipidemia

KEY POINTS

- Newer omega-3 fatty acid formulations have improved bioavailability and triglyceride-lowering efficacy.
- Omega-3 fatty acids have been shown to reduce cardiovascular risk in certain high-risk subgroups.
- Omega-3 fatty acids provide cardiovascular protection through multiple mechanisms, including lipid-lowering and non–lipid-altering pathways.
- Although there is no evidence of significant harm, data to suggest significant benefit in event reduction rates with omega-3 fatty acids are lacking.
- Ongoing large, randomized, controlled trials in high-risk patients are highly anticipated.

INTRODUCTION

The benefits of omega-3 fatty acids have been recognized since the beginning of the 20th century; however, the first US Federal Drug Administration (FDA)–approved formulation was not available until 2004. Since that time, newer formulations consisting of omega-3 carboxylic acids or pure eicosapentaenoic acid (EPA) ethyl esters have been developed. Omega-3 fatty acids are most recognized for their ability to reduce serum triglycerides; however, there has been debate regarding their role in the medical armamentarium for the treatment of hypertriglyceridemia or other forms of dyslipidemia. The most recent recommendations from the American College of Cardiology/American Heart Association (ACC/AHA) guidelines on cholesterol management[1] published in 2013 do not suggest a major role of omega-3 fatty acid therapy in the treatment of dyslipidemia. This diminished role is predominantly because large trials studying nonstatin cholesterol-lowering medications showed lack of significant benefit. Subgroup analyses of those trials looking at subjects with elevated triglycerides and low high-density

Disclosures: Dr M.H. Davidson was the Chief Medical Officer of Omthera until June 2015; omega-3 carboxylic acids were developed by Omthera Pharmaceuticals. L.B. Benes, N.S. Bassi, and M.A. Kalot have nothing to disclose.
[a] Section of Cardiology, The University of Chicago Medicine, 5841 South Maryland Avenue, MC 6080, Chicago, IL 60637, USA; [b] Section of Cardiology, University of California – Los Angeles, UCLA Cardiovascular Center (Westwood), 100 UCLA Medical Plaza, Suite 630, Los Angeles, CA 90095, USA; [c] Department of Medicine, American University of Beirut, Riad El Solh, Beirut 1107 2020, Lebanon
* Corresponding author.
E-mail address: mdavidso@bsd.uchicago.edu

lipoprotein cholesterol (HDL-C), an unfavorable pattern of dyslipidemia, suggest there may in fact be a benefit. Current trials are ongoing with newer omega-3 fatty acid formulations to determine if patients at increased risk for atherosclerotic cardiovascular disease derive benefit from therapy. This article discusses the evolution of omega-3 fatty acid therapy as well as its current and future role in the treatment of dyslipidemia.

AVAILABLE OMEGA-3 FATTY ACID FORMULATIONS

The first omega-3 fatty acid formulation, omega-3 acid ethyl esters, was approved by the FDA in 2004 under the trade name Omacor (Reliant Pharmaceuticals, Liberty Corner, NJ) for the treatment of triglyceride levels of 500 mg/dL or more. It was renamed to Lovaza in 2007 (GlaxoSmithKline, Brentford, UK); however, Omacor is still available outside of the United States. Icosapent ethyl (Vascepa, Amarin Pharmaceuticals, Bedminster, NJ) was approved in 2012 for the treatment of severe hypertriglyceridemia (triglycerides of $\geq$500 mg/dL). Icosapent ethyl differed from the initial omega-3 fatty acid formulation by containing pure EPA ethyl esters rather than both EPA and docosahexaenoic acid (DHA). In 2014, omega-3 carboxylic acids (Epanova, AstraZeneca, Wilmington, DE) gained approval for the treatment of severe hypertriglyceridemia (triglycerides of $\geq$500 mg/dL). Omega-3 carboxylic acids consist of free fatty acids rather than a prodrug form; they have improved bioavailability and can be taken independently of meals because they are not reliant on hydrolysis by pancreatic lipase for absorption.

Momentum for the development of supplemental omega-3 fatty acids came in part from the Gruppo Italiano per lo Studio della Sopravvivenza nell'Infarto miocardico (GISSI)-Prevenzione trial published in 1999[2] and further encouraged by the Japan EPA Lipid Intervention Study (JELIS) published in 2007.[3] The GISSI-Prevention trial showed that, in an Italian population, the administration of 1 g/d of polyunsaturated fatty acids to patients who experienced a myocardial infarction in the past 3 months reduced the primary endpoint of death, nonfatal myocardial infarction, and stroke by 10% to 15% at a follow-up of 3.5 years. The reduction in the primary endpoint was largely driven by a reduction in deaths.[2] JELIS suggested a benefit of adding omega-3 fatty acids to a statin, because there was a decrease in major adverse cardiovascular events (MACE) with a 19% risk reduction in those taking both compared with those only taking a statin over 5 years of follow-up, with more benefit seen in those on

therapy for secondary prevention.[3] More recently, the EpanoVa fOr Lowering Very high triglyceridEs (EVOLVE) trial has demonstrated the triglyceride-lowering ability of the omega-3 carboxylic acids, with a 25.5% to 30.9% reduction after 12 weeks compared with 4.3% in controls given olive oil in patients with severe hypertriglyceridemia (triglycerides of $\geq$500 mg/dL).[4]

Of the available formulations within the United States, omega-3 acids ethyl esters have been the most widely prescribed, in part because of their longer time on the market and generic options. In the last few years, studies comparing the ethyl esters and newer formulations suggest that greater benefit can be expected from the newer forms owing to their improved bioavailability. The Epanova compared to Lovaza in a pharmacokinetic single-dose evaluation (ECLIPSE) study demonstrated that omega-3 carboxylic acids, which are already in the free fatty acid form, result in about a 4-fold increase in bioavailability compared with omega-3 acid ethyl esters when taken with a low-fat meal.[5] ECLIPSE II similarly demonstrated greater EPA and DHA serum levels with omega-3 carboxylic acid use compared with omega-3 acids ethyl esters while on a low-fat diet over a longer observation period of 14 days.[6] Greater triglyceride-lowering ability was found with omega-3 carboxylic acids.

OMEGA-3 FATTY ACIDS' BENEFITS AND MECHANISM OF ACTION

Omega-3 fatty acids are best known for their triglyceride-lowering ability. Earlier formulations of EPA and DHA demonstrated about a 20% reduction,[7,8] whereas EVOLVE found closer to a 30% reduction in serum triglycerides with omega-3 carboxylic acids.[4,5] There are numerous proposed mechanisms to account for these findings, which include decreased hepatic very low-density lipoprotein (VLDL) synthesis and increased triglyceride clearance from the serum. One such mechanism is a decrease in VLDL triglyceride synthesis by altering transcription factors such as sterol regulatory element-binding proteins and peroxisome proliferator-activated receptors involved in triglyceride synthesis in the hepatocyte.[9,10] It is possible that EPA serves as a poor substrate for VLDL triglycerides, leading to lipid-poor VLDL rather than triglyceride-rich VLDL secretion into the serum.[11,12] Omega-3 fatty acids also increase serum clearance of triglyceride-rich lipoproteins by increased lipoprotein lipase activity.[10]

As demonstrated most recently in EVOLVE, omega-3 fatty acids induce favorable changes in other lipoproteins, including a reduction in non–HDL-C, VLDL, and remnantlike particle cholesterol.[4] EVOLVE showed significant reductions in lipoprotein-associated phospholipase A2 (Lp-PLA$_2$) and arachidonic acid levels, suggesting a decrease in inflammation and platelet activation.[4] Omega-3 fatty acids may lead to an increase in low-density lipoprotein cholesterol (LDL-C); however, it decreases the amount of small, dense LDL-C and is not accompanied by an increase in apolipoprotein B, suggesting that this represents a shift in LDL-C particle size instead of a true increase in LDL-C.[4,7,8,13,14] **Table 1** further details changes in lipid parameters observed in EVOLVE.

It is presently debated how much of the cardioprotection observed in some studies is due to the triglyceride-lowering effect versus other mechanisms. In JELIS, the cardioprotective benefits seen in the group taking EPA was not associated with changes in triglycerides, total cholesterol, HDL-C, or LDL-C, indicating the presence of non–lipid-altering pathways.[3] This may be due in part to cardiac arrhythmia suppression,[15,16] leading to decreased sudden cardiac death. Omega-3 fatty acids are incorporated into myocardial cell membranes and, therefore, may change ion channel properties.[17,18] Studies looking at arrhythmia suppression with omega-3 fatty

acid administration have been mixed; however, there seems to be more evidence of benefit in patients with ischemia-driven arrhythmias.[10] A meta-analysis published in 2009 consisting of 3 trials looking at ventricular arrhythmias and death in patients with implantable cardioverter-defibrillators and a prior history of ventricular tachycardia or ventricular fibrillation found no difference in the rates of appropriate implantable cardioverter-defibrillator therapy; however, a trend toward lower arrhythmia rate in those with a history of coronary artery disease (hazard ratio, 0.79; 95% confidence interval 0.60–1.06) taking omega-3 fatty acids.[19]

Omega-3 fatty acids improve endothelial function and modestly lower blood pressure.[20,21] Studies looking at peripheral artery flow-mediated dilatation, a clinical marker of improved endothelial function, show benefit with therapy.[22,23] A recent in vitro model using a proteomic approach found an upregulation of glutathione and a downregulation of vascular cell adhesion molecule 1 with endothelial cell exposure to EPA, supporting prior evidence that omega-3 fatty acids improve endothelial function and have antiinflammatory properties.[24] Similar to the Lp-PLA$_2$ lowering found with omega-3 carboxylic acid use in EVOLVE, the Multi-center, plAcebo-controlled,

Table 1
Median percent change from baseline in lipid levels in patients with severe hypertriglyceridemia (triglycerides ≥500 mg/dL) in the EVOLVE study

	OM3-CA 2 g/d		OM3-CA 4 g/d		Placebo (Olive Oil) 4 g/d	
	Baseline (mg/dL)	Percent Change	Baseline (mg/dL)	Percent Change	Baseline (mg/dL)	Percent Change
TG	717	−25.9[b]	655	−30.9[c]	682	−4.3
Non-HDL-C	205	−7.6[a]	225	−9.6[b]	215	2.5
HDL-C	27.3	7.4	28.7	5.8	28.1	1.9
Total C	241	−5.4[a]	254	−7.5[b]	246	3.2
LDL-C	77.3	19.2[b]	90.3	19.4[c]	78.2	3.0
VLDL	123	−26.6[b]	126	−33.0[c]	125	−8.5
RLP-C	44.5	−20.7[a]	43.0	−27.5[c]	52.3	3.4
Apo AI	130	0.0[b]	134	−0.9[b]	131	5.9
Apo B	114	3.8	118	3.8	110	0.9
Apo CIII	24.5	−10.9[a]	24.5	−14.4[c]	24.0	1.6
Lp-PLA$_2$	266	−14.9[c]	249	−17.2[c]	258	−1.9

Abbreviations: Apo, apolipoprotein; HDL-C, high-density lipoprotein cholesterol; LDL-C, low-density lipoprotein cholesterol; Lp-PLA$_2$, lipoprotein-associated phospholipase A$_2$; OM3-CA, omega-3 carboxylic acids; RLP-C, remnant-like particle cholesterol; TG, triglycerides; Total-C, total cholesterol; VLDL, very low-density lipoprotein cholesterol.
[a] $P<.05$ significantly different from placebo.
[b] $P<.01$ significantly different from placebo.
[c] $P<.001$ significantly different from placebo.
Data from Kastelein JJ, Maki KC, Susekov A, et al. Omega-3 free fatty acids for the treatment of severe hypertriglyceridemia: the EpanoVa fOr Lowering Very high triglyceridEs (EVOLVE) trial. J Clin Lipidol 2014;8(1):94–106.

Randomized, double-blINd, 12-week study with an open-label Extension (MARINE) and Effect of AMR101 (Icosapent Ethyl) on Triglyceride Levels in Patients on Statins with High Triglyceride Levels (ANCHOR) studies found a reduction in inflammatory markers including Lp-PLA$_2$ with icosapent ethyl use.[25]

Given the multitude of cardiovascular changes associated with omega-3 fatty acid use, the pathway(s) responsible for cardioprotection are difficult to delineate.

DYSLIPIDEMIA SUBGROUPS WITH THE GREATEST ANTICIPATED BENEFIT

Trials consisting of nonstatin therapies aimed at treating hypertriglyceridemia have failed to show a reduction in cardiovascular events. Most of these studies used fibrates in the treatment arm, including the Veterans Affairs HDL Intervention Trial (VA-HIT),[26] the Bezafibrate Infarction Prevention (BIP) study,[27] the Fenofibrate Intervention and Event Lowering in Diabetes (FIELD) study,[28] and the Action to Control Cardiovascular Risk in Diabetes (ACCORD) Lipid trial.[29] Subgroup analyses of these studies found that those in the highest group of baseline triglycerides with or without low HDL-C had a significant reduction in event rates. The unfavorable pattern of dyslipidemia consisting of hypertriglyceridemia and low HDL-C is common, especially in diabetic patients.[30,31] As discussed elsewhere in this article, outcome trials looking at newer formulations of omega-3 fatty acids are ongoing and may help to elucidate whether those with this unfavorable pattern of dyslipidemia or other markers of increased cardiovascular risk benefit from omega-3 fatty acid therapy. Given that omega-3 fatty acids have similar triglyceride-lowering efficacy as fibrates in addition to other cardiovascular benefits as described, it can be hypothesized that these studies will demonstrate benefit.

RESIDUAL RISK DESPITE STATIN THERAPY

Several studies have shown an association between increased triglycerides and cardiovascular disease.[32–34] Most patients with hypertriglyceridemia, defined as triglycerides of 150 mg/dL or greater, also have an indication for a statin, for which there is well-demonstrated cardiovascular benefit. Fortunately, statins provide a dose-dependent reduction in triglycerides, with an expected reduction of about 5% to 20%.[35] This means that patients with mildly increased triglycerides may achieve a triglyceride level of less than 150 mg/dL with statin therapy; however, as

demonstrated in a metaanalysis by Nicholls and colleagues,[35] only 0% to 24% of those with baseline triglyceride levels of greater than 300 mg/dL will achieve a level under the target of 150 mg/dL with a statin. Therefore, for many patients treated with a statin, residual risk remains.

Prior studies have demonstrated benefit of combination statin and omega-3 fatty acid therapy. The 2007 Combination of prescription Omega-3 Simvastatin (COMBOS) study[36] showed significant reductions in triglycerides and VLDL levels in those on combination therapy compared with simvastatin alone. The ANCHOR study followed in 2012,[37] demonstrating that when omega-3 icosapent ethyl was added to a statin there was greater reduction in triglycerides, LDL-C, apolipoprotein B, VLDL, Lp-PLA$_2$, and C-reactive protein compared with placebo plus statin in diabetic patients. Similarly, the Epanova Combined with a Statin in Patients with Hypertriglyceridemia to Reduce non-HDL Cholesterol (ESPRIT) study showed similar benefits in 2013 when omega-3 carboxylic acid therapy was added to a statin, resulting in significant reductions in triglycerides, VLDL, arachidonic acid, and non–HDL-C.[38] This finding was true when analyzed by statin type when looking at the 3 most commonly prescribed statins: rosuvastatin, atorvastatin, and simvastatin (Fig. 1). All 3 of these trials included patients with baseline triglycerides between 200 and 500 mg/dL. See Table 2 for trends observed in the COMBOS, ANCHOR, and ESPRIT trials.

Omega-3 fatty acids and statins have different mechanisms of action; therefore, the benefits provided by their combination may simply be additive from different pathways and/or owing to compensatory benefits. For example, statins have been shown to increase proprotein convertase subtilisin/kexin type 9[39] and arachidonic acid levels,[40] whereas omega-3 fatty acids lower them.[38,41] As discussed, JELIS found a decrease in MACE rates when omega-3 fatty acids were added to a statin; however, this change was independent of lipoprotein levels.[3] Therefore, although statins provide a large net benefit, the addition of omega-3 fatty acids might counteract the paradoxic effects while providing additional independent pathways of benefit, accounting for the further decrease in event rates observed.

CURRENT AND FUTURE ROLE OF OMEGA-3 FATTY ACID THERAPY

Approximately 31% of the United States' population has hypertriglyceridemia with a level of 150 mg/dL or greater and 16% have triglyceride

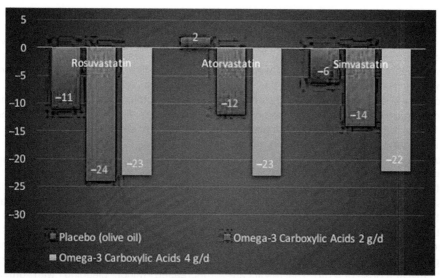

Fig. 1. Median percent change in triglycerides after adding omega-3 carboxylic acids to 3 commonly prescribed statins. For all 3 statins, the addition of omega-3 carboxylic acids at either 2 or 4 g/d led to a significant reduction in serum triglycerides in the ESPRIT study, which included patients with severe hypertriglyceridemia (triglycerides of ≥500 mg/dL).

levels of 200 mg/dL or greater.[42] The 2013 ACC/AHA guidelines on cholesterol management[1] do not provide specific recommendations on the treatment of hypertriglyceridemia, but rather reference the AHA 2011 guidelines on triglyceride management.[42] The 2011 AHA guidelines recommend achieving a triglyceride level of less than 100 mg/dL through diet (including dietary omega-3 fatty acids) and exercise and to consider medical therapy if levels remain greater than

500 mg/dL. Recently, the AHA published an advisory on omega-3 fatty acid use in different patient populations based on the currently available data. For all populations studied, there was no evidence of significant harm. For most populations, there was either lack of data or lack of convincing benefit. Exceptions found were the use of omega-3 fatty acids as secondary prevention for patients with prevalent coronary heart disease to reduce coronary heart disease–related death

Table 2
Percent change in lipid parameters with the addition of omega-3 fatty acids to statin therapy in patients with hypertriglyceridemia (triglycerides 200–500 mg/dL) in the COMBOS, ANCHOR, and ESPRIT trials

Lipid Parameter % Change from BL	COMBOS (N = 256)		ANCHOR (N = 702)		ESPRIT (N = 647)	
	Ethyl Esters		Icosapent Ethyl		Carboxylic Acids	
	4 g/d + Statin	Placebo (Corn Oil) + Statin	4 g/d + Statin	Placebo (Mineral Oil) + Statin	4 g/d + Statin	Placebo (Olive Oil) + Statin
TGs	−29.5[a]	−6.3	−17.5[a]	5.9	−21[b]	−6
Non-HDL-C	−9[a]	−2.2	−5[a]	9.8	−7[b]	−1
LDL-C	0.7	−2.8	1.5[a]	8.8	1.3	1.1
Apo-B	−4.2[a]	−1.9	−2.2[a]	7.1	−2.1[b]	0.3
HDL-C	3.4[a]	−1.2	−1[a]	4.8	3	2

Abbreviations: Apo, apolipoprotein; BL, baseline; HDL-C, high-density lipoprotein cholesterol; LDL-C, low-density lipoprotein cholesterol; TG, triglycerides; VLDL, very low-density lipoprotein cholesterol.
[a] $P<.05$ significantly different from placebo.
[b] $P<.01$ significantly different from placebo.
Data from Refs.[36–38]

(class IIa recommendation) and in patients with heart failure with reduced ejection fraction (ejection fraction of <40%) to reduce death and hospitalizations (class IIa recommendation).[43] The authors of this 2017 advisory note that with the exception of JELIS, the omega-3 fatty acids used in the randomized controlled trials were low doses.

Large, randomized, controlled trials using higher omega-3 fatty acid doses and newer formulations are currently underway to assess the effects on clinical outcomes. The Reduction of Cardiovascular Events with EPA-Intervention Trial (REDUCE-IT) is looking at 8000 patients with an increased risk of cardiovascular disease who are considered to have controlled LDL-C on statin therapy, but have persistent hypertriglyceridemia (available at: https://clinicaltrials.gov/ct2/show/NCT01492361). The omega-3 formulation used in REDUCE-IT is icosapent ethyl at a dose of 4 g/d. Trial results are anticipated towards the end of 2018. The Outcomes Study to Assess Statin Residual Risk Reduction with Epanova in High CV Risk Patients with Hypertriglyceridemia (STRENGTH; available at: https://clinicaltrials.gov/ct2/show/NCT02104817) enrolled approximately 13,000 patients at high risk of cardiovascular disease with hypertriglyceridemia and low HDL-C levels. The trial is designed to assess for a difference in MACE between statin and omega-3 carboxylic acid combination therapy versus statin alone. Estimated completion is the end of 2019. These 2 trials are highly anticipated because prior trials used older omega-3 fatty acid formulations at lower doses in patients who were at lower cardiovascular risk. The newer formulations are expected to demonstrate greater benefit given higher bioavailability and/or triglyceride lowering. Furthermore, because subgroup analyses of prior trials looking at triglyceride lowering showed benefit in those with higher baseline triglycerides with or without low HDL-C, it is welcomed that these higher risk patients will be studied in greater number. A Study of Cardiovascular Events in Diabetes (ASCEND) began enrollment in 2005 to study the rate of cardiovascular events in patients with diabetes given aspirin 100 mg/d for primary prevention versus placebo with or without omega-3 ethyl esters (available at: https://clinicaltrials.gov/ct2/show/NCT00135226). The trial is completed and results will be reported in 2018. If it demonstrates a reduction in MACE rates with omega-3 fatty acid use, it would be the first to show more convincing benefit for those with diabetes.

Given the lack of harm, the major limitation of stronger endorsement of omega-3 fatty acids has been unconvincing benefit; the results from these trials may very well change that. If a reduction in event rates is indeed found, greater emphasis can be placed on triglyceride lowering with omega-3 fatty acids in patients with any level of hypertriglyceridemia. This measure will help to reduce the residual risk that remains for patients on statin therapy. Additionally, some patients with hypertriglyceridemia do not have an indication for or tolerate a statin; omega-3 fatty acids may help to fill the void of cardiovascular risk reduction for such patients.

RISKS OF OMEGA-3 FATTY ACID THERAPY

Omega-3 fatty acids are generally well tolerated and felt to be safe. The most common adverse effect is gastrointestinal disturbance, including diarrhea, nausea, and eructation, seen at a rate of 19% to 27% compared with 7% in the placebo arm in EVOLVE.[4] There has been concern for increased minor bleeding with omega-3 fatty acid; however, no significant increased rates of major bleeding have been reported. Given the lack of evidence of significant risk of omega-3 fatty acid use, the AHA 2017 advisory reports no perceived harm with treatment.[43]

SUMMARY

In previous cardiovascular outcome trials with fenofibrate (ACCORD)[29] and niacin (AIM-HIGH),[44] the population with both elevated triglycerides paired with low HDL-C had a high residual risk despite statin therapy and there was a suggestion of benefit with triglyceride-lowering therapy. The ACCORD trial is especially relevant, finding that fenofibrate reduced major adverse cardiac events by 31% in the prespecified subgroup in the upper tertile of triglycerides (TG > 203 mg/dL) and the lower tertile of HDL-C (HDL-C < 32 mg/dL), but the P value for an interaction was .06 (not significant). Omega-3 fatty acids containing both EPA and DHA or EPA alone in combination with statins lowers triglycerides and non–HDL-C. The non–HDL-C reduction in patients with mixed dyslipidemia (triglycerides between 200 and 500 mg/dL) is due to a decrease in VLDL and remnant cholesterol with a modest decrease, neutral effect, or slight increase in LDL-C (depending on baseline LDL-C levels). Omega-3 fatty acids containing DHA also shift small dense LDL-C to large LDL-C and modestly improves HDL-C. The potential cardiovascular benefits of these compositional cholesterol changes are being tested in 2 large outcome trials, REDUCE-IT and STRENGTH. In addition, Omega-3 fatty acids are thought to provide cardioprotection via additional mechanisms beyond triglyceride lowering, and also may help to combat the paradoxic effects of statins such as increases in proprotein convertase subtilisin/kexin type 9 and arachidonic acid levels. Therefore, if the cardiovascular outcome trials with novel omega-3 fatty acids prove successful, there will be a significant shift in therapy from statin monotherapy to combination treatment for the management of patients with mixed dyslipidemia with high residual risk.

REFERENCES

1. Stone NJ, Robinson JG, Lichtenstein AH, et al. American College of Cardiology/American Heart Association Task Force on practice guidelines. 2013 ACC/AHA guideline on the treatment of blood cholesterol to reduce atherosclerotic cardiovascular risk in adults: a report of the American College of Cardiology/American Heart Association Task Force on practice guidelines. J Am Coll Cardiol 2014; 63(25 Pt B):2889–934.

2. Dietary supplementation with n-3 polyunsaturated fatty acids and vitamin E after myocardial infarction: results of the GISSI-Prevenzione trial. Gruppo Italiano per lo Studio della Sopravvivenza nell'Infarto miocardico. Lancet 1999;354(9177):447–55 [Erratum appears in Lancet 2001;357(9256):642; Erratum appears in Lancet 2007;369(9556):106].

3. Yokoyama M, Origasa H, Matsuzaki M, et al. Effects of eicosapentaenoic acid on major coronary events in hypercholesterolaemic patients (JELIS): a randomised open-label, blinded endpoint analysis. Lancet 2007;369(9567):1090–8 [Erratum appears in Lancet 2007;370(9583):220].

4. Kastelein JJ, Maki KC, Susekov A, et al. Omega-3 free fatty acids for the treatment of severe hypertriglyceridemia: the EpanoVa fOr Lowering Very high triglyceridEs (EVOLVE) trial. J Clin Lipidol 2014; 8(1):94–106.

5. Davidson MH, Johnson J, Rooney MW, et al. A novel omega-3 free fatty acid formulation has dramatically improved bioavailability during a low-fat diet compared with omega-3-acid ethyl esters: the ECLIPSE (Epanova compared to Lovaza in a pharmacokinetic single-dose evaluation) study. J Clin Lipidol 2012;6(6):573–84.

6. Offman E, Marenco T, Ferber S, et al. Steady-state bioavailability of prescription omega-3 on a low-fat diet is significantly improved with a free fatty acid formulation compared with an ethyl ester formulation: the ECLIPSE II study. Vasc Health Risk Manag 2013;9:563–73.

7. Mori TA, Burke V, Puddey IB, et al. Purified eicosapentaenoic and docosahexaenoic acids have differential effects on serum lipids and lipoproteins, LDL particle size, glucose, and insulin in mildly hyperlipidemic men. Am J Clin Nutr 2000;71(5): 1085–94.

8. Kelley DS, Siegel D, Vemuri M, et al. Docosahexaenoic acid supplementation improves fasting and postprandial lipid profiles in hypertriglyceridemic men. Am J Clin Nutr 2007;86(2):324–33.

9. Fisher EA, Pan M, Chen X, et al. The triple threat to nascent apolipoprotein B. Evidence for multiple, distinct degradative pathways. J Biol Chem 2001; 276(30):27855–63.

10. Harris WS, Miller M, Tighe AP, et al. Omega-3 fatty acids and coronary heart disease risk: clinical and mechanistic perspectives. Atherosclerosis 2008; 197(1):12–24.

11. Parks JS, Johnson FL, Wilson MD, et al. Effect of fish oil diet on hepatic lipid metabolism in nonhuman primates: lowering of secretion of hepatic triglyceride but not apoB. J Lipid Res 1990;31(3):455–66.

12. Parks JS, Wilson MD, Johnson FL, et al. Fish oil decreases hepatic cholesteryl ester secretion but not apoB secretion in African green monkeys. J Lipid Res 1989;30(10):1535–44.

13. Leigh-Firbank EC, Minihane AM, Leake DS, et al. Eicosapentaenoic acid and docosahexaenoic acid from fish oils: differential associations with lipid responses. Br J Nutr 2002;87(5):435–45.

14. Maki KC, Van Elswyk ME, McCarthy D, et al. Lipid responses to a dietary docosahexaenoic acid supplement in men and women with below average levels of high density lipoprotein cholesterol. J Am Coll Nutr 2005;24(3):189–99.

15. Mozaffarian D, Wu JH. Omega-3 fatty acids and cardiovascular disease: effects on risk factors, molecular pathways, and clinical events. J Am Coll Cardiol 2011;58(20):2047–67.

16. Reiffel JA, McDonald A. Antiarrhythmic effects of omega-3 fatty acids. Am J Cardiol 2006;98(4A): 50i–60i.

17. Harris WS, Sands SA, Windsor SL, et al. Omega-3 fatty acids in cardiac biopsies from heart transplantation patients: correlation with erythrocytes and response to supplementation. Circulation 2004; 110(12):1645–9.

18. Leaf A, Kang JX, Xiao YF, et al. Clinical prevention of sudden cardiac death by n-3 polyunsaturated fatty acids and mechanism of prevention of arrhythmias by n-3 fish oils. Circulation 2003;107(21):2646–52.

19. Brouwer IA, Raitt MH, Dullemeijer C, et al. Effect of fish oil on ventricular tachyarrhythmia in three studies in patients with implantable cardioverter defibrillators. Eur Heart J 2009;30(7):820–6.

20. Dangardt F, Osika W, Chen Y, et al. Omega-3 fatty acid supplementation improves vascular function and reduces inflammation in obese adolescents. Atherosclerosis 2010;212(2):580–5.

21. Geleijnse JM, Giltay EJ, Grobbee DE, et al. Blood pressure response to fish oil supplementation: meta-regression analysis of randomized trials. J Hypertens 2002;20(8):1493–9.

22. Sawada T, Tsubata H, Hashimoto N, et al. Effects of 6-month eicosapentaenoic acid treatment on post-prandial hyperglycemia, hyperlipidemia, insulin secretion ability, and concomitant endothelial dysfunction among newly-diagnosed impaired glucose metabolism patients with coronary artery disease. An open label, single blinded, prospective randomized controlled trial. Cardiovasc Diabetol 2016;15(1):121.

23. Casanova MA, Medeiros F, Trindade M, et al. Omega-3 fatty acids supplementation improves endothelial function and arterial stiffness in hypertensive patients with hypertriglyceridemia and high cardiovascular risk. J Am Soc Hypertens 2017; 11(1):10–9.

24. Zhang L, Xiao K, Zhao X, et al. Quantitative proteomics reveals key proteins regulated by eicosapentaenoic acid in endothelial activation. Biochem Biophys Res Commun 2017;487(2):464–9.

25. Bays HE, Ballantyne CM, Braeckman RA, et al. Icosapent ethyl, a pure ethyl ester of eicosapentaenoic acid: effects on circulating markers of inflammation from the MARINE and ANCHOR studies. Am J Cardiovasc Drugs 2013;13(1):37–46.

26. Robins SJ, Collins D, Wittes JT, et al, VA-HIT Study Group. Veterans Affairs High-Density Lipoprotein Intervention Trial. Relation of gemfibrozil treatment and lipid levels with major coronary events: VA-HIT: a randomized controlled trial. JAMA 2001;285(12): 1585–91.

27. Bezafibrate Infarction Prevention (BIP) study. Secondary prevention by raising HDL cholesterol and reducing triglycerides in patients with coronary artery disease. Circulation 2000;102(1):21–7.

28. Scott R, O'Brien R, Fulcher G, et al, Fenofibrate Intervention and Event Lowering in Diabetes (FIELD) Study Investigators. Effects of fenofibrate treatment on cardiovascular disease risk in 9,795 individuals with type 2 diabetes and various components of the metabolic syndrome: the Fenofibrate Intervention and Event Lowering in Diabetes (FIELD) study. Diabetes Care 2009;32(3):493–8.

29. ACCORD Study Group, Ginsberg HN, Elam MB, Lovato LC, et al. Effects of combination lipid therapy in type 2 diabetes mellitus. N Engl J Med 2010; 362(17):1563–74.

30. UK Prospective Diabetes Study (UKPDS). XI: biochemical risk factors in type 2 diabetic patients at diagnosis compared with age-matched normal subjects. Diabet Med 1994;11(6):534–44.

31. Soran H, Schofield JD, Adam S, et al. Diabetic dyslipidaemia. Curr Opin Lipidol 2016;27(4):313–22.

32. Hokanson JE, Austin MA. Plasma triglyceride level is a risk factor for cardiovascular disease independent of high-density lipoprotein cholesterol level: a meta-analysis of population-based prospective studies. J Cardiovasc Risk 1996;3(2):213–9.

33. Nordestgaard BG, Benn M, Schnohr P, et al. Non-fasting triglycerides and risk of myocardial infarction, ischemic heart disease, and death in men and women. JAMA 2007;298(3):299–308.

34. Sarwar N, Danesh J, Eiriksdottir G, et al. Triglycerides and the risk of coronary heart disease: 10,158 incident cases among 262,525 participants in 29 Western prospective studies. Circulation 2007; 115(4):450–8.

35. Nicholls SJ, Brandrup-Wognsen G, Palmer M, et al. Meta-analysis of comparative efficacy of increasing dose of Atorvastatin versus Rosuvastatin versus Simvastatin on lowering levels of atherogenic lipids (from VOYAGER). Am J Cardiol 2010; 105(1):69–76.

36. Davidson MH, Stein EA, Bays HE, et al. Efficacy and tolerability of adding prescription omega-3 fatty acids 4 g/d to simvastatin 40 mg/d in hypertriglyceridemic patients: an 8-week, randomized, double-blind, placebo-controlled study. Clin Ther 2007; 29(7):1354–67.

37. Ballantyne CM, Bays HE, Kastelein JJ, et al. Efficacy and safety of eicosapentaenoic acid ethyl ester (AMR101) therapy in statin-treated patients with persistent high triglycerides (from the ANCHOR study). Am J Cardiol 2012;110(7):984–92.

38. Maki KC, Orloff DG, Nicholls SJ, et al. A highly bioavailable omega-3 free fatty acid formulation improves the cardiovascular risk profile in high-risk, statin-treated patients with residual hypertriglyceridemia (the ESPRIT trial). Clin Ther 2013;35(9): 1400–11.e1-3.

39. Guo YL, Zhang W, Li JJ. PCSK9 and lipid lowering drugs. Clin Chim Acta 2014;437:66–71.

40. Nakamura N, Hamazaki T, Jokaji H, et al. Effect of HMG-CoA reductase inhibitors on plasma polyunsaturated fatty acid concentrations in patients with hyperlipidemia. Int J Clin Lab Res 1998; 28(3):192–5.

41. Graversen CB, Lundbye-Christensen S, Thomsen B, et al. MARINE n-3 polyunsaturated fatty acids lower plasma proprotein convertase subtilisin kexin type 9 levels in pre- and postmenopausal women: a randomized study. Vascul Pharmacol 2016;76:37–41.

42. Miller M, Stone NJ, Ballantyne C, et al, American Heart Association Clinical Lipidology, Thrombosis, and Prevention Committee of the Council on Nutrition, Physical Activity, and Metabolism, Council on Arteriosclerosis, Thrombosis and Vascular Biology, Council on Cardiovascular Nursing, Council on the Kidney in Cardiovascular Disease. Triglycerides and cardiovascular disease: a scientific statement from the American Heart Association. Circulation 2011;123(20): 2292–333.

43. Siscovick DS, Barringer TA, Fretts AM, et al, American Heart Association Nutrition Committee

of the Council on Lifestyle and Cardiometabolic Health; Council on Epidemiology and Prevention; Council on Cardiovascular Disease in the Young; Council on Cardiovascular and Stroke Nursing; and Council on Clinical Cardiology. Omega-3 polyunsaturated fatty acid (fish oil) supplementation and the prevention of clinical cardiovascular disease: a science advisory from the American Heart Association. Circulation 2017;135(15):e867–84.

44. AIM-HIGH Investigators, Boden WE, Probstfield JL, Anderson T, et al. Niacin in patients with low HDL cholesterol levels receiving intensive statin therapy. N Engl J Med 2011;365(24):2255–67.

Is Lipoprotein(a) Ready for Prime-Time Use in the Clinic?

Katrina L. Ellis, PhD[a,b], Gerald F. Watts, MD, DSc[a,c,*]

KEYWORDS

- Lipoprotein(a) • Atherosclerotic cardiovascular disease • Pharmacotherapy • Risk assessment
- Models of care

KEY POINTS

- Lipoprotein(a), a polymorphic lipoprotein, is a potent heritable risk factor for atherosclerotic cardiovascular disease and aortic stenosis.
- The causal role for lipoprotein(a) in atherosclerotic cardiovascular disease is well-supported by genetic, epidemiologic, and experimental studies.
- Several therapies can lower Lipoprotein(a), but none have been tested for their effects on cardiovascular disease outcomes in patients selected for having elevated plasma Lipoprotein(a).
- There is only a moderate level of evidence supporting routine screening for elevated Lipoprotein(a), but conditional recommendations can be made for testing certain groups of patients.
- Whether Lipoprotein(a) remains a risk factor for atherosclerotic cardiovascular disease after low-density lipoprotein cholesterol is decreased to very low levels remains an issue.

INTRODUCTION

Lipoprotein(a) [Lp(a)] is a low-density lipoprotein (LDL)-like particle covalently bound to a hydrophilic glycoprotein called apolipoprotein(a) [apo(a)] that is under potent genetic control. Plasma levels of Lp(a) vary by up to 1000-fold among individuals, with 1 in 4 having levels that may increase the risk of atherosclerotic cardiovascular disease (ASCVD; **Fig. 1**).[1] Several new sources of evidence support a causal role for Lp(a) in (ASCVD) and aortic valve stenosis (reviewed in[2]). Individuals with elevated Lp(a) have a high life-time burden of ASCVD. This notion is important for coronary prevention. However, is Lp(a) ready for prime-time use in coronary prevention clinics?

BIOLOGY AND EPIDEMIOLOGY OF LIPOPROTEIN(a)

For full details of this topic the reader is referred to a recent review.[2] The structure of the Lp(a) particle is shown in **Fig. 2**. The LDL-like moiety contains 1 apoB-100 molecule indistinguishable from LDL per se, with apo(a) linked to apoB-100 by a single disulphide bond.[3] The apo(a) gene (*LPA*) has sequence homology with plasminogen.[4] Plasma Lp(a) concentration and isoform size are highly heritable, and largely determined by genetic variation in the *LPA* gene. The kringle 4 type-2 (KIV_2) copy number variant gives rise to at least 40 different sized apo(a) isoforms and explains on average between 30% and 70% of the variation in Lp(a) concentration. Mendelian randomization and genome-wide association studies

Disclosure Statement: K.L. Ellis was supported by a Royal Perth Hospital Medical Research Foundation Fellowship. G.F. Watts has received honoraria for advisory groups and research grants from Amgen, Sanofi, and Regeneron, as well as honoraria for consulting from Kowa and Gemphire.

[a] School of Medicine, University of Western Australia, 35 Stirling Highway, Crawley, WA 6009, Australia; [b] School of Biomedical Sciences, University of Western Australia, 35 Stirling Highway, Crawley, WA 6009, Australia; [c] Department of Cardiology, Lipid Disorders Clinic, Royal Perth Hospital, GPO Box X2213, Perth, WA 6001, Australia
* Corresponding author. Department of Cardiology, Lipid Disorders Clinic, Royal Perth Hospital, PO Box X2213, Perth, Western Australia 6847, Australia.
E-mail address: gerald.watts@uwa.edu.au

Cardiol Clin 36 (2018) 287–298
https://doi.org/10.1016/j.ccl.2017.12.010
0733-8651/18/© 2017 Elsevier Inc. All rights reserved.

cardiology.theclinics.com

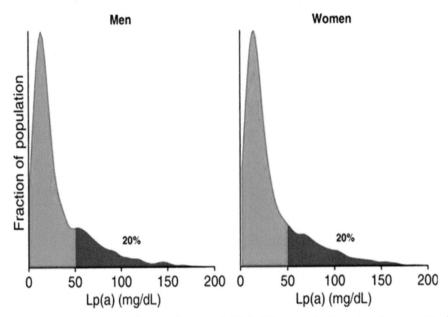

Fig. 1. The population distribution of serum lipoprotein(a) (Lp[a]) concentrations. Levels are positively skewed, with approximately 20% of individuals have elevated Lp(a) of 50 mg/dL or greater. (*From* Nordestgaard BG, Chapman MJ, Ray K, et al. Lipoprotein(a) as a cardiovascular risk factor: current status. Eur Heart J 2010;31(23):2845; with permission.)

have elucidated the role of Lp(a) in ASCVD and aortic stenosis.[2] Although the main site of Lp(a) catabolism is the liver, several distinct cellular receptors have been proposed to mediate Lp(a) clearance, including the LDL receptor (LDLR) and other members of the LDLR family, scavenger receptor class B type 1

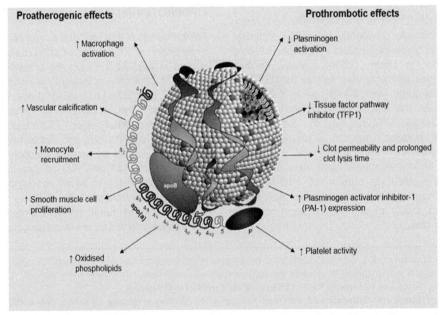

Fig. 2. Structure and pathobiology of lipoprotein(a) (Lp[a]). Lp(a) consists of a low-density lipoprotein (LDL)-like moiety bound to apo(a). Apo(a) contains 10 types of KIV, followed by a kringle 5-linke sequence (KV) and an inactive protease-like domain (P). The number of kringle 4 type-2 repeats determines Lp(a) isoform size. Many potential pathogenic effects have been ascribed to Lp(a), largely from in vitro studies, and almost all of which have been directly ascribed to apo(a). The majority of these functions must be considered speculative at present. (*From* Boffa MB, Koschinsky ML. Update on lipoprotein(a) as a cardiovascular risk factor and mediator. Curr Atheroscler Rep 2013;15(10):360; with permission.)

(SR-BI) and the plasminogen receptor.[2] Lp(a) levels vary greatly between individuals of different ethnicity, with higher plasma Lp(a) levels detected in South Asians compared with Chinese and non-Hispanic whites; Lp(a) concentrations are 2- to 3-fold higher in blacks compared with whites. Ethnic variability in plasma Lp(a) levels implies the need for defining population-specific Lp(a) thresholds for assessing ASCVD risk. Elevated Lp(a) can promote thrombosis, inflammation, oxidative stress, and calcification, and can impair fibrinolysis. **Fig. 2** summarizes the potential pathogenic mechanisms of Lp(a), but these are at present speculative. Further research is required into the structure/function relationships of Lp(a) and their role in ASCVD and calcific aortic valve disease.

CAUSAL ROLE OF LIPOPROTEIN(a) IN ATHEROSCLEROTIC CARDIOVASCULAR DISEASE

The causal role of elevated Lp(a) in ASCVD is supported by several coherent strands of evidence that may be judged according to the Bradford-Hill criteria.[2] Epidemiology supports a biological gradient, temporality, and a strong association between elevated Lp(a) and ASCVD outcomes.[5] Consistent associations have been demonstrated across multiple populations. The specificity of associations are well-emphasized by Mendelian randomization studies (for example[6]). Biological plausibility is underpinned by experimental data that confirm that elevated Lp(a) can induce atherosclerosis, inflammation, oxidative stress, and atherothrombosis (see **Fig. 2**).[2] Transgenic animal experiments show that Lp(a) induces atherosclerosis, with reversal of process with an intervention, according with Kochs postulates for causality.[2] There is also a clear analogy between the evidence for elevated Lp(a) and LDL cholesterol (for which there is a solid causal association with ASCVD). The key divergence is the lack of evidence showing that specific reduction in Lp(a) leads to a reduction in cardiovascular events.[2] As reviewed elsewhere in this article, this evidence should accrue with trials of specific new interventions that potently lower Lp(a). A positive outcome may be expected from observations made in patients undergoing lipoprotein apheresis (LA).[7]

THERAPEUTIC LOWERING OF LIPOPROTEIN(a): TOWARD WIDER CLINICAL USE OR CLINICAL TRIALS?

Despite compelling evidence for the role of Lp(a) in ASCVD, the justification for its clinical use requires a review of older and newer therapies for lowering Lp(a), which are summarized elsewhere in this article and in **Table 1**. It should be noted that there

Table 1
Treatments for lowering lipoprotein(a)

Therapy	Putative Primary Mechanism of Action	Predicted Relative Mean Reduction in Lp(a) Concentration (%)
Niacin	Decreases mobilization of free fatty acids from peripheral adipocytes and hepatic production of apo(a)	↓20–25
Estrogen	Effect on the *LPA* promoter	↓25
Lipoprotein apheresis	Extracorporeal removal of atherogenic lipoproteins	↓30[a] to 75[b]
PCSK9 inhibitors	Decreases PCSK9 binding to the LDL receptor	↓30
APOB antisense oligonucleotides	Decreases hepatic production of apo B-100	↓30
MTP Inhibitors	Decreases hepatic secretion and assembly of VLDL	↓15–20
CETP Inhibitors	Decreases exchange of neutral lipids among lipoproteins	↓30
THR agonists	Activation of β isoform proposed to reduce apoB synthesis	↓40
IL-6R mAbs	Decrease in interleukin-6 induced *LPA* messenger RNA and protein expression	↓35
LPA antisense oligonucleotides	Decreases hepatic production of apo(a)	↓80

Abbreviations: apo(a), apolipoprotein(a); LDL, low-density lipoprotein; *LPA*, apo(a) gene; mAbs, monoclonal antibodies; PCSK9, proprotein convertase subtilisin/kexin type 9; THR, thyroid hormone receptor; VLDL, very low-density lipoprotein.
[a] Interval mean reduction.
[b] Acute reduction.

are no clinical trial data that have selected patients for having elevated plasma concentrations of Lp(a). Accordingly, no drugs have been approved by regulatory agencies for selectively lowering Lp(a).

Niacin, Aspirin, and Estrogen

Niacin dose-dependently decreases Lp(a). In the AIM-HIGH trial (Atherothrombosis Intervention in Metabolic Syndrome with Low HDL/High Triglyceride and Impact on Global Health Outcomes), high-dose niacin (1.5-2.0 g/d) added to a statin reduced Lp(a) by 19%,[8] but had no effect on CVD events. In HPS-2-Thrive (Heart Protection Study 2-Treatment of HDL to Reduce the Incidence of Vascular Events), niacin also reduced Lp(a) by 24% but also had no effect on CVD events[9]; drug adverse effects (including hyperglycemia, hyperuricemia, and skin flushing) were common.[10] Neither trial selected patients for having elevated Lp(a), noting that reduction in Lp(a) of at least 30% would be required to achieve a reduction in cardiovascular outcomes.

Aspirin therapy (81 mg/d) can lower Lp(a) by up to 20% in Japanese patients with an Lp(a) of greater than 30 mg/dL, possibly by reducing the transcription of the apo(a) gene.[11] Whether aspirin consistently lowers Lp(a) in different racial groups and the impact on cardiovascular events remains unclear.

Hormone replacement therapy containing estrogens can also lower Lp(a) levels. However, this therapy can also increase triglycerides, smaller LDL and HDL particles, and inflammation, partly accounting for increased risk of CVD in older women.[12] It is unlikely estrogens will be used to specifically lower Lp(a).[12]

Lipoprotein Apheresis

LA, an extracorporeal method for removal of LDL and other atherogenic apoB-containing lipoproteins from the circulation, can reduce Lp(a) between 46% and 75%.[7] With the exception of the POCARD system,[13] none of the existing LA methods are specific for Lp(a). It is, therefore, difficult to unbundle the factors responsible for improvement in CVD outcomes after unselective apheresis. LA also lowers LDL cholesterol and apoB, and improves inflammation, cell adhesion molecules, endothelial function, and red blood cell deformability.[14] According to the American Society for Apheresis,[15] LA qualifies as a second-line treatment either as a monotherapy or combination therapy, to treat elevated Lp(a) levels.[14] An international consensus recommends that nicotinic acid (1–3 g/d) be used as first line to treat elevated Lp(a) in patients with premature coronary disease, with weekly selective apheresis as second line if a Lp(a) concentration remains greater than 30 mg/dL (>45 nmol/L).

In an investigation of patients with high Lp(a) and progressive ASCVD on maximally tolerated lipid-lowering therapy, LA was associated with a significant and sustained decline (over 5 years) in the mean annual rate of major adverse coronary events (MACE).[16] However, because LA is nonspecific, it is difficult to determine whether the decreases in coronary artery disease (CAD) events in these studies is due to the reduction in Lp(a), LDL, triglyceride-rich lipoproteins, or in all of these lipoproteins. A subgroup analysis stratified by LDL cholesterol concentration suggested that the decrease in MACE could in the main be attributed to the effect of apheresis on Lp(a).[17] Specific Lp(a) lowering with apheresis is possible with a column containing a sheep antibody against Lp(a). In patients with ASCVD and Lp(a) of 50 mg/dL or greater (with LDL cholesterol of ≤2.6 mmol/L) on long-term statin therapy, specific Lp(a) apheresis can regress carotid intima media thickness[13] and angiographically defined coronary atherosclerosis over 2 years.[18] The use of LA to treat elevated Lp(a) in high-risk patients has level 3 evidence (expert opinion and clinical experience) with a grade C recommendation (useful to guide practice, but care should be taken in application). Several newer therapies reviewed elsewhere in this article can also reduce Lp(a) concentrations, but their use in combination with apheresis to lower Lp(a) has not been tested rigorously. Despite its effectiveness in lowering atherogenic lipoproteins, including Lp(a), apheresis places a significant burden on health care services and patients. However, impairment of quality of life among survivors seems to be related to the underlying severity of ASCVD rather than to the LA procedure itself.[19]

Newer Therapies, Nonspecific Lowering of Lipoprotein(a): Proprotein Convertase Subtilisin/Kexin Type 9 Inhibitors, Mipomersen, Microsomal Triglyceride Transfer Protein Inhibitors, Cholesteryl Ester Transfer Protein Inhibitors, and Other Agents

Proprotein convertase subtilisin/kexin type 9 inhibitors

The most promising approaches for inhibiting proprotein convertase subtilisin/kexin type 9 (PCSK9) clinically involve the use of small interfering RNA or monoclonal antibodies (mAbs). In patients at high CVD risk or with elevated LDL cholesterol on maximally tolerated statin therapy, inclisiran, a small interfering RNA against PCSK9 reduced LDL cholesterol by up to 52.6% and Lp(a) by

25.6%.[20] The PCSK9 mAbs evolocumab and alirocumab are approved by regulatory agencies for lowering LDL cholesterol, but they can also both reduce plasma Lp(a) by approximately 30%.[2] Evolocumab lowers Lp(a) in homozygous familial hypercholesterolemia (FH) patients with at least one a defective LDLR mutation (2%–25% of normal LDL uptake), the extent of Lp(a) lowering correlating with that of LDL cholesterol.[21] In homozygous LDLR-negative patients (<2% of LDL uptake), variable effects have been reported on Lp(a) concentration with evolocumab therapy.[21] Given that PCSK9 mAbs work primarily through the LDLR, it is likely that the LDLR is required for the Lp(a) lowering effect.

Alirocumab can reduce the need for apheresis in heterozygous FH,[22] but whether this also applies to patients being treated for high Lp(a) remains to be demonstrated. In the landmark FOURIER trial (Further Cardiovascular Outcomes Research with PCSK9 Inhibition in Subjects with Elevated Risk), evolocumab significantly reduced the incidence of a triple MACE endpoint over a median 2.2 years of follow-up without an increase in treatment-related adverse events in high-risk subjects on statin therapy.[23] This trial did not specifically select patients for having high Lp(a), and further analyses in relation to baseline Lp(a) levels are awaited. The investigation of alirocumab in the ODYSSEY Outcomes trial is ongoing with results expected in 2018.

Mipomersen
Mipomersen, an antisense oligonucleotide (ASO) against apoB-100, reduces LDL cholesterol as well as apoB-100 and Lp(a) by approximately 30%.[24] It seems that mipomersen somewhat paradoxically increases the clearance of apoB-100–containing lipoproteins so that associated reductions in Lp(a) may be a result of the diminished availability of apoB-100 for coupling with apo(a).[25] Several adverse effects of mipomersen therapy have been described; the most common include injection site reactions, flulike symptoms, and an increase in both hepatic fat and liver transaminases.[26] A number of risk evaluation and mitigation strategies are required for its use in the United States, where it has been approved for the treatment of homozygous FH; the drug is not approved in Europe, and mipomersen is not indicated for specifically lowering Lp(a).

Microsomal triglyceride transfer protein inhibitors
Inhibition of microsomal triglyceride transfer protein decreases the assembly and secretion of apoB-containing lipoproteins, potentially lowering Lp(a) concentration by decreasing the coupling of apoB-100 with apo(a). However, the reductions in Lp(a) with lomitapide in clinical trials have been modest with loss of effect over time.[27] Hence, it seems unlikely that this agent will be specifically valuable for treating high Lp(a), noting also concerns about hepatic steatosis. Studies of the synergistic effect with apheresis in lowering Lp(a) merit consideration.[2,14]

Cholesteryl ester transfer protein inhibitors
Cholesteryl ester transfer protein (CETP) inhibitors increase HDL cholesterol and robustly lower LDL cholesterol and Lp(a) as monotherapy or combined with a statin. Three CETP inhibitors have failed in clinical trials owing to futility or adverse effects.[2] Anacetrapib can reduce Lp(a) by approximately 30% with few drug-related adverse events in high cardiovascular risk patients, including FH.[28,29] The recent findings from the REVEAL Trial (Randomized EVAluation of the Effects of Anacetrapib Through Lipid-modification) demonstrated that, in patients with ASCVD, the addition of anacetrapib to background intensive statin therapy lowered the incidence of major coronary events compared with placebo over a median 4.1 years of follow-up.[30] The absolute benefit in this trial was incrementally small, but comparable to IMPROVE-IT (IMProved Reduction of Outcomes: Vytorin Efficacy International Trial) with ezetimibe; the benefit was considered to be related to the reduction in non-HDL cholesterol as opposed to the increase in HDL cholesterol.[30] The reduction in non-HDL cholesterol includes a component from Lp(a), which per se decreased by an average of 25%; there was also a trend to greater coronary benefit in patients with a baseline Lp(a) above the top tertile (>55 nmol/L). The CETP inhibitor AMG 899, a new highly potent CETP inhibitor that markedly increases cellular cholesterol efflux, has an acceptable safety profile and remains under development.[31]

Others agents: thyromimetics, interleukin-6 receptor monoclonal antibodies, and farnesoid X receptor agonists
Thyromimetics may lower Lp(a) by approximately 40% in combination with statins or ezetimibe.[32] Clinical reports of impaired hepatic function and cartilage damage in dogs led to premature termination of eprotirome.[33] A clinical trial in patients with heterozygous FH is investigating the effects of MGL-3196 (a liver targeted selective agonist of the thyroid hormone) on LDL cholesterol, Lp(a), and other atherogenic lipoproteins.[34] Tocilizumab, a mAb that blocks the interleukin-6 receptor, can lower Lp(a) by 37%, but can adversely increase LDL cholesterol and triglycerides by up to 28%.[35] Farnesoid X receptor agonists can also

lower Lp(a) by repressing hepatic *LPA* gene expression.[36] The mechanism of action and safety of the above drugs require further study.

Selective lowering of lipoprotein(a): apolipoprotein(a) antisense and silencing agents

Selective apo(a) antisense therapy targets hepatic apo(a) messenger RNA, inhibiting the translation of the *LPA* gene. This prevents the production of the apo(a) protein and the subsequent coupling of apo(a) to apoB-100. Current second-generation apo(a) ASOs have superior messenger RNA affinity and potency compared with first-generation molecules.[37]

Initial investigations of an apo(a) antisense (IONIS 144367) in *LPA* transgenic mice showed an 85% reduction in plasma Lp(a) levels and plasma-OxPL concentrations.[37] Further studies in cynomolgus monkeys provided validation for IONIS-APO(a)$_{RX}$, an ASO that binds to the exon 24 to 25 splice site of apo(a), as a potent apo(a)-lowering agent where efficacy is independent of apo(a) isoform size and plasma Lp(a) concentration.[37] The unique efficacy and safety of this ASO in reducing Lp(a) and OxPL by up to 78% was demonstrated in early controlled clinical trials in human subjects, including those with elevated Lp(a).[38,39] A reduction in Lp(a) and OxPL concentration was also associated with a reduction in monocyte inflammatory activation.[39]

To increase specificity and limit off-target effects, a new ligand-conjugated ASO therapy has been developed. IONIS-APO(a)-L$_{RX}$ consists of modified IONIS-APO(a)$_{RX}$ that is conjugated to a tri-antennary *N*-acetyl galactosamine (GalNAc$_3$) complex.[39] Because the ligands for GalNAc$_3$ are expressed exclusively on hepatocytes,[37] such an approach significantly increases the efficacy of ASO's targeting hepatic messenger RNA, enabling significant reductions in both dose and dosing frequency.[37] In a first-in-man controlled trial, IONIS-APO(a)-L$_{RX}$ was shown to be 30 times more potent than IONIS-APO(a)$_{RX}$; in the subjects receiving the highest dose of IONIS-APO(a)-L$_{RX}$ (approximately 1/10th of the dose of IONIS-APO[a]-$_{RX}$), Lp(a) concentration was reduced by 92.4% compared with placebo, with no adverse effects reported.[39]

Because apo(a) antisense is the only therapy that can reduce Lp(a) by more than 50%, it will theoretically be the preferred treatment for patients with very high Lp(a) levels. Another approach for decreasing the production of apo(a) uses small interfering RNA therapeutics, such as ARC-LPA. This agent is being developed for clinical use.[40] Preliminary and clinical trials are awaited with interest. The long-term efficacy, safety, and cost efficiency in preventing cardiovascular events in patients with high Lp(a) needs to be demonstrated before new biologics targeting the expression of the apo(a) protein can be used clinically.

PRACTICAL CONSIDERATIONS FOR A FUTURE MODEL OF CARE

International Guidelines: Is There Consensus and How Strong Is the Evidence?

The first guideline on the detection and management of elevated Lp(a) was from the European Atherosclerosis Society.[1] More recent guidelines have been from the National Lipid Association,[41] European Atherosclerosis Society/European Society of Cardiology,[42] Canadian Cardiovascular Society,[43] and Mighty Medic Group.[14] **Table 2** summarizes their collective recommendations. Evidence levels are moderate and strengths of recommendations conditional or guarded.

Detection: Targeted and Systematic Screening

Because there are no therapies that specifically lower Lp(a), and hence no clinical trial data supporting a reduction in ASCVD risk with specific intervention, the case for screening for high Lp(a) has been questioned by certain expert bodies, particularly in the United States.[44] With a more patient-orientated approach, other authorities recommend Lp(a) testing in certain clinical situations, such as in individuals with a personal or family history of premature CAD or at intermediate/high risk of CAD. Testing for high Lp(a) is also recommended in younger patients with recurrent cardiovascular events despite the use of high-intensity statins and good control of other risk cardiovascular factors, as well as in patients whose LDL cholesterol remains refractory to treatment with high-intensity statins plus ezetimibe.[1,45] Patients with FH merit being tested for elevated Lp(a).[2,46]

The strong heritability of Lp(a), the imminently available novel therapeutic agents targeting Lp(a), and the ability to correct other traditional cardiovascular risk factors, can provide a rationale for cascade testing family members of index cases with elevated Lp(a) (above the 90th centile). However, the cost effectiveness of such an approach remains to be demonstrated before formal recommendations on cascade testing for Lp(a) can be made.[46]

Analytical caveats: a thorny issue

Most immunoassays for Lp(a) are not isoform independent. Hence, Lp(a) concentration will be overestimated in individuals with a high KIV$_2$ copy number, and underestimated in those with a low KIV$_2$ copy number. Isoform independent assays with calibrators traceable to a World Health

Table 2
International recommendations for the measurement and treatment of lipoprotein(a)

	EAS 2010[1]	NLA 2015[41]	EAS/ESC 2016[42]	Canadian Cardiovascular Society 2016[43]	Mighty Medic Group 2017[14]
Measurement	Lp(a) should be measured once in individuals at intermediate or high risk of CVD using an isoform-insensitive assay: i. Premature CVD ii. FH iii. Family history of premature CVD and/or elevated Lp(a) iv. Recurrent CVD despite statin treatment v. ≥3% 10-y risk of fatal CVD according to European guidelines vi. ≥10% 10-y risk of fatal and/or nonfatal CHD according to the US guidelines	Lp(a) ≥50 mg/dL using an isoform-insensitive assay is an additional risk indicator (other than major atherosclerotic cardiovascular disease risk factors) that might be considered for risk refinement.	Lp(a) screening should be considered in individuals with high CVD risk or a strong family history of premature atherothrombotic disease: i. Premature CVD ii. FH iii. A family history of premature CVD and/or elevated Lp(a) iv. Recurrent CVD despite optimal lipid-lowering treatment v. ≥5% 10-y risk of fatal CVD according to SCORE	Lp(a) might aid risk assessment in subjects with intermediate Framingham Risk Score or with a family history of premature CAD. Particular attention should be given to individuals with Lp(a) >30 mg/dL.	Lp(a) mass should be measured once in all subjects at intermediate or high risk of CVD/CHD who present with: i. Premature CVD ii. FH iii. A family history of premature CVD without elevated LDL-C levels or recurrent CVD despite statin treatment.
Treatment	Recommend Lp(a) <80th percentile (<~50 mg/dL) as a secondary priority after reduction in LDL-C and total cholesterol in patients with CVD and/or diabetes, and in those without CVD or diabetes but at intermediate or high absolute risk.	Focus on more intensive LDL-C lowering if Lp(a) is ≥50 mg/dL.	In patients at risk with high Lp(a), a reasonable option is an intensified treatment of modifiable risk factors including LDL-C.	Nonspecific recommendation to use Lp(a) to facilitate shared decision making regarding treatment for other risk factors.	Lp(a) mass <30 mg/dL (<45 nmol/L) is considered normal. Nicotinic acid (1–3 g/d) used to be first-line treatment, but is no longer available in Europe. If refractory, weekly selective LA is effective to reduce Lp(a) mass when administered on long-term basis.

Abbreviations: CAD, coronary artery disease; CHD, coronary heart disease; CVD, cardiovascular disease; EAS, European Atherosclerosis Society; ESC, European Society of Cardiology; FH, familial hypercholesterolaemia; LA, lipoprotein apheresis; LDL-C, low-density lipoprotein cholesterol; Lp(a), lipoprotein(a); NLA, National Lipid Association; SCORE, Systematic Coronary Risk Evaluation.

Organization/International Federation of Clinical Chemistry and Laboratory Medicine reference (107 μmol/L) are recommended.[47] Because protein alone is being measured, Lp(a) should be expressed as molar concentrations that reflect the number of Lp(a) particles. Of all immunoassays investigated, the Denka Seiken latex-enhanced turbidimetric method is most concordant with the "reference" enzyme-linked immunosorbent assay.[47] This enzyme-linked immunosorbent assay has been extensively evaluated, uses different size calibrators, and has been shown to be insensitive to apo(a) isoform size heterogeneity. We stress the importance of using a precise Lp(a) assay that is insensitive to apo(a) isoform size and using a recognized Lp(a) standard.[47]

Risk Assessment: Toward Precision Medicine

Selected studies suggest the potential value of Lp(a) in risk assessment. In the Bruneck study, a 15-year prospective investigation in the general population, Lp(a) was an independent risk factor for CAD and improved both risk discrimination and reclassification when added to Framingham and Reynolds Risk Scores; the most pronounced reclassification improvement was 39.6% in the intermediate risk group.[48] In the EPIC (European Prospective Investigation of Cancer)-Norfolk cohort, adding Lp(a) (<30 mg/dL vs ≥30 mg/dL) to the American College of Cardiology/American Heart Association and Systematic Coronary Risk Evaluation (SCORE) algorithms resulted in a net reclassification index of 15.9% and 16.8%, respectively, in intermediate risk individuals.[49] In the Copenhagen City Heart Study, addition of elevated Lp(a) (≥50 mg/dL) to conventional CVD risk factors yielded an net reclassification index of 16% for myocardial infarction and 3% for coronary heart disease.[50] The Brisighella Heart Study found that Lp(a) was a significant predictor of CVD over 25 years in individuals at intermediate or high CVD risk, as determined by Italian-specific risk charts.[51]

However, these findings do not concord with an earlier metaanalysis,[52] or with the BiomarCaRE (Biomarkers for Cardiovascular Risk Assessment in Europe) project in which the addition of Lp(a) to conventional risk factors resulted in a reclassification rate of only approximately 1% for major coronary events and incident CVD events.[53] Importantly, these studies might have been confounded by analytical issues related to types of Lp(a) assays, sample storage conditions, and heterogeneity of the sample population.

Significantly, Lp(a) seems to be an independent predictor of CVD in patients with established CAD.[54] In symptomatic patients with nonobstructive CAD, Lp(a) was an independent predictor of MACE and enabled risk stratification of such patients.[54] Higher Lp(a) was additionally identified as an independent predictor of mortality in patients undergoing coronary angiography and percutaneous coronary intervention.[55] Similarly, in statin treated patients undergoing a first percutaneous coronary intervention, elevated Lp(a) was an independent predictor of MACE over approximately 5 years follow-up.[56] Whether Lp(a) remains a risk factor for ASCVD after LDL cholesterol is decreased with a statin to low levels is a critical issue referred to elsewhere in this article.[2,57]

Elevated Lp(a) has been shown to be independently associated with increased CAD risk in some but not all studies of FH.[2] Cross-sectional study design, lack of accurate diagnosis of FH, and analytical issues with the Lp(a) assay might have confounded the negative findings. In the most comprehensive, prospective study of molecularly defined FH, Lp(a) (>50 mg/dL) was an independent predictor of incident ASCVD risk over 5 and 10 years; the strength of this study is the genetic diagnosis of FH, the relatively large sample size, and the duration of follow-up.[58]

Lifestyle and Pharmacotherapy: Is It All About Low-Density Lipoprotein Cholesterol?

The management of patients with elevated Lp(a) starts by correcting conventional cardiovascular risk factors with diet, exercise, smoking cessation, weight regulation, and stress management. The importance of lifestyle factors was emphasized in the EPIC-Norfolk study, in which ideal cardiovascular health, defined by an American Heart Association metric, was associated with a 75% reduction in cardiovascular risk in people with high Lp(a).[59]

The most efficacious therapies for lowering Lp(a) include apheresis, PCSK9 mAbs, and apo(a) antisense therapy. There is no convincing argument at present for the use of nicotinic acid in patients with elevated Lp(a). A critical issue is whether Lp(a) remains a risk factor for ASCVD after LDL cholesterol is lowered to recommended targets.[57] Prediction of recurrent events may be confounded by the statistical phenomenon of index event bias. The notion that Lp(a) is not a risk factor for progression of ASCVD after LDL cholesterol is at target also derives principally from angiographic and intravascular ultrasound studies.[60,61] Recent analyses from AIM-HIGH,[8] LIPID (Long-Term Intervention with Pravastatin in Ischaemic Disease),[62] and JUPITER (Justification for the Use of Statins in Prevention: an Intervention Trial Evaluating Rosuvastatin),[63] however, demonstrate that, in treated patients with average LDL cholesterol, Lp(a) greater than the top quartile (>0.5 g/L) may increase risk of recurrent CVD events by up to 60%. A post hoc analysis from the AIM-HIGH trial[8] also suggests that future trials need to select patients for having plasma concentration of Lp(a) of greater than 0.5 g/L and lower Lp(a) with an intervention by more than 50%. Hence, Lp(a) seems to be an independent risk factor for CVD events after LDL cholesterol is lowered with a statin, but it remains unclear whether this applies to very low LDL cholesterol concentrations.[23]

SUMMARY: PRIME-TIME USE?

Recent genetic epidemiology provides the most persuasive evidence supporting the causal role of Lp(a) in ASCVD. Lp(a) has several properties that can induce atherothrombosis, but no clinical trial has demonstrated that selective reduction in elevated Lp(a) reduces the incidence of CVD. The inability to meet this crucial Bradford-Hill criterion diminishes the level of evidence and strength

of recommendation for the routine measurement of Lp(a) in the primary and secondary prevention of coronary disease. One must, therefore, strictly conclude that Lp(a) is not ready for prime-time use in primary care and specialist clinics.

However, because the quality of evidence is at least moderate, in our view a conditional recommendation for using Lp(a) in the clinic can be made. This recommendation implies that further research, in particular a large clinical endpoint trial, is likely to impact on the confidence of the estimate of the effect of using Lp(a) in clinical practice. Knowledge of Lp(a) could be particularly useful in reclassification of subjects at intermediate risk of CVD, as assessed by conventional and new risk algorithms. Lp(a) should be measured in individuals with a personal family history of premature coronary disease, FH, and possibly those with recurrent coronary events despite optimal cholesterol-lowering therapy. Information on Lp(a) may further point to more aggressive treatment of conventional CVD risk factors, or to searching for subclinical atherosclerosis with cardiac

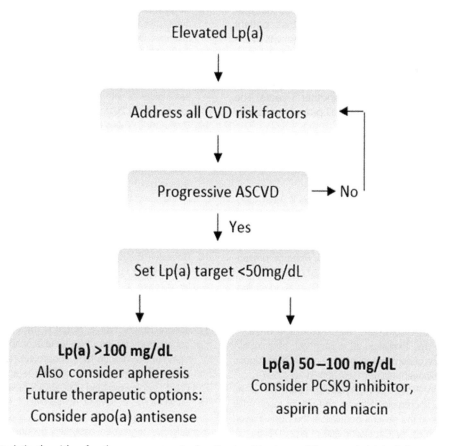

Fig. 3. Futuristic algorithm for the management of patients with elevated lipoprotein(a) (Lp[a]). ASCVD, atherosclerotic cardiovascular disease; CVD, cardiovascular disease; PCSK9, proprotein convertase subtilisin/kexin type 9. (*From* Ellis KL, Hooper AJ, Burnett JR, et al. Progress in the care of common inherited atherogenic disorders of apolipoprotein B metabolism. Nat Rev Endocrinol 2016;12(8):477; with permission.)

computed tomography scanning. Measurement of Lp(a) should use an assay that is, well-standardized and isoform independent. The value of cascade testing first-degree relatives of an index case has not been demonstrated, but could be motivational for the successful implementation of healthy lifestyles in primary prevention. Elevated Lp(a) with multigenic hypercholesterolemia or familial combined hyperlipidemia may mimic FH, and should always be considered in patients who return a negative genetic test for FH.[64]

The selective use of Lp(a) in the clinic will evidently require good judgment calls, and balanced and shared decision making. The evidence levels and strength of recommendation for more extended measurement of Lp(a) will accrue from clinical outcome trials using specific therapies (such as apo[a] antisense and silencing RNA) targeted at high-risk patients (eg, with ASCVD, FH, diabetes) with elevated Lp(a). A futuristic algorithm for the management of patients with elevated Lp(a)[64] is shown in **Fig. 3**, but the realization of this protocol needs to wait for evidence from the clinical intervention trials, as discussed. As with FH, standardized models of care, registries, patient support groups, and codification for Lp(a) will eventually be required.[2] The prime time use of Lp(a) in clinical practice mandates that all of the Bradford-Hill criteria for causality be met, a requirement that may not be achieved for another 5 years. The priorities for future research into Lp(a) were recently communicated.[2,65]

REFERENCES

1. Nordestgaard BG, Chapman MJ, Ray K, et al. Lipoprotein(a) as a cardiovascular risk factor: current status. Eur Heart J 2010;31(23):2844–53.
2. Ellis KL, Boffa MB, Sahebkar A, et al. The renaissance of lipoprotein(a): brave new world for preventive cardiology? Prog Lipid Res 2017;68:57–82.
3. Koschinsky ML, Cote GP, Gabel B, et al. Identification of the cysteine residue in apolipoprotein(a) that mediates extracellular coupling with apolipoprotein B-100. J Biol Chem 1993;268(26):19819–25.
4. McLean JW, Tomlinson JE, Kuang WJ, et al. cDNA sequence of human apolipoprotein(a) is homologous to plasminogen. Nature 1987;330(6144):132–7.
5. Kamstrup PR, Benn M, Tybjaerg-Hansen A, et al. Extreme lipoprotein(a) levels and risk of myocardial infarction in the general population: the Copenhagen City Heart Study. Circulation 2008;117(2):176–84.
6. Kamstrup PR, Tybjaerg-Hansen A, Steffensen R, et al. Genetically elevated lipoprotein(a) and increased risk of myocardial infarction. JAMA 2009;301(22):2331–9.

7. Waldmann E, Parhofer KG. Lipoprotein apheresis to treat elevated lipoprotein (a). J Lipid Res 2016; 57(10):1751–7.
8. Albers JJ, Slee A, O'Brien KD, et al. Relationship of apolipoproteins A-1 and B, and lipoprotein(a) to cardiovascular outcomes: the AIM-HIGH trial (Atherothrombosis Intervention in Metabolic Syndrome with Low HDL/High Triglyceride and Impact on Global Health Outcomes). J Am Coll Cardiol 2013; 62(17):1575–9.
9. Boden WE, Sidhu MS, Toth PP. The therapeutic role of niacin in dyslipidemia management. J Cardiovasc Pharmacol Ther 2014;19(2):141–58.
10. HPS2-THRIVE Collaborative Group. HPS2-THRIVE randomized placebo-controlled trial in 25 673 high-risk patients of ER niacin/laropiprant: trial design, pre-specified muscle and liver outcomes, and reasons for stopping study treatment. Eur Heart J 2013;34(17):1279–91.
11. Akaike M, Azuma H, Kagawa A, et al. Effect of aspirin treatment on serum concentrations of lipoprotein (a) in patients with atherosclerotic diseases. Clin Chem 2002;48(9):1454–9.
12. Howard BV, Rossouw JE. Estrogens and cardiovascular disease risk revisited: the Women's Health Initiative. Curr Opin Lipidol 2013;24(6):493–9.
13. Ezhov M, Safarova M, Afanasieva O, et al. Specific lipoprotein (a) apheresis attenuates progression of carotid intima-media thickness in coronary heart disease patients with high lipoprotein (a) levels. Atheroscler Suppl 2015;18:163–9.
14. Stefanutti C, Julius U, Watts GF, et al. Towards an international consensus–integrating lipoprotein apheresis and new lipid-lowering drugs. J Clin Lipidol 2017;11(4):858–71.
15. Schwartz J, Padmanabhan A, Aqui N, et al. Guidelines on the use of therapeutic apheresis in clinical practice–evidence-based approach from the writing committee of the American Society for Apheresis: the seventh special issue. J Clin Apher 2016;31(3):149–338.
16. Roeseler E, Julius U, Heigl F, et al. Lipoprotein apheresis for lipoprotein(a)-associated cardiovascular disease: prospective 5 years of follow-up and apolipoprotein(a) characterization. Arterioscler Thromb Vasc Biol 2016;36(9):2019–27.
17. Jaeger BR, Richter Y, Nagel D, et al. Longitudinal cohort study on the effectiveness of lipid apheresis treatment to reduce high lipoprotein (a) levels and prevent major adverse coronary events. Nat Clin Pract Cardiovasc Med 2009;6(3):229–39.
18. Safarova MS, Ezhov MV, Afanasieva OI, et al. Effect of specific lipoprotein (a) apheresis on coronary atherosclerosis regression assessed by quantitative coronary angiography. Atheroscler Suppl 2013;14(1):93–9.
19. Rosada A, Kassner U, Banisch D, et al. Quality of life in patients treated with lipoprotein apheresis. J Clin Lipidol 2016;10(2):323–9.e6.

20. Ray KK, Landmesser U, Leiter LA, et al. Inclisiran in patients at high cardiovascular risk with elevated LDL cholesterol. N Engl J Med 2017;376(15):1430–40.

21. Raal FJ, Honarpour N, Blom DJ, et al. Inhibition of PCSK9 with evolocumab in homozygous familial hypercholesterolaemia (TESLA Part B): a randomised, double-blind, placebo-controlled trial. Lancet 2015; 385(9965):341–50.

22. Moriarty PM, Parhofer KG, Babirak SP, et al. Alirocumab in patients with heterozygous familial hypercholesterolaemia undergoing lipoprotein apheresis: the ODYSSEY ESCAPE trial. Eur Heart J 2016;37(48): 3588–95.

23. Sabatine MS, Giugliano RP, Keech AC, et al. Evolocumab and clinical outcomes in patients with cardiovascular disease. N Engl J Med 2017;376(18):1713–22.

24. Stein EA, Raal FJ. New therapies for reducing low-density lipoprotein cholesterol. Endocrinol Metab Clin North Am 2014;43(4):1007–33.

25. Reyes-Soffer G, Moon B, Hernandez-Ono A, et al. Complex effects of inhibiting hepatic apolipoprotein B100 synthesis in humans. Sci Transl Med 2016; 8(323):323ra312.

26. Thomas GS, Cromwell WC, Ali S, et al. Mipomersen, an apolipoprotein B synthesis inhibitor, reduces atherogenic lipoproteins in patients with severe hypercholesterolemia at high cardiovascular risk: a randomized, double-blind, placebo-controlled trial. J Am Coll Cardiol 2013;62(23):2178–84.

27. Cuchel M, Meagher EA, du Toit Theron H, et al. Efficacy and safety of a microsomal triglyceride transfer protein inhibitor in patients with homozygous familial hypercholesterolaemia: a single-arm, open-label, phase 3 study. Lancet 2013;381(9860):40–6.

28. Cannon CP, Shah S, Dansky HM, et al. Safety of anacetrapib in patients with or at high risk for coronary heart disease. N Engl J Med 2010;363(25):2406–15.

29. Kastelein JJ, Besseling J, Shah S, et al. Anacetrapib as lipid-modifying therapy in patients with heterozygous familial hypercholesterolaemia (REALIZE): a randomised, double-blind, placebo-controlled, phase 3 study. Lancet 2015;385(9983):2153–61.

30. The HPS3/TIMI55-REVEAL Collaborative Group. Effects of anacetrapib in patients with atherosclerotic vascular disease. N Engl J Med 2017;377(13): 1217–27.

31. Hovingh GK, Kastelein JJ, van Deventer SJ, et al. Cholesterol ester transfer protein inhibition by TA-8995 in patients with mild dyslipidaemia (TULIP): a randomised, double-blind, placebo-controlled phase 2 trial. Lancet 2015;386(9992):452–60.

32. Shoemaker TJ, Kono T, Mariash CN, et al. Thyroid hormone analogues for the treatment of metabolic disorders: new potential for unmet clinical needs? Endocr Pract 2012;18(6):954–64.

33. Sjouke B, Langslet G, Ceska R, et al. Eprotirome in patients with familial hypercholesterolaemia (the AKKA trial): a randomised, double-blind, placebo-controlled phase 3 study. Lancet Diabetes Endocrinol 2014;2(6):455–63.

34. Madrigal Pharmaceuticals. 2017. Madrigal Pharmaceuticals announces the initiation of a phase 2 study of MGL-3196 in patients with heterozygous familial hypercholesterolemia (HeFH). Available at: https://globenewswire.com/news-release/2017/02/23/926994/0/en/Madrigal-Pharmaceuticals-Announces-the-Initiation-of-a-Phase-2-Study-of-MGL-3196-in-Patients-with-Heterozygous-Familial-Hypercholesterolemia-HeFH.html. Accessed September 25, 2017.

35. McInnes IB, Thompson L, Giles JT, et al. Effect of interleukin-6 receptor blockade on surrogates of vascular risk in rheumatoid arthritis: MEASURE, a randomised, placebo-controlled study. Ann Rheum Dis 2015;74(4):694–702.

36. Ghosh Laskar M, Eriksson M, Rudling M, et al. Treatment with the natural FXR agonist chenodeoxycholic acid reduces clearance of plasma LDL whilst decreasing circulating PCSK9, lipoprotein(a) and apolipoprotein C-III. J Intern Med 2017;281(6): 575–85.

37. Graham MJ, Viney N, Crooke RM, et al. Antisense inhibition of apolipoprotein (a) to lower plasma lipoprotein (a) levels in humans. J Lipid Res 2016; 57(3):340–51.

38. Tsimikas S, Viney NJ, Hughes SG, et al. Antisense therapy targeting apolipoprotein(a): a randomised, double-blind, placebo-controlled phase 1 study. Lancet 2015;386(10002):1472–83.

39. Viney NJ, van Capelleveen JC, Geary RS, et al. Antisense oligonucleotides targeting apolipoprotein(a) in people with raised lipoprotein(a): two randomised, double-blind, placebo-controlled, dose-ranging trials. Lancet 2016;388(10057):2239–53.

40. Amgen. Amgen and Arrowhead Pharmaceuticals announce two cardiovascular collaborations. Available at: http://www.amgen.com/media/news-releases/2016/09/amgen-and-arrowhead-pharmaceuticals-announce-two-cardiovascular-collaborations/. Accessed September 25, 2017.

41. Jacobson TA, Maki KC, Orringer CE, et al. National lipid association recommendations for patient-centered management of dyslipidemia: part 2. J Clin Lipidol 2015;9:S1–122.

42. Catapano AL, Graham I, De Backer G, et al. 2016 ESC/EAS guidelines for the management of dyslipidaemias: the task force for the management of dyslipidaemias of the European Society of Cardiology (ESC) and European Atherosclerosis Society (EAS) Developed with the special contribution of the European Asscocciation for Cardiovascular Prevention & Rehabilitation (EACPR). Atherosclerosis 2016;253:281–344.

43. Anderson TJ, Gregoire J, Pearson GJ, et al. 2016 Canadian Cardiovascular Society guidelines for the

management of dyslipidemia for the prevention of cardiovascular disease in the adult. Can J Cardiol 2016;32(11):1263–82.

44. Stone NJ, Robinson JG, Lichtenstein AH, et al. 2013 ACC/AHA guideline on the treatment of blood cholesterol to reduce atherosclerotic cardiovascular risk in adults: a report of the American College of Cardiology/American Heart Association Task Force on Practice Guidelines. Circulation 2014;129(25 Suppl 2):S1–45.

45. Reiner Z, Catapano AL, De Backer G, et al. ESC/EAS guidelines for the management of dyslipidaemias: the task force for the management of dyslipidaemias of the European Society of Cardiology (ESC) and the European Atherosclerosis Society (EAS). Eur Heart J 2011;32(14):1769–818.

46. Alonso R, Andres E, Mata N, et al. Lipoprotein(a) levels in familial hypercholesterolemia: an important predictor of cardiovascular disease independent of the type of LDL receptor mutation. J Am Coll Cardiol 2014;63(19):1982–9.

47. Marcovina SM, Albers JJ, Scanu AM, et al. Use of a reference material proposed by the international federation of clinical chemistry and laboratory medicine to evaluate analytical methods for the determination of plasma lipoprotein(a). Clin Chem 2000; 46(12):1956–67.

48. Willeit P, Kiechl S, Kronenberg F, et al. Discrimination and net reclassification of cardiovascular risk with lipoprotein(a): prospective 15-year outcomes in the Bruneck Study. J Am Coll Cardiol 2014;64(9):851–60.

49. Verbeek R, Sandhu MS, Hovingh GK, et al. Lipoprotein(a) improves cardiovascular risk prediction based on established risk algorithms. J Am Coll Cardiol 2017;69(11):1513–5.

50. Kamstrup PR, Tybjaerg-Hansen A, Nordestgaard BG. Extreme lipoprotein(a) levels and improved cardiovascular risk prediction. J Am Coll Cardiol 2013; 61(11):1146–56.

51. Fogacci F, Cicero AFG, D'Addato S, et al. Serum lipoprotein(a) level as long-term predictor of cardiovascular mortality in a large sample of subjects in primary cardiovascular prevention: data from the Brisighella Heart Study. Eur J Intern Med 2017;37: 49–55.

52. Emerging Risk Factors Collaboration, Di Angelantonio E, Gao P, Pennells L, et al. Lipid-related markers and cardiovascular disease prediction. JAMA 2012;307(23): 2499–506.

53. Waldeyer C, Makarova N, Zeller T, et al. Lipoprotein(a) and the risk of cardiovascular disease in the European population: results from the BiomarCaRE consortium. Eur Heart J 2017;38(32):2490–8.

54. Xie H, Chen L, Liu H, et al. Long-term prognostic value of lipoprotein(a) in symptomatic patients with nonobstructive coronary artery disease. Am J Cardiol 2017;119(7):945–50.

55. Feng Z, Li HL, Bei WJ, et al. Association of lipoprotein(a) with long-term mortality following coronary angiography or percutaneous coronary intervention. Clin Cardiol 2017;40(9):674–8.

56. Suwa S, Ogita M, Miyauchi K, et al. Impact of lipoprotein (a) on long-term outcomes in patients with coronary artery disease treated with statin after a first percutaneous coronary intervention. J Atheroscler Thromb 2017;24(11):1125–31.

57. Tsimikas S. A test in context: lipoprotein(a): diagnosis, prognosis, controversies, and emerging therapies. J Am Coll Cardiol 2017;69(6):692–711.

58. Perez de Isla L, Alonso R, Mata N, et al. Predicting cardiovascular events in familial hypercholesterolemia: the SAFEHEART Registry (Spanish Familial Hypercholesterolemia Cohort Study). Circulation 2017; 135(22):2133–44.

59. Perrot N, Verbeek R, Sandhu M, et al. Ideal cardiovascular health influences cardiovascular disease risk associated with high lipoprotein(a) levels and genotype: the EPIC-Norfolk prospective population study. Atherosclerosis 2017;256:47–52.

60. Maher VG, Brown B, Marcovina SM, et al. Effects of lowering elevated LDL cholesterol on the cardiovascular risk of lipoprotein(a). JAMA 1995;274(22):1771–4.

61. Puri R, Ballantyne CM, Hoogeveen RC, et al. Lipoprotein(a) and coronary atheroma progression rates during long-term high-intensity statin therapy: insights from SATURN. Atherosclerosis 2017;263:137–44.

62. Nestel PJ, Barnes EH, Tonkin AM, et al. Plasma lipoprotein(a) concentration predicts future coronary and cardiovascular events in patients with stable coronary heart disease. Arterioscler Thromb Vasc Biol 2013;33(12):2902–8.

63. Khera AV, Everett BM, Caulfield MP, et al. Lipoprotein(a) concentrations, rosuvastatin therapy, and residual vascular risk: an analysis from the JUPITER Trial (Justification for the Use of Statins in Prevention: an Intervention Trial Evaluating Rosuvastatin). Circulation 2014;129(6):635–42.

64. Ellis KL, Hooper AJ, Burnett JR, et al. Progress in the care of common inherited atherogenic disorders of apolipoprotein B metabolism. Nat Rev Endocrinol 2016;12(8):467–84.

65. Tsimikas S, Fazio S, Ferdinand KC, et al. NHLBI Working Group recommendations to reduce Lipoprotein(a)-mediated risk of cardiovascular disease and aortic stenosis. JACC 2018;71(2):177–92.

Cholesteryl Ester Transfer Protein Inhibitors as Agents to Reduce Coronary Heart Disease Risk

Philip J. Barter, MBBS, PhD, FRACP*, Kerry-Anne Rye, PhD

KEYWORDS

- Cholesteryl ester transfer protein • Inhibitor • High density lipoprotein
- Atherosclerotic cardiovascular disease • Clinical trial

KEY POINTS

- Cholesteryl ester transfer protein (CETP) promotes a net mass transfer of cholesteryl esters from the nonatherogenic high density lipoprotein (HDL) fraction to the potentially proatherogenic non-HDL fractions.
- Inhibition of CETP in rabbits is antiatherogenic.
- A genetic deficiency of CETP in people results in a reduced risk of having an atherosclerotic cardiovascular event.
- Inhibition of CETP in people reduces the risk of having a coronary event.
- Inhibition of CETP in people has the potential to prevent statin-induced new-onset diabetes.

INTRODUCTION

Results of the REVEAL trial[1] establish that inhibition of the cholesteryl ester transfer protein (CETP) by treatment with anacetrapib reduces the risk of having a coronary event in high-risk, statin-treated patients. This result contrasts with an absence of benefit (or even harm) observed in previous human clinical outcome trials of small molecule CETP inhibitors.[2–4]

This article addresses several key issues related to CETP and its inhibition, including

- What is CETP, and what does it do?
- Effects of CETP on plasma lipoproteins
- Impact of CETP activity on atherosclerotic cardiovascular disease (ASCVD)
- Effect of CETP inhibitors in human clinical trials

- Conflicting results in human clinical outcome trials of CETP inhibitors
- Effect of CETP inhibition on the risk of new onset diabetes

WHAT IS CHOLESTERYL ESTER TRANSFER PROTEIN, AND WHAT DOES IT DO?

CETP promotes a net mass transfer of cholesteryl esters from the nonatherogenic high density lipoprotein (HDL) fraction to the potentially proatherogenic non-HDL fractions.

The presence in human plasma of CETP was first reported in 1978.[5] CETP has since been characterized as an hydrophobic glycoprotein[6] that is synthesized mainly in the liver.[7,8] Activity of CETP varies widely between different species,[9] being present in people, nonhuman primates,

Disclosure Statement: P.J. Barter has received a research grant from Pfizer. He has also received honoraria received from Amgen, AstraZeneca, Merck, Pfizer and Sanofi, and Regeneron. Additionally, he is a member of the advisory boards for Amgen, Merck, Pfizer and Sanofi, and Regeneron. K-A. Rye has received a research grant from Merck, as well as honoraria from CSL Behring.
School of Medical Sciences, University of New South Wales, Sydney, New South Wales 2052, Australia
* Corresponding author.
E-mail addresses: pbarter@ozemail.com.au; p.barter@unsw.edu.au

Cardiol Clin 36 (2018) 299–310
https://doi.org/10.1016/j.ccl.2017.12.011
0733-8651/18/© 2017 Elsevier Inc. All rights reserved.

rabbits, and hamsters but absent in most other species, including rodents, the animals used most commonly in studies of atherosclerosis.

CETP promotes bidirectional transfers and thus an equilibration of neutral lipids (cholesteryl esters and triglyceride) between plasma lipoprotein particles.[10,11] Two models have been proposed to account for these transfers (**Fig. 1**). One is a shuttle model,[12–14] in which CETP binds transiently to a lipoprotein particle, during which there is an exchange of neutral lipids (cholesteryl esters and triglyceride) between CETP and the lipoprotein. CETP and its neutral lipid cargo then dissociates from the lipoprotein before binding transiently to and exchanging neutral lipids with another lipoprotein particle. Multiple interactions of CETP with lipoprotein particles result ultimately in the equilibration of neutral lipids between all lipoproteins in plasma. The second proposed model is a tunnel model, in which CETP forms a bridge between 2 lipoprotein particles[15,16] with neutral lipids exchanging between the lipoproteins through a tunnel in the CETP molecule. The end result of the tunnel model is again an equilibration of neutral lipids between all plasma lipoproteins. It is probable that both models operate in human plasma, although the relative contribution of the 2 mechanisms is not known.

Most of the cholesteryl esters in plasma are generated in HDLs as a product of the reaction catalyzed by lecithin:cholesterol acyltransferase (LCAT), while the majority of plasma triglyceride enters the circulation as a component of the triglyceride-rich chylomicrons and very low density lipoproteins (VLDLs). Thus, the CETP-mediated equilibration of these neutral lipids between plasma lipoproteins results in a net mass transfer of cholesteryl esters from the HDL fraction to the non-HDL fractions and of triglyceride from non-HDLs to HDLs (**Fig. 2**).

EFFECTS OF CHOLESTERYL ESTER TRANSFER PROTEIN ON PLASMA LIPOPROTEINS

Evidence that CETP impacts on plasma lipoproteins in people is provided by observations in people with a genetic deficiency of CETP.[17–21] Such people have increased levels of HDL cholesterol and apoA-I (the major HDL apolipoprotein) and decreased concentrations of non-HDL cholesterol

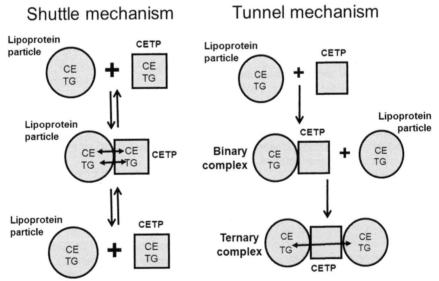

Fig. 1. Mechanism of action of CETP. Shuttle model. CETP in plasma collides randomly with particles in all lipoprotein fractions to form transient complexes that facilitate an exchange of both cholesteryl esters (CEs) and triglyceride (TG) between the lipoprotein particles and the CETP molecules. CETP subsequently dissociates from the lipoprotein particle to circulate in plasma in a free state until it collides with another lipoprotein particle (either in the same or in a different lipoprotein fraction) to form a new transient complex with further exchange of CE and TG between lipoprotein particle and CETP molecule. In this way, CETP promotes an equilibration of both CE and TG between all lipoprotein particles. Tunnel model. CETP in plasma collides randomly a lipoprotein particle to form a binary complex. This binary complex then collides with another lipoprotein particle to form a ternary complex. A tunnel in the CETP molecule then enables an exchange of both CEs and TG between the lipoprotein particles contained in the ternary complex. The ternary complex then dissociates to release the lipoprotein particles and the CETP molecule to repeat the process. The end result is an equilibration of both CEs and TG between all lipoprotein particles as occurs with the shuttle model.

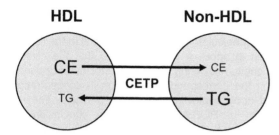

Fig. 2. Net effect of activity of CETP. Because most of the CEs in plasma originate in HDLs in the LCAT reaction, and the majority of the TG in plasma enters plasma as a component of non-HDL particles, the net effect of the equilibration promoted by CETP is a net mass transfer of CEs from HDLs to non-HDLs and of TG from non-HDLs to HDLs.

and apoB (the major protein component of the non-HDL fractions). Studies using CETP inhibitors in people have confirmed the conclusions drawn from the genetic studies.

Inhibition of CETP leads to retention of cholesteryl esters in HDL particles where they are synthesized by LCAT. This increases the HDL core volume, which is accompanied by a compensatory increase in HDL surface constituents, including apoA-I.

A reduction in the level of non-HDL cholesterol is the consequence not only of the reduced transfer of cholesteryl esters from HDLs but also to an up-regulation of the LDL receptor and a consequent enhanced rate of removal of non-HDL particles from plasma.[22,23] The mechanism by which CETP inhibition up-regulates the LDL receptor is not known but may relate to an increase in the efflux of cholesterol from cells to HDLs,[24,25] resulting in a transient depletion of cell cholesterol, which increases synthesis of the LDL receptor. Regardless of the mechanism, an enhanced removal of non-HDL particles from plasma explains why CETP inhibition not only reduces the concentration of non-HDL cholesterol but also reduces the concentration of apoB. Because there is 1 molecule of apoB per particle in the non-HDL fractions, the CETP inhibitor-mediated reduction in apoB levels indicates that CETP inhibition also reduces in the number of non-HDL particles.

Inhibiting activity of CETP has potentially beneficial effects beyond the observed changes in lipid and lipoprotein concentrations. For example, in studies conducted in vivo, inhibition of CETP reduces intimal thickening and regenerates functional endothelium in the damaged aortas of rabbits.[26] Inhibition of CETP also results in increased collateral blood vessel formation in rabbits with hind-limb ischemia.[27] In human studies

conducted ex vivo, HDLs isolated from patients treated with a CETP inhibitor have an enhanced ability to promote the efflux of cholesterol from macrophages.[24,25]

CETP also plays a role in the remodeling of HDLs in plasma. CETP mediates the transfer of cholesteryl esters from HDLs to triglyceride-rich lipoproteins (TRLs) and the transfer of triglyceride from TRLs to HDLs. This results in the formation of HDL particles that are depleted of cholesteryl esters and enriched in triglyceride. Subsequent activity of hepatic lipase hydrolyses the HDL triglycerides, resulting in HDL particles that are depleted of cholesteryl esters and no longer enriched in triglycerides. This loss of core lipids is accompanied by a reduction in HDL particle size.[28]

IMPACT OF CHOLESTERYL ESTER TRANSFER PROTEIN ACTIVITY ON ATHEROSCLEROTIC CARDIOVASCULAR DISEASE
Studies in Animals

Rodents lack activity of CETP and are naturally resistant to the development of atherosclerosis. Transgenic expression of the *CETP* gene in mice and rats has, in most studies, resulted in an increased susceptibility to the development of atherosclerosis. This has been observed in mice fed an atherogenic diet,[29] in apoE knock-out mice,[30] in LDL receptor knock-out mice,[30] in apoE3-Leiden mice,[31] and in hypertensive rats.[32] However, in a study of SR-B1 knockout mice, expression of CETP had no effect on atherosclerosis.[33] In studies of some mouse models, expression of the *CETP* gene has an antiatherogenic rather than a proatherogenic effect. These include studies in *db/db* mice,[34] in LCAT transgenic mice,[35] in ovariectomized mice,[36] in testosterone-deficient mice,[37] and in apoC-III transgenic mice with hypertriglyceridemia.[38] In the last study, however, it was also reported that expression of the *CETP* gene was proatherogenic in normotriglyceridemic mice.[38] So, the results in rodents appear to be model dependent.

In contrast to mice, rabbits have a high level of CETP activity[9] and are extremely susceptible to the development of diet-induced atherosclerosis. Inhibiting CETP in rabbits, whether by the use of antisense oligodeoxynucleotides,[39] by an anti-CETP vaccine[40] or by administration of small-molecule CETP inhibitors,[41,42] inhibits development of atherosclerosis. There is no evidence in any rabbit study that atherosclerosis is increased when CETP is inhibited. The studies in rabbits provide strong support for the hypothesis that CETP inhibition is antiatherogenic.

Genetic Studies in People

Results of small genetic studies in people have been conflicting and confusing and have been consistent with CETP being both proatherogenic and antiatherogenic. The results of larger genetic studies, however, have been consistent and have led to the conclusion that CETP is proatherogenic and that its inhibition is potentially antiatherogenic.

In a large meta-analysis of 92 studies involving 113,833 participants, it was concluded that CETP gene polymorphisms that are associated with decreased CETP activity and mass are accompanied by an elevated concentration of HDL cholesterol, a lower concentration of LDL cholesterol, and a significantly decreased risk of having a coronary event.[43] A similar conclusion was drawn from analysis of a cohort of 18,245 healthy Americans in the Women's Genome Health Study.[44] This conclusion was further supported in another meta-analysis in which a common variation of the CETP gene was accompanied by higher levels of HDL cholesterol, lower levels of LDL cholesterol, and a reduced risk of myocardial infarction, comparable to that reported in the earlier meta-analysis.[45]

Perhaps the most compelling genetic evidence suggesting that activity of CETP may be proatherogenic is provided by the Copenhagen City Heart Study[46] and by a study of the effect of protein-truncating variants at the CETP gene.[47] In the Copenhagen City Heart Study, 10,261 people were followed for up to 34 years.[46] More than 3000 of these people had a cardiovascular event, and 3807 people died. In this study, 2 common CETP gene polymorphisms known to be associated with low CETP activity were associated with significant reductions in the risk of ischemic heart disease, myocardial infarction, ischemic cerebrovascular disease, and ischemic stroke. People with these polymorphisms also had increased longevity, with no evidence of adverse effects.

In a study of protein-truncating variants in the CETP gene, it was found that the HDL cholesterol level was 22.6 mg/dL higher, and the LDL cholesterol level was 12.2 mg/dL lower than in those without the variants. These lipoprotein changes were accompanied by a significant 30% lower risk of having a coronary event.[47]

Another genetic study investigated the association between changes in levels of LDL cholesterol and the risk of cardiovascular events related to variants in the CETP gene and the 3-hydroxy-3-methylglutaryl-CoA reductase (HMGCR) gene.[48] It was found that in people who had the combination of variants in the CETP gene and the HMGCR gene (the target of statins), there were discordant reductions in levels of LDL cholesterol and apoB. The reduction in risk of cardiovascular events was significantly less than expected per unit change in LDL cholesterol but was proportional to the reduction in apoB. It was concluded that the clinical benefit of lowering LDL cholesterol levels depends on the corresponding reduction in concentration of apoB-containing lipoprotein particles. The results of REVEAL[1] support this conclusion by showing that when activity of CETP is reduced there are problems with assaying LDL cholesterol levels. Under such conditions, levels of apoB and non-HDL cholesterol (rather than LDL cholesterol) provide a more reliable measure of the concentration of atherogenic lipoproteins.

Collectively, these human genetic studies provide strong support for the proposition that CETP inhibition will be antiatherogenic.

EFFECT OF CHOLESTERYL ESTER TRANSFER PROTEIN INHIBITORS IN HUMAN CLINICAL TRIALS

Five CETP inhibitors have been investigated in humans. These include torcetrapib, dalcetrapib, evacetrapib, anacetrapib and TA-8995 (also known as AMG-8995). The precise mechanism of action of these inhibitors is uncertain. All but TA-8995 have been investigated in large, randomized, double-blind, cardiovascular clinical outcome trials.

Torcetrapib

Treatment with torcetrapib increased the concentration of HDL cholesterol and apoA-I by 70% and 25%, respectively, and decreased levels of LDL cholesterol and apoB by 25% and 12.5%, respectively.[2] The effect of torcetrapib on atherosclerosis in people was investigated in 3 imaging trials. ILLUSTRATE[49] used intravascular ultrasound (IVUS) to assess the effect of torcetrapib on coronary atheroma burden, while RADIANCE 1[50] and RADIANCE 2[51] used B-mode ultrasound to assess the effects of torcetrapib on carotid intima-media thickness. Treatment with torcetrapib had no effect (positive or negative) on either atheroma burden in the coronary arteries or on carotid artery intima-media thickness in these studies.

The effect of torcetrapib on clinical cardiovascular events was also investigated. The ILLUMINATE trial[2] (Fig. 3) included 15,067 people with manifest cardiovascular disease or type-2 diabetes. All participants received effective doses of atorvastatin. Torcetrapib increased HDL cholesterol levels by 72% and decreased LDL cholesterol levels by 25%. This trial was terminated after 18 months because of a statistically significant excess of deaths (93 vs 59) in the participants treated with

ILLUMINATE Trial

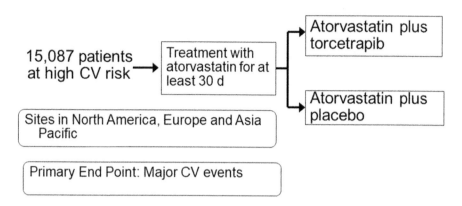

15,087 patients at high CV risk → Treatment with atorvastatin for at least 30 d → Atorvastatin plus torcetrapib

Atorvastatin plus placebo

Sites in North America, Europe and Asia Pacific

Primary End Point: Major CV events

Trial terminated early after median follow-up of 18 mo because of a significant increase in both mortality and CV events in torcetrapib-treated participants

Fig. 3. Design of the ILLUMINATE trial with torcetrapib.

torcetrapib.[2] No single cause of death explained the harm caused by torcetrapib. There was also a statistically significant 25% increase in ASCVD events in those taking torcetrapib.

The explanation for the harm caused by torcetrapib is not known, but may relate to off-target effects of the drug that are unrelated to CETP inhibition. However, there was also circumstantial evidence that the increase in HDL cholesterol may have reduced the adverse effects of torcetrapib in the ILLUMINATE trial. In a post-hoc analysis of the group treated with torcetrapib, the level of HDL cholesterol achieved in the torcetrapib-treated patients was an inverse predictor of events.[52] Furthermore, in a post-hoc analysis of the ILLUSTRATE trial, there was significant regression of coronary atheroma in the torcetrapib-treated patients who achieved the highest on-treatment level of HDL cholesterol.[53]

Dalcetrapib

Dalcetrapib is a weak CETP inhibitor that decreases CETP activity by 30% to 50% and increases the concentration of HDL cholesterol by up to 30%, with little effect on the level of LDL cholesterol or any other atherogenic lipoproteins. Treatment with dalcetrapib had no effect on human atherosclerotic plaques[54] and did not improve endothelial function.[55]

The effect of dalcetrapib on clinical ASCVD events was investigated in the dal-OUTCOMES study[3] (**Fig. 4**), which included 15,871 participants

who were recruited soon after an acute coronary syndrome (ACS) event. Treatment with dalcetrapib in this trial increased the concentration of HDL cholesterol by about 30% and the concentration of apoA-I by 9% but had a minimal effect on the levels of LDL cholesterol and apoB. At the second prespecified interim analysis conducted after a median follow-up period of 31 months, the independent data and safety monitoring board recommended termination of the trial for futility. It was concluded that treatment with dalcetrapib neither reduced ASCVD events nor caused harm.[3]

In an interesting genetic study of the dal-OUTCOMES trial, it was reported that effects of dalcetrapib on cardiovascular outcomes were influenced by a polymorphism in the *ADCY9* (adenylate cyclase type 9) gene (rs1967309). Patients with the AA genotype had a significant 39% reduction in cardiovascular events when treated with dalcetrapib compared with a 27% increase in events in those with the GG genotype.[56] Whether an impact of polymorphisms in the *ADCY9* gene is also apparent with other CETP inhibitors is currently not known. A clinical outcome trial of treatment with dalcetrapib in people with the AA genotype is currently under way.

Evacetrapib

Evacetrapib is a CETP inhibitor that appears to have none of the serious adverse effects of torcetrapib.[4] It was reported to reduce the level of LDL cholesterol by about 30% over and above that

dal-OUTCOMES Trial

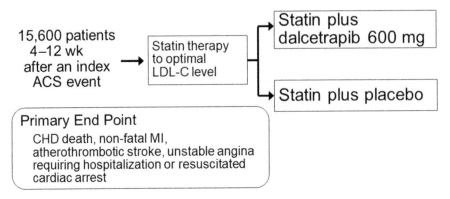

Fig. 4. Design of the Dal-OUTCOMES trial with dalcetrapib.

achieved by a statin and to double the concentration of HDL cholesterol.[4]

The effect of evacetrapib on ASCVD events was evaluated in the Assessment of Clinical Effects of Cholesteryl Ester Transfer Protein Inhibition With Evacetrapib (ACCELERATE) trial[4] (**Fig. 5**). Approximately 12,500 high-risk, statin-treated patients were randomized to receive evacetrapib or placebo with a planned follow-up of about 3 years. However, the study was terminated after just over 2 years when it became apparent that there could not be a positive outcome even if the trial had continued for its planned 3-year follow-up.

There was no evidence that evacetrapib caused harm, but also, despite a significant reduction in concentrations of LDL cholesterol and apoB and a substantial increase in concentrations of HDL cholesterol and apoA-I, there was no reduction in ASCVD events.[4]

Anacetrapib

Like dalcetrapib and evacetrapib, anacetrapib is a CETP inhibitor that appears not to have the serious adverse effects observed with torcetrapib. Its effects on plasma lipoproteins are similar to those

ACCELERATE trial

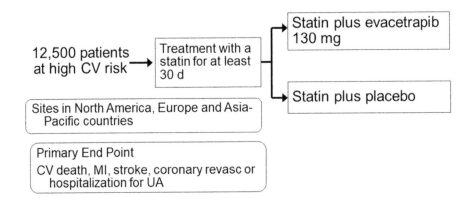

Fig. 5. Design of the ACCELERATE trial with evacetrapib.

induced by evacetrapib. The safety and lipid efficacy of anacetrapib were investigated in the DEFINE trial.[57]

DEFINE was a randomized, double-blind, placebo-controlled, 18-month trial in patients (n = 1623) with manifest coronary heart disease or at high risk of developing coronary heart disease[57] (**Fig. 6**). All participants were taking a statin to achieve optimal levels of LDL cholesterol prior to being randomized to receive anacetrapib (100 mg/d) or placebo. Anacetrapib decreased the level of LDL cholesterol from 81 mg/dL to 45 mg/dL, an apparent 40% reduction compared with that seen with the placebo, although the use of the Friedwald equation to assay LDL cholesterol in this study may have resulted in an overestimation of the true reduction that was probably closer to 30%. The concentration of non-HDL cholesterol was reduced by 32%, and that of apoB was reduced by 21%. Treatment with anacetrapib increased HDL cholesterol levels from 41 mg/dL at baseline to 101 mg/dL in the anacetrapib group (an increase of 138% beyond that seen with placebo) and increased levels of apoA-I by 45%. Treatment with anacetrapib had no observable effect on blood pressure or on levels of electrolytes or aldosterone, effects that had been seen in people treated with torcetrapib. Prespecified, adjudicated cardiovascular events occurred in 16 patients treated with anacetrapib (2.0%) and 21 patients receiving placebo (2.6%) (P = .40). Significantly fewer patients in the anacetrapib group than in the placebo group underwent revascularization (8 vs 28, P = .001).[57] The prespecified Bayesian analysis indicated that this event distribution provided a predictive probability of 94% that anacetrapib would not be associated with the increase in cardiovascular events that was seen with torcetrapib in the ILLUMINATE trial. It was concluded that treatment with anacetrapib had robust, favorable effects on plasma lipoprotein levels, an acceptable safety profile, and, within the limits of the power of the study, it did not result in the adverse cardiovascular effects observed with torcetrapib.

In a long-term follow-up of participants in the DEFINE trial, it was found that anacetrapib had accumulated in adipose tissue and remained detectable in the body for 2 years or more after receiving the last dose of the drug.[58] There was no evidence, however, that this retention of anacetrapib was associated with any adverse effects.

The results of DEFINE provided the basis for proceeding with a study to test the hypothesis that anacetrapib-induced inhibition of CETP in people will inhibit development of atherosclerosis and reduce the risk of having a cardiovascular event. The validity of this hypothesis has now been substantiated by the results of REVEAL.[1]

The REVEAL trial included 30,449 adults with atherosclerotic vascular disease[1] (**Fig. 7**). Baseline cholesterol levels on intensive atorvastatin therapy were mean LDL cholesterol 61 mg/dL (1.58 mmol/L), mean nonHDL cholesterol 92 mg/dL (2.38 mmol/L), and mean HDL cholesterol 40 mg/dL (1.03 mmol/L). After a run-in period on atorvastatin, participants were continued on atorvastatin and randomly assigned to receive anacetrapib 100 mg daily or placebo in a double-blind design. The primary endpoint was major coronary events, defined as coronary death, myocardial infarction, or coronary revascularization. The median follow-up was 4.1 years.

DEFINE trial

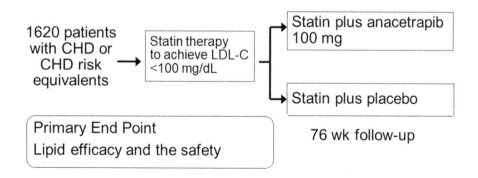

Lipid efficacy confirmed; no safety issues

Fig. 6. Design of the DEFINE trial with anacetrapib.

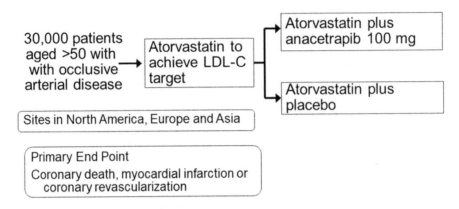

REVEAL trial

30,000 patients aged >50 with with occlusive arterial disease → Atorvastatin to achieve LDL-C target → Atorvastatin plus anacetrapib 100 mg / Atorvastatin plus placebo

Sites in North America, Europe and Asia

Primary End Point
Coronary death, myocardial infarction or coronary revascularization

Median follow-up of 4.1 y

Significant reduction in coronary events; no harm

Fig. 7. Design of the REVEAL trial with anacetrapib.

Compared with placebo, anacetrapib reduced non-HDL cholesterol level by 17 mg/dL (0.43 mmol/L, 17%) and increased HDL cholesterol level by 43 mg/dL (1.11 mmol/L, 104%).[1] Treatment with anacetrapib reduced the number of patients who had a major coronary event by 9% (P = .004). There was no apparent effect on the risk of having an ischemic stroke. Compared with placebo, treatment with anacetrapib had no significant effects on mortality or cancer and did not result in any other serious adverse events.

As has been observed with other CETP inhibitors,[2,4] treatment with anacetrapib was accompanied by in a small increase in both systolic (0.7 mm Hg) and diastolic (0.3 mm Hg) blood pressure.[1] There was no evidence, however, of any blood pressure-related adverse effects resulting from treatment with anacetrapib.[1]

In REVEAL, there was virtually no effect of anacetrapib treatment on coronary events during the first 2 years of the trial.[1] However, in years 3 and 4 of treatment with anacetrapib, there was a reduction in the primary endpoint of about 14%. In the period beyond 4 years, there was a statistically significant 17% reduction in the primary endpoint. The observed delay in clinical outcome benefit, with no effect in the first 2 years of treatment, raises the possibility that a reduction in coronary events may have been even greater had the trial continued for 5 or 6 years, as in most of the early statin trials.

There were several prespecified subgroups investigated in REVEAL. Although there was no evidence of statistically significant heterogeneity in any of the subgroups, there was a trend toward a greater reductions in the primary endpoint in those with higher baseline levels of both LDL and non-HDL cholesterol. There was a statistically significant 17% reduction in the primary endpoint in those whose baseline non-HDL cholesterol levels were greater than 101 mg/dL.[1]

There was evidence that the assay of LDL cholesterol in those treated with anacetrapib was influenced by the assay method used. As a consequence, it was decided that LDL cholesterol levels in anacetrapib-treated people cannot be reliably determined and that non-HDL-cholesterol and apoB levels (that are not assay dependent) should be used.

The observed reduction of 9.1% in the primary endpoint accompanied by a 17 mg/dL reduction in non-HDL cholesterol[1] was greater than predicted from the results of the IMPROVE-IT trial with ezetimibe in which a reduction in non-HDL cholesterol of 20 mg/dL was accompanied by a 6.1% reduction in risk of having a major cardiovascular event.[59] Whether this result in REVEAL reflects a benefit beyond the reduction in non-HDL cholesterol remains to be determined. The only conclusion that can be drawn with confidence is that anacetrapib-induced inhibition of CETP reduces the risk of having a coronary event in people who are well-treated with a statin. Whether reduced coronary risk is related to a reduction in non-HDL cholesterol, an increase in HDL, or a combination of the two will be the subject of much debate but cannot be determined from this trial.

One issue of possible concern with anacetrapib relates to its long-term retention in the body after treatment has been terminated. Its accumulation in adipose tissue with slow release into plasma explains why there is an effect on plasma lipoproteins that persists for up to 2 years after cessation of treatment.[58] It will be important to follow REVEAL participants after the trial to monitor not only potential benefits, but also whether any adverse effects of the treatment emerge after therapy has been terminated.

TA-8995 (AMG-8995)

The most recently reported CETP inhibitor is TA-8995 (also known as AMG-8995). Its safety and tolerability were assessed in a 12-week randomized, double-blind, placebo-controlled trial in patients with baseline LDL cholesterol levels between 2·5 mmol/L and 4·5 mmol/L, HDL cholesterol levels between 0·8 and 1·8 mmol/L, and triglyceride levels below 4·5 mmol/L (ClinicalTrials. gov, number NCT01970215).[60] Treatment with TA8995 reduced LDL cholesterol levels by up to 45% whether given alone or on top of a statin, and increased HDL cholesterol levels by up to 180%. No serious adverse events were observed.[60] A cardiovascular clinical outcome trial will be needed to determine whether these effects will translate into a reduction of ASCVD events.

REASONS FOR THE CONFLICTING RESULTS IN HUMAN CLINICAL OUTCOME TRIALS OF CHOLESTERYL ESTER TRANSFER PROTEIN INHIBITORS
Harm Caused by Torcetrapib

Studies conducted after the ILLUMINATE trial was terminated found that torcetrapib had several serious off-target adverse effects. These included an increase in blood pressure[2]; synthesis, secretion, and the plasma level of aldosterone[61,62]; and in endothelin-1.[63] These off-target effects meant that the hypothesis that CETP inhibition reduces ASCVD risk could not be tested in the ILLUMINATE trial.

No Reduction in Cardiovascular Events with Dalcetrapib

The reason for an absence of any beneficial effect of dalcetrapib in the dal-OUTCOMES trial is not known. It is possible that the neutral result reflected an absence of a reduction in the level of non-HDL cholesterol in the participants in the dal-cetrapib arm of the study.[3] Another possibility is that CETP inhibition is not effective in patients treated soon after an ACS event. This is supported by reports of an impairment of some of the cardioprotective functions of HDLs isolated from patients after an ACS event,[64] and by the unexpected observation in dal-OUTCOMES that the level of HDL cholesterol in the placebo group did not predict the risk of having a cardiovascular event.[3] The latter result is in conflict with multiple human population studies that show an inverse relationship between HDL cholesterol and CV events. So, with hindsight, it is possible that, in the absence of a reduction in the levels of LDL cholesterol or apoB and in the presence of a possibly dysfunctional HDL fraction, the lack of any effect on ASCVD events in dal-OUTCOMES may have been predictable. Another possible explanation for the absence of cardiovascular benefit in dal-OUTCOMES is that the median follow-up of 31 months[3] may have been insufficient to detect a reduction in ASCVD events.

No Reduction in Cardiovascular Events with Evacetrapib

The reason for the failure of evacetrapib to reduce ASCVD events is uncertain, but it may simply have been that the trial was too short to detect benefit. Indeed, in several of the early statin trials conducted in people with existing ASCVD, the benefits of treatment were not apparent until treatment had been continued for more than 2 years.[65] This was also the case in the REVEAL trial.[1] If REVEAL had terminated at the same time as ACCELERATE, the conclusion would have been the same as that drawn from ACCELERATE.

EFFECT OF CHOLESTERYL ESTER TRANSFER PROTEIN INHIBITION ON THE RISK OF DEVELOPING DIABETES

The observation that CETP inhibition improves glycemic control[66] and reduces the risk of developing type 2 diabetes[1] in statin-treated patients is of potentially major importance. Treatment with statins for 4 years is known to be associated with a 9% increase in the risk for developing type 2 diabetes.[67] Although this risk of statin-induced diabetes is low in absolute terms, and very low when compared with the statin-induced reduction in coronary events in people with diabetes, this observation has led to concern among many physicians and patients and has impacted both on decisions to initiate statin therapy and to ensure continued adherence to therapy in many already taking a statin. The addition of a CETP inhibitor to a statin has the potential not only to further reduce the risk of having a coronary event but also to neutralize the statin-induced increase in new onset diabetes.

The mechanism by which CETP inhibition exerts an antidiabetic effect is not known but may relate to the increase in concentration of HDLs and apoA-I.

There is evidence that HDLs enhance the uptake of glucose by skeletal muscle[68] and also stimulate the synthesis and secretion of insulin from pancreatic beta cells.[69]

SUMMARY

In conclusion, inhibition of CETP reduces the concentration of non-HDL cholesterol and the number of non-HDL particles, enhances HDL functionality, and increases the concentration of HDL cholesterol and apoA-I. Despite an absence of benefit in earlier trials of CETP inhibition, the REVEAL trial has now shown that treatment with the CETP inhibitor, anacetrapib, reduces the risk of having a coronary event in high-risk, statin-treated patients. The mechanism by which CETP inhibition reduces coronary events is currently uncertain. The role of CETP inhibition in clinical practice remains to be determined, although it may have an important place in those at risk of developing diabetes.

REFERENCES

1. The HPS3/TIMI55–REVEAL Collaborative Group. Effects of anacetrapib in patients with atherosclerotic vascular disease. N Engl J Med 2017;377(13): 1217–27.
2. Barter PJ, Caulfield M, Eriksson M, et al. Effects of torcetrapib in patients at high risk for coronary events. N Engl J Med 2007;357(21):2109–22.
3. Schwartz GG, Olsson AG, Abt M, et al. Effects of dalcetrapib in patients with a recent acute coronary syndrome. N Engl J Med 2012;367(22):2089–99.
4. Lincoff AM, Nicholls SJ, Riesmeyer JS, et al. Evacetrapib and cardiovascular outcomes in high-risk vascular disease. N Engl J Med 2017;376(20):1933–42.
5. Barter PJ, Lally JI. The activity of an esterified cholesterol transferring factor in human and rat serum. Biochim Biophys Acta 1978;531(2):233–6.
6. Hesler CB, Swenson TL, Tall AR. Purification and characterization of a human plasma cholesteryl ester transfer protein. J Biol Chem 1987;262(5): 2275–82.
7. Drayna D, Jarnagin AS, McLean J, et al. Cloning and sequencing of human cholesteryl ester transfer protein cDNA. Nature 1987;327(6123):632–4.
8. Jiang XC, Moulin P, Quinet E, et al. Mammalian adipose tissue and muscle are major sources of lipid transfer protein mRNA. J Biol Chem 1991;266(7):4631–9.
9. Ha YC, Barter PJ. Differences in plasma cholesteryl ester transfer activity in sixteen vertebrate species. Comp Biochem Physiol B 1982;71(2):265–9.
10. Barter PJ, Jones ME. Kinetic studies of the transfer of esterified cholesterol between human plasma low and high density lipoproteins. J Lipid Res 1980;21(2):238–49.
11. Barter PJ, Rye KA. Cholesteryl ester transfer protein inhibition as a strategy to reduce cardiovascular risk. J Lipid Res 2012;53(9):1755–66.
12. Barter PJ, Hopkins GJ, Calvert GD. Transfers and exchanges of esterified cholesterol between plasma lipoproteins. Biochem J 1982;208(1):1–7.
13. Swenson TL, Brocia RW, Tall AR. Plasma cholesteryl ester transfer protein has binding sites for neutral lipids and phospholipids. J Biol Chem 1988; 263(11):5150–7.
14. Tall AR. Plasma cholesteryl ester transfer protein. J Lipid Res 1993;34(8):1255–74.
15. Ihm J, Quinn DM, Busch SJ, et al. Kinetics of plasma protein-catalyzed exchange of phosphatidylcholine and cholesteryl ester between plasma lipoproteins. J Lipid Res 1982;23(9):1328–41.
16. Zhang L, Yan F, Zhang S, et al. Structural basis of transfer between lipoproteins by cholesteryl ester transfer protein. Nat Chem Biol 2012;8(4):342–9.
17. Maruyama T, Sakai N, Ishigami M, et al. Prevalence and phenotypic spectrum of cholesteryl ester transfer protein gene mutations in Japanese hyperalphalipoproteinemia. Atherosclerosis 2003;166(1):177–85.
18. Brown ML, Inazu A, Hesler CB, et al. Molecular basis of lipid transfer protein deficiency in a family with increased high-density lipoproteins. Nature 1989; 342(6248):448–51.
19. Nagano M, Yamashita S, Hirano K, et al. Two novel missense mutations in the CETP gene in Japanese hyperalphalipoproteinemic subjects: high-throughput assay by Invader assay. J Lipid Res 2002;43(7): 1011–8.
20. Ritsch A, Drexel H, Amann FW, et al. Deficiency of cholesteryl ester transfer protein. Description of the molecular defect and the dissociation of cholesteryl ester and triglyceride transport in plasma. Arterioscler Thromb Vasc Biol 1997;17(12):3433–41.
21. Teh EM, Dolphin PJ, Breckenridge WC, et al. Human plasma CETP deficiency: identification of a novel mutation in exon 9 of the CETP gene in a Caucasian subject from North America. J Lipid Res 1998;39(2): 442–56.
22. Millar JS, Brousseau ME, Diffenderfer MR, et al. Effects of the cholesteryl ester transfer protein inhibitor torcetrapib on apolipoprotein B100 metabolism in humans. Arterioscler Thromb Vasc Biol 2006;26(6): 1350–6.
23. Millar JS, Reyes-Soffer G, Jumes P, et al. Anacetrapib lowers LDL by increasing ApoB clearance in mildly hypercholesterolemic subjects. J Clin Invest 2015;125(6):2510–22.
24. Nicholls SJ, Ruotolo G, Brewer HB, et al. Cholesterol efflux capacity and pre-beta-1 HDL concentrations

are increased in dyslipidemic patients treated with evacetrapib. J Am Coll Cardiol 2015;66(20):2201–10.

25. Yvan-Charvet L, Matsuura F, Wang N, et al. Inhibition of cholesteryl ester transfer protein by torcetrapib modestly increases macrophage cholesterol efflux to HDL. Arterioscler Thromb Vasc Biol 2007;27(5):1132–8.

26. Wu BJ, Shrestha S, Ong KL, et al. Cholesteryl ester transfer protein inhibition enhances endothelial repair and improves endothelial function in the rabbit. Arterioscler Thromb Vasc Biol 2015;35(3):628–36.

27. Wu BJ, Shrestha S, Ong KL, et al. Increasing HDL levels by inhibiting cholesteryl ester transfer protein activity in rabbits with hindlimb ischemia is associated with increased angiogenesis. Int J Cardiol 2015;199:204–12.

28. Rye KA, Bursill CA, Lambert G, et al. The metabolism and anti-atherogenic properties of HDL. J Lipid Res 2009;50(Suppl):S195–200.

29. Marotti KR, Castle CK, Boyle TP, et al. Severe atherosclerosis in transgenic mice expressing simian cholesteryl ester transfer protein. Nature 1993; 364(6432):73–5.

30. Plump AS, Masucci-Magoulas L, Bruce C, et al. Increased atherosclerosis in ApoE and LDL receptor gene knock-out mice as a result of human cholesteryl ester transfer protein transgene expression. Arterioscler Thromb Vasc Biol 1999;19(4):1105–10.

31. Westerterp M, van der Hoogt CC, de Haan W, et al. Cholesteryl ester transfer protein decreases high-density lipoprotein and severely aggravates atherosclerosis in APOE*3-Leiden mice. Arterioscler Thromb Vasc Biol 2006;26(11):2552–9.

32. Herrera VL, Makrides SC, Xie HX, et al. Spontaneous combined hyperlipidemia, coronary heart disease and decreased survival in Dahl salt-sensitive hypertensive rats transgenic for human cholesteryl ester transfer protein. Nat Med 1999;5(12):1383–9.

33. Hildebrand RB, Lammers B, Meurs I, et al. Restoration of high-density lipoprotein levels by cholesteryl ester transfer protein expression in scavenger receptor class B type I (SR-BI) knockout mice does not normalize pathologies associated with SR-BI deficiency. Arterioscler Thromb Vasc Biol 2010; 30(7):1439–45.

34. MacLean PS, Bower JF, Vadlamudi S, et al. Cholesteryl ester transfer protein expression prevents diet-induced atherosclerotic lesions in male db/db mice. Arterioscler Thromb Vasc Biol 2003;23(8):1412–5.

35. Foger B, Chase M, Amar MJ, et al. Cholesteryl ester transfer protein corrects dysfunctional high density lipoproteins and reduces aortic atherosclerosis in lecithin cholesterol acyltransferase transgenic mice. J Biol Chem 1999;274(52):36912–20.

36. Cazita PM, Berti JA, Aoki C, et al. Cholesteryl ester transfer protein expression attenuates atherosclerosis in ovariectomized mice. J Lipid Res 2003; 44(1):33–40.

37. Casquero AC, Berti JA, Salerno AG, et al. Atherosclerosis is enhanced by testosterone deficiency and attenuated by CETP expression in transgenic mice. J Lipid Res 2006;47(7):1526–34.

38. Hayek T, Masucci-Magoulas L, Jiang X, et al. Decreased early atherosclerotic lesions in hypertriglyceridemic mice expressing cholesteryl ester transfer protein transgene. J Clin Invest 1995; 96(4):2071–4.

39. Sugano M, Makino N, Sawada S, et al. Effect of antisense oligonucleotides against cholesteryl ester transfer protein on the development of atherosclerosis in cholesterol-fed rabbits. J Biol Chem 1998; 273(9):5033–6.

40. Rittershaus CW, Miller DP, Thomas LJ, et al. Vaccine-induced antibodies inhibit CETP activity in vivo and reduce aortic lesions in a rabbit model of atherosclerosis. Arterioscler Thromb Vasc Biol 2000;20(9):2106–12.

41. Okamoto H, Yonemori F, Wakitani K, et al. A cholesteryl ester transfer protein inhibitor attenuates atherosclerosis in rabbits. Nature 2000; 406(6792):203–7.

42. Morehouse LA, Sugarman ED, Bourassa PA, et al. Inhibition of CETP activity by torcetrapib reduces susceptibility to diet-induced atherosclerosis in New Zealand White rabbits. J Lipid Res 2007; 48(6):1263–72.

43. Thompson A, Di Angelantonio E, Sarwar N, et al. Association of cholesteryl ester transfer protein genotypes with CETP mass and activity, lipid levels, and coronary risk. JAMA 2008;299(23):2777–88.

44. Ridker PM, Pare G, Parker AN, et al. Polymorphism in the CETP gene region, HDL cholesterol, and risk of future myocardial infarction: genomewide analysis among 18 245 initially healthy women from the Women's Genome Health Study. Circ Cardiovasc Genet 2009;2(1):26–33.

45. Voight BF, Peloso GM, Orho-Melander M, et al. Plasma HDL cholesterol and risk of myocardial infarction: a mendelian randomisation study. Lancet 2012;380(9841):572–80.

46. Johannsen TH, Frikke-Schmidt R, Schou J, et al. Genetic inhibition of CETP, ischemic vascular disease and mortality, and possible adverse effects. J Am Coll Cardiol 2012;60(20):2041–8.

47. Nomura A, Won HH, Khera AV, et al. Protein-Truncating variants at the cholesteryl ester transfer protein gene and risk for coronary heart disease. Circ Res 2017;121(1):81–8.

48. Ference BA, Kastelein JJP, Ginsberg HN, et al. Association of genetic variants related to CETP inhibitors and statins with lipoprotein levels and cardiovascular risk. JAMA 2017;318(10):947–56.

49. Nissen SE, Tardif JC, Nicholls SJ, et al. Effect of torcetrapib on the progression of coronary atherosclerosis. N Engl J Med 2007;356(13):1304–16.

50. Kastelein JJ, van Leuven SI, Burgess L, et al. Effect of torcetrapib on carotid atherosclerosis in familial hypercholesterolemia. N Engl J Med 2007;356(16):1620–30.

51. Bots ML, Visseren FL, Evans GW, et al. Torcetrapib and carotid intima-media thickness in mixed dyslipidaemia (RADIANCE 2 study): a randomised, double-blind trial. Lancet 2007;370(9582):153–60.

52. Barter P. Lessons learned from the Investigation of Lipid Level Management to Understand its Impact in Atherosclerotic Events (ILLUMINATE) trial. Am J Cardiol 2009;104(10 Suppl):10E-5E.

53. Nicholls SJ, Tuzcu EM, Brennan DM, et al. Cholesteryl ester transfer protein inhibition, high-density lipoprotein raising, and progression of coronary atherosclerosis: insights from ILLUSTRATE (Investigation of Lipid Level Management Using Coronary Ultrasound to Assess Reduction of Atherosclerosis by CETP Inhibition and HDL Elevation). Circulation 2008;118(24):2506–14.

54. Fayad ZA, Mani V, Woodward M, et al. Safety and efficacy of dalcetrapib on atherosclerotic disease using novel non-invasive multimodality imaging (dal-PLAQUE): a randomised clinical trial. Lancet 2011;378(9802):1547–59.

55. Luscher TF, Taddei S, Kaski JC, et al. Vascular effects and safety of dalcetrapib in patients with or at risk of coronary heart disease: the dal-VESSEL randomized clinical trial. Eur Heart J 2012;33(7):857–65.

56. Tardif JC, Rheaume E, Lemieux Perreault LP, et al. Pharmacogenomic determinants of the cardiovascular effects of dalcetrapib. Circ Cardiovasc Genet 2015;8(2):372–82.

57. Cannon CP, Shah S, Dansky HM, et al. Safety of anacetrapib in patients with or at high risk for coronary heart disease. N Engl J Med 2010;363(25):2406–15.

58. Gotto AM Jr, Kher U, Chatterjee MS, et al. Lipids, safety parameters, and drug concentrations after an additional 2 years of treatment with anacetrapib in the DEFINE study. J Cardiovasc Pharmacol Ther 2014;19(6):543–9.

59. Cannon CP, Blazing MA, Giugliano RP, et al. Ezetimibe added to statin therapy after acute coronary syndromes. N Engl J Med 2015;372(25):2387–97.

60. Hovingh GK, Kastelein JJ, van Deventer SJ, et al. Cholesterol ester transfer protein inhibition by TA-8995 in patients with mild dyslipidaemia (TULIP): a randomised, double-blind, placebo-controlled phase 2 trial. Lancet 2015;386(9992):452–60.

61. Clerc RG, Stauffer A, Weibel F, et al. Mechanisms underlying off-target effects of the cholesteryl ester transfer protein inhibitor torcetrapib involve L-type calcium channels. J Hypertens 2010;28(8):1676–86.

62. Hu X, Dietz JD, Xia C, et al. Torcetrapib induces aldosterone and cortisol production by an intracellular calcium-mediated mechanism independently of cholesteryl ester transfer protein inhibition. Endocrinology 2009;150(5):2211–9.

63. Simic B, Hermann M, Shaw SG, et al. Torcetrapib impairs endothelial function in hypertension. Eur Heart J 2012;33(13):1615–24.

64. Besler C, Heinrich K, Rohrer L, et al. Mechanisms underlying adverse effects of HDL on eNOS-activating pathways in patients with coronary artery disease. J Clin Invest 2011;121(7):2693–708.

65. Sacks FM, Pfeffer MA, Moye LA, et al. The effect of pravastatin on coronary events after myocardial infarction in patients with average cholesterol levels. Cholesterol and recurrent events trial investigators. N Engl J Med 1996;335(14):1001–9.

66. Barter PJ, Rye KA, Tardif JC, et al. Effect of torcetrapib on glucose, insulin, and hemoglobin A1c in subjects in the Investigation of Lipid Level Management to Understand its Impact in Atherosclerotic Events (ILLUMINATE) trial. Circulation 2011;124(5):555–62.

67. Sattar N, Preiss D, Murray HM, et al. Statins and risk of incident diabetes: a collaborative meta-analysis of randomised statin trials. Lancet 2010;375(9716):735–42.

68. Drew BG, Duffy SJ, Formosa MF, et al. High-density lipoprotein modulates glucose metabolism in patients with type 2 diabetes mellitus. Circulation 2009;119(15):2103–11.

69. Fryirs MA, Barter PJ, Appavoo M, et al. Effects of high-density lipoproteins on pancreatic beta-cell insulin secretion. Arterioscler Thromb Vasc Biol 2010;30(8):1642–8.

High-Density Lipoprotein Infusions

Kohei Takata, MD, PhD, Belinda A. Di Bartolo, PhD, Stephen J. Nicholls, MBBS, PhD*

KEYWORDS

- High-density lipoproteins • Lipids • Cardiovascular risk • Atherosclerosis

KEY POINTS

- High-density lipoproteins (HDLs) have presented an attractive target for development of new therapies in cardiovascular prevention on the basis of epidemiology and preclinical studies demonstrating their protective properties.
- Infusion of HDL mimetics has advanced to clinical development.
- Despite promising results of early clinical studies, more recent trials have failed to demonstrate a beneficial effect of infusing HDL mimetics in statin-treated patients.

INTRODUCTION

The consistent benefit of lowering levels of low-density lipoprotein cholesterol (LDL-C) with statins on cardiovascular events in large outcomes trials has led to widespread use of these agents in preventive approaches for treatment of patients determined to be at high cardiovascular risk.[1–3] However, as many clinical events continue to occur, despite use of statin therapy, there has been increasing interest in developing additional approaches that target other factors to achieve greater risk reduction.[4] By virtue of reports suggesting that HDLs play a protective role against atherosclerotic cardiovascular disease, there has been considerable interest in the development of therapies targeting HDL functionality.[5] Among these approaches, infusion of HDL mimetics has advanced to clinical development. The progress of these studies will be reviewed.

HIGH-DENSITY LIPOPROTEIN AND PROTECTION

Epidemiology studies consistently demonstrate an inverse relationship between HDL-C levels and the prospective risk of cardiovascular disease.[6] This is further evidenced within clinical trials, in which low HDL-C levels continue to be associated with an increase in cardiovascular risk in patients with low LDL-C levels.[7,8] Animal studies demonstrate that targeting HDL functionality via direct infusion or transgenic expression of its major apolipoproteins exerts favorable effects on the burden and composition of atherosclerotic plaque.[9–13] In addition to the central role of HDL in promotion of cholesterol efflux and reverse cholesterol transport, laboratory studies have also demonstrated that HDL impacts favorable effects on inflammatory, oxidative, apoptotic, and thrombotic factors implicated in atherosclerosis.[14] Systemic measures of cholesterol efflux capacity and paroxonase, as a measure of anti-inflammatory activity, are associated with the risk of cardiovascular events.[15–17] More recently, factors such as inflammation, smoking, and dysglycemia have been reported to impair HDL functionality, with potential consequences for cardiovascular risk.[18–20] These observations suggest that therapeutic approaches promoting HDL functionality may be a useful strategy for

Disclosure: Nicholls disclosures are research support from AstraZeneca, Amgen, Anthera, Eli Lilly, Esperion, Novartis, Cerenis, The Medicines Company, Resverlogix, InfraReDx, Roche, Sanofi-Regeneron and LipoScience and a consultant for AstraZeneca, Eli Lilly, Anthera, Omthera, Merck, Takeda, Resverlogix, Sanofi-Regeneron, CSL Behring, Esperion, Boehringer Ingelheim. Other authors have no disclosures.
South Australian Health and Medical Research Institute, University of Adelaide, PO Box 11060, Adelaide, SA 5001, Australia
* Corresponding author.
E-mail address: stephen.nicholls@sahmri.com

Cardiol Clin 36 (2018) 311–315
https://doi.org/10.1016/j.ccl.2017.12.012
0733-8651/18/© 2017 Elsevier Inc. All rights reserved.

treatment of high-risk patients in addition to statins.

HIGH-DENSITY LIPOPROTEIN EFFECTS OF EXISTING LIPID THERAPIES

The challenge to date has been the ability to demonstrate that favorably targeting HDL translates to cardiovascular benefit. Some evidence has emerged from study of current lipid-modifying therapies to suggest that HDL effects are associated with their benefit. Modest HDL-C raising is associated with the ability of statins to slow disease progression and reduce cardiovascular events.[21] Elevating small HDL particles is associated as an independent predictor of the ability of gemfibrozil to reduce cardiovascular events.[22] Niacin, the most effective HDL-C raising agent currently used in clinical practice, has been reported to produce regression of angiographic disease in the setting prior to use of more intensive statin therapy.[23] The failure to demonstrate benefit of adding niacin to more contemporary statin therapy has raised concerns with regards to its clinical utility for reducing cardiovascular risk.[24,25]

The development of cholesteryl ester transfer protein (CETP) inhibitors was primarily based on their ability to substantially raise HDL-C levels more than current therapies. However, the findings of these agents in clinical trials have been largely disappointing, with reports of toxicity and clinical futility.[6] Even when anacetrapib was demonstrated to have a modest clinical benefit, it was uncertain whether this had anything to do with HDL-C raising, and the agent was not moving forward to regulatory approval.[26] Considerable interest has focused on the potential to use HDL infusions as a treatment for patients with established atherosclerotic disease. Translating reports in animal studies, early human studies have demonstrated that infusing HDL-related mimetics increases fecal sterol excretion, a surrogate measure of reverse cholesterol transport, and improves endothelial function, suggesting potentially favorable effects on the artery wall.[27–29] These findings have provided the impetus for clinical development of a range of HDL mimetics in human studies.

ApoA-I MILANO

Variants of apoA-I have been reported to be of potential clinical utility in HDL therapeutics. In the Italian hamlet of Limone sul Garda, the naturally occurring apoA-I Milano (AIM) variant has been reported to associate with prolonged life expectancy despite the presence of low HDL-C levels.[30,31] This mutant involves an arginine-to-cysteine mutation, generating a protein that can form heterodimers and exert cholesterol efflux and anti-inflammatory properties in preclinical studies.[32,33] When incorporated into an HDL mimetic containing phospholipid (ETC-216), this has been demonstrated to have favorable effects on vascular function, atherosclerosis, and in stent neointimal hyperplasia in mouse and rabbit models.[34–36]

A small early human study demonstrated that infusing either 15 or 45 mg/kg of ETC-216 produced rapid regression of coronary atherosclerosis on serial intravascular ultrasound imaging in patients following an acute coronary syndrome.[37] The lack of difference in therapeutic effect between the 2 doses suggested a potential ability to saturate cholesterol transport pathways at the lower dose. Subsequent reports found greater regression in lesions containing the highest plaque burden at baseline and that regression was accompanied by reverse remodeling of the artery wall.[38] Although this mimetic was well tolerated within the course of this study, it became apparent that it was difficult to generate large quantities in a standardized manner required to perform larger clinical trials. Refinement of the manufacturing process produced a mimetic (MDCO-216) that retained the favorable effects on cholesterol efflux and anti-inflammatory activity.[39–41] However, a repeat imaging study in patients following an acute coronary syndrome failed to replicate evidence of plaque regression.[42] Whether this represents an inability of MDCO-216 to regress disease in patients treated with more intensive statin therapy than used in the earlier study remains unknown. Nevertheless, the inability to demonstrate a favorable impact on atherosclerosis in addition to standard medical therapy suggests that clinical development of this mimetic will not advance.

CER

CER-001 is an HDL mimetic containing wild-type apoA-I and sphingomyelin as its predominant lipid species. This particle is negatively charged in a similar manner to native pre-β HDL, distinguishing it from other HDL mimetics in clinical development.[43] This may underscore the observation of greater cholesterol transport activity in vivo, with favorable impacts on atherosclerotic plaque in animal models.[44,45] Small, single-center studies demonstrated beneficial effects on carotid atherosclerotic plaque burden using magnetic resonance and inflammatory activity using positron emission tomography.[46,47] The Can HDL Infusions

Significantly Quicken Atherosclerosis Regression (CHI-SQUARE) study evaluated the impact of 6 weekly infusions of CER-001 (3, 6, or 12 mg/kg) compared with placebo in patients following an acute coronary syndrome.[48] Although the primary analysis of this study suggested no significant impact on plaque burden, a subsequent analysis using anatomically matched arterial segments demonstrated significant plaque regression at the lowest CER-001 dose. Additional reports found even greater regression with this dose in patients harboring a greater plaque burden at baseline.[49] This provided the rationale for performing a second clinical trial, directly comparing the 3 mg/kg dose and placebo, administered as 10 infusions, in patients with a minimal plaque burden.[50] However, this study failed to replicate these findings, suggesting that short-term administration of CER-001 in the period following an acute coronary syndrome is unlikely to be of clinical utility.[51] Development of this mimetic continues to undergo evaluation in more stable atherosclerotic states.

CSL

CSL-111 is an HDL mimetic containing wild-type apolipoprotein A-I and phospholipid, with early evidence of a nonsignificant trend toward regression of coronary atherosclerosis in patients following an acute coronary syndrome in the Effect of rHDL on Atherosclerosis-Safety and Efficacy (ERASE) trial.[52] This was associated with beneficial effects on angiographic stenoses and ultrasonic measures of plaque composition. During the course of this study, the higher dose was discontinued because of an incidence of liver enzyme elevations. This favorable impact on coronary atherosclerosis complemented reports that CSL-111 infusions reduced the lipid and inflammatory content of femoral plaque in patients treated prior to undergoing percutaneous intervention.[53] Subsequent refinement of the manufacturing process yielded a new mimetic (CSL-112), which has progressed in clinical development. The ApoA-I Event Reducing in Ischemic Syndromes (AEGIS-1) trial evaluated the impact of infusing CSL-112 at a dose of 2 or 4 g, administered intravenously on a weekly basis for 4 weeks compared with placebo in patients following a myocardial infarction.[54] This study, primarily designed as a safety evaluation, demonstrated no adverse effects on liver and kidney function.[54] In addition, predictable dose-dependent increases in ABCA1-mediated cholesterol efflux by more than fourfold were observed with CSL-112.[54] This has given considerable support for advancing development of this mimetic to a larger cardiovascular outcomes trial.

IMPLICATIONS OF THESE FINDINGS

Despite the optimism that infusing HDL mimetics exerts favorable effects on lipid transport and inflammatory mediators of atherosclerosis, this has not, to date, proven to result in convincing evidence of clinical benefit in statin-treated patients. Whether the positive results of the first imaging trial using ETC-216 reflected a small cohort and use of less intensive statin therapy is uncertain. It also is unknown what is the optimal dose, frequency of administration, or clinical setting for use. The disappointing results have been observed, despite favorable effects on cholesterol efflux capacity.[55,56] Although this measure has been reported to be associated with cardiovascular risk,[57] the clinical significance of therapeutic changes in efflux capacity is unknown. Ultimately, the impact of HDL infusions can only be determined by assessing their effect on cardiovascular events in a large-scale clinical trial.

SUMMARY

HDL mimetics present an attractive approach to promoting HDL functionality without increasing HDL-C levels. Despite promising results of early clinical studies, more recent trials have failed to demonstrate a beneficial effect of infusing HDL mimetics in statin-treated patients. There remain considerable uncertainties about the optimal clinical setting for administration of these agents. Nevertheless, until mimetics produce a beneficial effect on clinical events, they remain an unfulfilled promise in cardiovascular prevention.

REFERENCES

1. Baigent C, Blackwell L, Emberson J, et al. Efficacy and safety of more intensive lowering of LDL cholesterol: a meta-analysis of data from 170,000 participants in 26 randomised trials. Lancet 2010; 376(9753):1670–81.
2. Sacks FM, Pfeffer MA, Moye LA, et al. The effect of pravastatin on coronary events after myocardial infarction in patients with average cholesterol levels. Cholesterol and recurrent events trial investigators. N Engl J Med 1996;335(14):1001–9.
3. Shepherd J, Cobbe SM, Ford I, et al. Prevention of coronary heart disease with pravastatin in men with hypercholesterolemia. West of Scotland coronary prevention study group. N Engl J Med 1995; 333(20):1301–7.
4. Fruchart JC, Sacks F, Hermans MP, et al. The residual risk reduction initiative: a call to action to reduce residual vascular risk in patients with dyslipidemia. Am J Cardiol 2008;102(10 Suppl):1K–34K.

5. Rye KA, Barter PJ. Cardioprotective functions of HDLs. J Lipid Res 2014;55(2):168–79.

6. Karathanasis SK, Freeman LA, Gordon SM, et al. The changing face of HDL and the best way to measure it. Clin Chem 2017;63(1):196–210.

7. Gordon T, Castelli WP, Hjortland MC, et al. High density lipoprotein as a protective factor against coronary heart disease. The Framingham study. Am J Med 1977;62(5):707–14.

8. Barter P, Gotto AM, LaRosa JC, et al. HDL cholesterol, very low levels of LDL cholesterol, and cardiovascular events. N Engl J Med 2007;357(13):1301–10.

9. Badimon JJ, Badimon L, Fuster V. Regression of atherosclerotic lesions by high density lipoprotein plasma fraction in the cholesterol-fed rabbit. J Clin Invest 1990;85(4):1234–41.

10. Shah PK, Yano J, Reyes O, et al. High-dose recombinant apolipoprotein A-I(Milano) mobilizes tissue cholesterol and rapidly reduces plaque lipid and macrophage content in apolipoprotein e-deficient mice. Potential implications for acute plaque stabilization. Circulation 2001;103(25):3047–50.

11. Nicholls SJ, Cutri B, Worthley SG, et al. Impact of short-term administration of high-density lipoproteins and atorvastatin on atherosclerosis in rabbits. Arterioscler Thromb Vasc Biol 2005;25(11):2416–21.

12. Plump AS, Scott CJ, Breslow JL. Human apolipoprotein A-I gene expression increases high density lipoprotein and suppresses atherosclerosis in the apolipoprotein E-deficient mouse. Proc Natl Acad Sci U S A 1994;91(20):9607–11.

13. Rubin EM, Krauss RM, Spangler EA, et al. Inhibition of early atherogenesis in transgenic mice by human apolipoprotein AI. Nature 1991;353(6341):265–7.

14. Navab M, Reddy ST, Van Lenten BJ, et al. HDL and cardiovascular disease: atherogenic and atheroprotective mechanisms. Nat Rev Cardiol 2011;8(4):222–32.

15. Khera AV, Cuchel M, de la Llera-Moya M, et al. Cholesterol efflux capacity, high-density lipoprotein function, and atherosclerosis. N Engl J Med 2011;364(2):127–35.

16. Saleheen D, Scott R, Javad S, et al. Association of HDL cholesterol efflux capacity with incident coronary heart disease events: a prospective case-control study. Lancet Diabetes Endocrinol 2015;3(7):507–13.

17. Bhattacharyya T, Nicholls SJ, Topol EJ, et al. Relationship of paraoxonase 1 (PON1) gene polymorphisms and functional activity with systemic oxidative stress and cardiovascular risk. JAMA 2008;299(11):1265–76.

18. Vaisar T, Tang C, Babenko I, et al. Inflammatory remodeling of the HDL proteome impairs cholesterol efflux capacity. J Lipid Res 2015;56(8):1519–30.

19. Takata K, Imaizumi S, Kawachi E, et al. Impact of cigarette smoking cessation on high-density lipoprotein functionality. Circ J 2014;78(12):2955–62.

20. Morgantini C, Natali A, Boldrini B, et al. Anti-inflammatory and antioxidant properties of HDLs are impaired in type 2 diabetes. Diabetes 2011;60(10):2617–23.

21. Nicholls SJ, Tuzcu EM, Sipahi I, et al. Statins, high-density lipoprotein cholesterol, and regression of coronary atherosclerosis. JAMA 2007;297(5):499–508.

22. Otvos JD, Collins D, Freedman DS, et al. Low-density lipoprotein and high-density lipoprotein particle subclasses predict coronary events and are favorably changed by gemfibrozil therapy in the veterans affairs high-density lipoprotein intervention trial. Circulation 2006;113(12):1556–63.

23. Brown BG, Zhao XQ, Chait A, et al. Simvastatin and niacin, antioxidant vitamins, or the combination for the prevention of coronary disease. N Engl J Med 2001;345(22):1583–92.

24. Boden WE, Probstfield JL, Anderson T, et al. Niacin in patients with low HDL cholesterol levels receiving intensive statin therapy. N Engl J Med 2011;365(24):2255–67.

25. Landray MJ, Haynes R, Hopewell JC, et al. Effects of extended-release niacin with laropiprant in high-risk patients. N Engl J Med 2014;371(3):203–12.

26. Bowman L, Hopewell JC, Chen F, et al. Effects of anacetrapib in patients with atherosclerotic vascular disease. N Engl J Med 2017;377(13):1217–27.

27. Eriksson M, Carlson LA, Miettinen TA, et al. Stimulation of fecal steroid excretion after infusion of recombinant proapolipoprotein A-I. Potential reverse cholesterol transport in humans. Circulation 1999;100(6):594–8.

28. Angelin B, Parini P, Eriksson M. Reverse cholesterol transport in man: promotion of fecal steroid excretion by infusion of reconstituted HDL. Atheroscler Suppl 2002;3(4):23–30.

29. Spieker LE, Sudano I, Hurlimann D, et al. High-density lipoprotein restores endothelial function in hypercholesterolemic men. Circulation 2002;105(12):1399–402.

30. Gualandri V, Franceschini G, Sirtori CR, et al. AIMilano apoprotein identification of the complete kindred and evidence of a dominant genetic transmission. Am J Hum Genet 1985;37(6):1083–97.

31. Sirtori CR, Calabresi L, Franceschini G, et al. Cardiovascular status of carriers of the apolipoprotein A-I(Milano) mutant: the Limone sul Garda study. Circulation 2001;103(15):1949–54.

32. Favari E, Gomaraschi M, Zanotti I, et al. A unique protease-sensitive high density lipoprotein particle containing the apolipoprotein A-I(Milano) dimer effectively promotes ATP-binding Cassette A1-mediated cell cholesterol efflux. J Biol Chem 2007;282(8):5125–32.

33. Calabresi L, Sirtori CR, Paoletti R, et al. Recombinant apolipoprotein A-IMilano for the treatment of

cardiovascular diseases. Curr Atheroscler Rep 2006;8(2):163–7.

34. Ibanez B, Vilahur G, Cimmino G, et al. Rapid change in plaque size, composition, and molecular footprint after recombinant apolipoprotein A-I Milano (ETC-216) administration: magnetic resonance imaging study in an experimental model of atherosclerosis. J Am Coll Cardiol 2008;51(11):1104–9.

35. Parolini C, Marchesi M, Lorenzon P, et al. Dose-related effects of repeated ETC-216 (recombinant apolipoprotein A-I Milano/1-palmitoyl-2-oleoyl phosphatidylcholine complexes) administrations on rabbit lipid-rich soft plaques: in vivo assessment by intravascular ultrasound and magnetic resonance imaging. J Am Coll Cardiol 2008;51(11):1098–103.

36. Nicholls SJ, Uno K, Kataoka Y, et al. ETC-216 for coronary artery disease. Expert Opin Biol Ther 2011; 11(3):387–94.

37. Nissen SE, Tsunoda T, Tuzcu EM, et al. Effect of recombinant ApoA-I Milano on coronary atherosclerosis in patients with acute coronary syndromes: a randomized controlled trial. JAMA 2003;290(17): 2292–300.

38. Nicholls SJ, Tuzcu EM, Sipahi I, et al. Relationship between atheroma regression and change in lumen size after infusion of apolipoprotein A-I Milano. J Am Coll Cardiol 2006;47(5):992–7.

39. Kallend DG, Reijers JA, Bellibas SE, et al. A single infusion of MDCO-216 (ApoA-1 Milano/POPC) increases ABCA1-mediated cholesterol efflux and pre-beta 1 HDL in healthy volunteers and patients with stable coronary artery disease. Eur Heart J Cardiovasc Pharmacother 2016;2(1):23–9.

40. Kempen HJ, Asztalos BF, Moerland M, et al. High-density lipoprotein subfractions and cholesterol efflux capacities after infusion of MDCO-216 (Apolipoprotein A-IMilano/Palmitoyl-Oleoyl-Phosphatidyl-choline) in healthy volunteers and stable coronary artery disease patients. Arterioscler Thromb Vasc Biol 2016;36(4):736–42.

41. Reijers JAA, Kallend DG, Malone KE, et al. MDCO-216 does not induce adverse immunostimulation, in contrast to its predecessor ETC-216. Cardiovasc Drugs Ther 2017;31(4):381–9.

42. Amaki M, Konagai N, Fujino M, et al. Report of the American Heart Association (AHA) scientific sessions 2016, New Orleans. Circ J 2016;81(1):22–7.

43. Barbaras R. Non-clinical development of CER-001. Front Pharmacol 2015;6:220.

44. Tardy C, Goffinet M, Boubekeur N, et al. CER-001, a HDL-mimetic, stimulates the reverse lipid transport and atherosclerosis regression in high cholesterol diet-fed LDL-receptor deficient mice. Atherosclerosis 2014;232(1):110–8.

45. Tardy C, Goffinet M, Boubekeur N, et al. HDL and CER-001 inverse-dose dependent inhibition of atherosclerotic plaque formation in apoE-/- mice:

evidence of ABCA1 down-regulation. PLoS One 2015;10(9):e0137584.

46. Hovingh GK, Smits LP, Stefanutti C, et al. The effect of an apolipoprotein A-I-containing high-density lipoprotein-mimetic particle (CER-001) on carotid artery wall thickness in patients with homozygous familial hypercholesterolemia: the Modifying Orphan Disease Evaluation (MODE) study. Am Heart J 2015; 169(5):736–42.e1.

47. Zheng KH, van der Valk FM, Smits LP, et al. HDL mimetic CER-001 targets atherosclerotic plaques in patients. Atherosclerosis 2016;251:381–8.

48. Tardif JC, Ballantyne CM, Barter P, et al. Effects of the high-density lipoprotein mimetic agent CER-001 on coronary atherosclerosis in patients with acute coronary syndromes: a randomized trial. Eur Heart J 2014;35(46):3277–86.

49. Kataoka Y, Andrews J, Duong M, et al. Regression of coronary atherosclerosis with infusions of the high-density lipoprotein mimetic CER-001 in patients with more extensive plaque burden. Cardiovasc Diagn Ther 2017;7(3):252–63.

50. Andrews J, Janssan A, Nguyen T, et al. Effect of serial infusions of reconstituted high-density lipoprotein (CER-001) on coronary atherosclerosis: rationale and design of the CARAT study. Cardiovasc Diagn Ther 2017;7(1):45–51.

51. Yilmaz MB, Sahin M. Highlights from ACC.17 scientific sessions. Anatol J Cardiol 2017;17(5):351–2.

52. Tardif JC, Gregoire J, L'Allier PL, et al. Effects of reconstituted high-density lipoprotein infusions on coronary atherosclerosis: a randomized controlled trial. JAMA 2007;297(15):1675–82.

53. Shaw JA, Bobik A, Murphy A, et al. Infusion of reconstituted high-density lipoprotein leads to acute changes in human atherosclerotic plaque. Circ Res 2008;103(10):1084–91.

54. Michael Gibson C, Korjian S, Tricoci P, et al. Safety and tolerability of CSL112, a reconstituted, infusible, plasma-derived apolipoprotein A-I, after acute myocardial infarction: the AEGIS-I trial (ApoA-I event reducing in ischemic syndromes I). Circulation 2016; 134(24):1918–30.

55. Nicholls SJ, Ruotolo G, Brewer HB, et al. Cholesterol efflux capacity and pre-beta-1 HDL concentrations are increased in dyslipidemic patients treated with evacetrapib. J Am Coll Cardiol 2015;66(20): 2201–10.

56. Ronsein GE, Hutchins PM, Isquith D, et al. Niacin therapy increases high-density lipoprotein particles and total cholesterol efflux capacity but not ABCA1-specific cholesterol efflux in statin-treated subjects. Arterioscler Thromb Vasc Biol 2016;36(2): 404–11.

57. Rohatgi A, Khera A, Berry JD, et al. HDL cholesterol efflux capacity and incident cardiovascular events. N Engl J Med 2014;371(25):2383–93.

High-Density Lipoproteins
Effects on Vascular Function and Role in the Immune Response

Arash Haghikia, MD[a,b,]*, Ulf Landmesser, MD[a,b,c]

KEYWORDS

- HDL function • Immune response • Endothelial function • Atherosclerosis • Coronary disease

KEY POINTS

- Results of recent clinical trials and translational/genetic studies have led to a refined understanding of the role of high-density lipoproteins in coronary disease.
- Findings cumulatively suggest that plasma high-density lipoprotein cholesterol is likely not a causal cardiovascular risk factor and therefore is not an adequate therapeutic target in cardiovascular prevention.
- More recent data suggest that the functional properties of HDL and its effects on vascular cells are importantly altered in patients with high cardiovascular risk.
- Among pathologic conditions that promote high-density lipoprotein dysfunction, enhanced inflammation, for example, in chronic kidney disease, has been identified as a potential underlying mechanism.

HIGH-DENSITY LIPOPROTEIN CHOLESTEROL HYPOTHESIS

The "high-density lipoprotein (HDL) cholesterol (HDL-C) hypothesis" was suggested largely by epidemiologic studies demonstrating an inverse relationship between HDL-C and the incidence of coronary heart disease.[1] Initial results of the Framingham Heart study also considered HDL-C as a potent predictor of death owing to coronary heart disease. These results were later supported by the Emerging Risk Factors Collaboration study, which was adjusted for other cardiovascular risk factors.[2] Importantly, however, in these studies the link between cardiovascular risk and HDL-C was only noticeable in patients with low HDL-C levels during 2.79 million person-years of follow-up, whereas in patients with higher HDL-C levels (>50 mg/dL), no significant relationship between HDL-C levels and coronary disease is found.

POTENTIAL ATHEROPROTECTIVE EFFECTS OF HIGH-DENSITY LIPOPROTEIN IN ENDOTHELIAL CELLS

As a key player of the so-called reverse cholesterol transport, HDL can transport excess cholesterol from peripheral cells either to the liver for excretion into the bile or to adrenals, testes, and ovaries for steroid hormone synthesis. In particular, cholesterol in macrophages from atherosclerotic lesions is thought to be taken up by HDL particles.[3] This so-called cholesterol efflux involves distinct transporters on macrophages, such as ATP-binding cassette subfamily G1 (ABCG1), ATP binding cassette transporter A1 (ABCA1), and scavenger receptor class B type 1.[4] Importantly, the cholesterol efflux capacity of HDL is not reflected by the absolute HDL-C plasma levels. This finding has been demonstrated by experimental studies using mice with genetic deletion of ABCG1 and

Disclosure: The authors have nothing to disclose.
[a] Department of Cardiology, Charité Universitätsmedizin Berlin, Campus Benjamin Franklin, Hindenburgdamm 30, Berlin 12203, Germany; [b] German Center for Cardiovascular Research (DZHK), Partner Site Berlin, Postfach 65 21 33, Berlin 13316, Germany; [c] Berlin Institute of Health (BIH), Anna-Louisa-Karsch-Straße 2, Berlin 10178, Germany
* Corresponding author. Department of Cardiology, Charité Universitätsmedizin Berlin, Campus Benjamin Franklin, Hindenburgdamm 30, Berlin 12203, Germany.
E-mail address: arash.haghikia@charite.de

ABCA1 in macrophages leading to increased atherosclerosis without alteration of HDL-C plasma levels.[5]

However, beyond its cholesterol transportation functions, direct vascular protective and potentially antiatherogenic effects have been ascribed to HDL under physiologic conditions based on mechanistic studies.[6] In particular, HDL from healthy subjects is known to promote the release of nitric oxide from endothelial cells and endothelial nitric oxide synthase (eNOS).[7] Moreover, by downregulating the expression of leukocyte adhesion molecules, such as vascular cell adhesion molecule 1, HDL from healthy subjects is capable of inhibiting the adhesion of leukocytes.[8]

In addition, the antithrombotic effects of HDL from healthy subjects have been described, such as limiting tissue factor expression in endothelial cells.[9] Importantly, these potential vasoprotective effects of HDL have been observed by using HDL from healthy subjects. The underlying molecular mechanisms of potential protective vascular effects of HDL have been identified over the past years, among which the scavenger receptor class B type 1 receptor seems to be a major mediator of HDL effects on the endothelial cells, including stimulation of endothelial NO production.[10,11] Other mechanisms involving the transporter ABCG1 (releasing endothelial oxysterols) and sphingosine 1-phosphate (S1P) 3 receptors on endothelial cells have also been identified.[12,13]

POTENTIAL REGULATORY FUNCTIONS OF HIGH-DENSITY LIPOPROTEIN IN INFECTION CONTROL AND (AUTO-) IMMUNE DISORDERS

HDL has been suggested to exert innate defense functions, for example, on bacterial infection. These functions include suppression of proinflammatory effects of bacterial lipopolysaccharide and lipoteichoic acid, which are toxic components of bacterial cell membranes. These properties have been particularly noticeable in animal models of sepsis using either apolipoprotein (apo)A-I knockout mice with very low HDL-C, which resulted in an exaggerated inflammatory cytokine release,[14] or apoA-I transgenic mice with high HDL levels showing increased survival rate under septic conditions as compared with controls. This property of HDL is thought to be based on the interaction of lipopolysaccharide with lipopolysaccharide-binding protein with subsequent binding with the HDL receptor scavenger receptor class B type I promoting its clearance.[15]

Interestingly, also in humans, low HDL-C levels have been inversely correlated with the severity of sepsis and an amplified systemic inflammatory response.[16]

A role of HDL-C for autoimmune disorders has also been suggested based on studies on LDLR[−/−] and apoA-I[−/−] mice, which develop an autoimmune phenotype with enlarged peripheral lymph nodes and spleens, compared with LDLR2/2 mice, with a high expansion of all classes of lymph node immune cells, such as T and B cells, macrophages, and dendritic cells.[17] Moreover, mice deficient of scavenger receptor class B type I demonstrate excessive proliferation of T and B lymphocytes with increased proinflammatory cytokine production in lymphocytes and macrophages, circulating autoantibodies, deposition of immune complexes in glomeruli, and infiltration of leukocytes in the kidneys.[18] Cumulatively, these observations point to a protective role of HDL and HDL-related proteins and functional circuits against infectious and autoimmune diseases, although detailed mechanisms still need to be explored further.

REGULATORY PROPERTIES OF HIGH-DENSITY LIPOPROTEIN IN INNATE AND ADAPTIVE IMMUNITY: THE ROLE OF LIPID RAFTS

Accumulating evidence suggest a critical role of HDL and in particular its main structural and functional apoA-I in regulating immunologic functions of both innate and adaptive immune responses.[19] An underlying mechanism of HDL-regulated immune functions is the modulation of specific membrane microdomains enriched in cholesterol and sphingolipids called lipid rafts in which numerous receptors of immune cells are localized, such as Toll-like receptors (TLRs)[20] and T-cell receptors and B-cell receptors[21,22] **(Fig. 1)**.

For example, HDL is capable to decrease lipid raft abundance on apoA-I/ABCA1–mediated cholesterol efflux of monocyte plasma membranes,[23] thereby

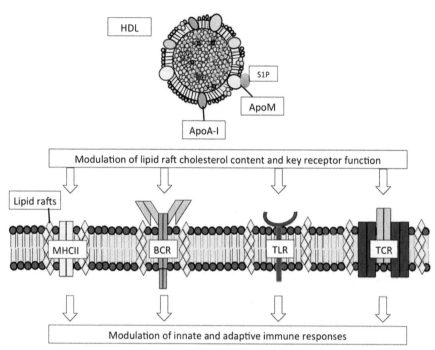

Fig. 1. Schematic illustration of how lipid rafts, in which key receptors of cells of both the innate and adaptive immunity are located, are modified by HDL. BCR, B-cell receptor; MHCII, major histocompatibility complex II; S1P, sphingosine-1-phosphate; TCR, T-cell receptor; TLR, toll-like receptor.

regulating the balance between the classically activated M1 macrophages that promote inflammation and M2 macrophages known to decrease immune reactions.[24]

Moreover, the activity of T-cell receptor and BCR, which are also membrane proteins localized within lipid rafts, can be modulated by HDL-dependent alteration of the composition and structure of lipid rafts, which is of particular relevance for autoimmunity and the development and progression of autoimmunologic diseases.[21] By modulating lipid rafts of T-cell receptors and BCRs in an S1P-dependent manner, HDL may impact trafficking of lymphocytes in the lymph node and circulation as well as the differentiation of T-cell subsets.[25,26] HDL has also been suggested to interfere with major histocompatibility complex II–dependent antigen presentation of monocytes and lymphocytes by modulating lipid rafts in which major histocompatibility complex II is embedded.[22]

Conclusively, apos and specific HDL-associated molecules, such as S1P, have been considered to impact signaling pathways of both the innate and adaptive immunity, particularly by modulating the lipid content of lipid rafts in which major receptors of immune cells are localized.

Although, under physiologic conditions, HDL promotes antiinflammatory pathways with potential atheroprotective effects, these properties are markedly altered in patients with manifest atherosclerotic cardiovascular diseases or renal failure, as described elsewhere in this article.

HIGH-DENSITY LIPOPROTEIN CHOLESTEROL AS THERAPEUTIC TARGET: RESULTS FROM RANDOMIZED, CONTROLLED CLINICAL TRIALS

In particular, the observations from epidemiologic studies pointing to an inverse relationship between HDL-C levels and cardiovascular risk have encouraged the testing of therapeutic strategies to increase HDL-C levels (**Table 1**). This concept was supported by experimental studies in transgenic mice expressing high amounts of human apoA-I and HDL that were protected from the development of diet-induced atherosclerotic lesions.[27] The first clinical trials aiming at raising HDL-C tested the effect of niacin therapy, which achieved a 29% increase in HDL-C[28] and prevented the progression of coronary disease when combined with simvastatin.[29] In this trial, however, niacin and simvastatin were tested together.

Subsequent prospective, randomized, controlled trials failed to demonstrate an incremental clinical benefit from the addition of niacin to statin therapy, despite a significant increase in HDL-C levels, such as the AIM-HIGH (Atherothrombosis Intervention in Metabolic Syndrome With Low HDL/High Triglycerides: Impact on Global Health) study, which

Table 1
Overview of major trials evaluating the effects of raising HDL-cholesterol

Trial	Major Finding	Ref
The Arterial Disease Multiple Intervention Trial (ADMIT)	Niacin therapy achieved 29% increase in HDL-C.	Elam et al,[28] 2000
The HDL-Atherosclerosis Treatment Study (HATS)	Reduction of 60%–90% in the rate of major coronary events with combination of simvastatin and niacin therapy.	Brown et al,[29] 2001
The AIM-HIGH study (Atherothrombosis Intervention in Metabolic Syndrome With Low HDL/High Triglycerides: Impact on Global Health)	In 3414 patients with established CV disease and low HDL-C levels extended-release niacin therapy did not improve CV outcome during a 3-y follow-up	AIM-HIGH Investigators,[30] 2011
The Heart Protection Study 2–Treatment of HDL to Reduce the Incidence of Vascular Events study (HPS2-THRIVE)	Trial involving more than 25,000 patients showed that extended-release niacin therapy with laropiprant in addition to statin therapy did not significantly reduce the risk of major vascular events but increased the risk of serious adverse events during a median follow-up period of 3.9 y.	Parish et al,[31] 2014
ILLUMINATE trial (Investigation of Lipid Level Management to Understand Its Impact in Atherosclerotic Events)	Trial involving more than 15,000 patients at high CV risk who received either the CETP inhibitor torcetrapib plus atorvastatin or atorvastatin alone. Torcetrapib therapy increased HDL-C by 72% and reduced LDL-C by 25%. However, it resulted in an increased risk of mortality and morbidity.	Barter et al,[32] 2007
Dal-Outcomes trial	A phase III trial to evaluate the effects of dalcetrapib on CV risk among patients with a recent acute coronary syndrome. Addition of dalcetrapib to standard therapy after an acute coronary syndrome raised the levels of HDL cholesterol and apolipoprotein A1, but the risk of major CV outcomes was not significantly altered.	Schwartz et al,[33] 2012
ACCELERATE trial (Assessment of the clinical effects of cholesteryl ester transfer protein inhibition with evacetrapib)	Phase III trial to evaluate the effect of the CETP inhibitor evacetrapib on major adverse CV outcomes in patients with high-risk vascular disease. Although evacetrapib lead to an increase of more than 130% in the mean HDL-C level, it did not result in a lower rate of CV events than placebo among patients with high-risk vascular disease.	Lincoff et al,[34] 2017
The HPS3/TIMI55–REVEAL trial	Trial tested the effects of anacetrapib in patients with atherosclerotic vascular disease. The so far largest outcome trial with a CETP inhibitor involved 30,449	HPS3/TIMI55-REVEAL Collaborative Group,[35] 2017

(continued on next page)

Trial	Major Finding	Ref
	adults with atherosclerotic vascular disease who were receiving intensive atorvastatin therapy. Anacetrapib lowered incidence of major coronary events as compared with placebo during a median follow-up period of 4.1 y. This effect may, however, also be attributable to the LDL-C lowering with the compound.	

Table 1
(continued)

Abbreviations: CETP, cholesterol ester transfer protein; CV, cardiovascular; HDL-C, high-density lipoprotein cholesterol; LDL-C, low-density lipoprotein cholesterol.

was terminated prematurely.[30] Moreover, in a recent very large outcome trial (HPS2-THRIVE [The Heart Protection Study 2–Treatment of HDL to Reduce the Incidence of Vascular Events study]) randomizing more than 25,000 patients, niacin in addition to statin therapy failed to lower the risk of major vascular events, but increased the risk of serious adverse events.[31]

Another approach to increasing HDL-C levels is inhibition of the cholesterol ester transfer protein (CETP), which was first tested by the ILLUMINATE trial (Investigation of Lipid Level Management to Understand Its Impact in Atherosclerotic Events)[32] involving more than 15,000 patients at high cardiovascular risk. In this trial, patients received either the CETP inhibitor torcetrapib plus atorvastatin or atorvastatin alone. Although torcetrapib therapy increased HDL-C by 72% and reduced low-density lipoprotein (LDL) cholesterol (LDL-C) by 25%, it resulted in an increased risk of mortality and morbidity. However, further analyses of torcetrapib pointed to off-target toxic effects of this compound as the underlying cause of the detrimental effects. However, another moderately active CETP inhibitor, dalcetrapib, that only increased HDL-C also failed to reduce the risk of recurrent cardiovascular events in patients with recent acute coronary syndrome in the Dal-Outcomes trial (A Study of RO4607381 in Stable Coronary Heart Disease Patients With Recent Acute Coronary Syndrome),[33] despite increasing HDL-C by 31%. Importantly, unlike torcetrpib, dalcetrapib had only a minimal effect on LDL-C.

Another outcome trial testing a different CETP inhibitor, evacetrapib, was terminated early in 2015 owing to a lack of prognostic benefit,[34] further questioning the HDL hypothesis. Last, another CETP inhibitor, anacetrapib was tested in the so far largest outcome trial with a CETP inhibitor involving 30,449 adults with atherosclerotic vascular disease and a long-term follow-up who were receiving intensive atorvastatin therapy.[35] The results were recently reported and demonstrated a lower incidence of major coronary events as compared with placebo during a median follow-up period of 4.1 years. However, because anacetrapib also reduced LDL-C levels by about 20%, it is possible that the beneficial effects of anacetrapib are, at least partly, owing to a reduction of LDL-C levels.

Furthermore, strategies to selectively stimulate production of apoA-I, for example, with the agent RVX-208 in the ASSERT trial (Efficacy and Safety of a Novel Oral Inducer of Apolipoprotein A-I Synthesis in Statin-Treated Patients With Stable Coronary Artery Disease) failed to achieve change in plaque regression in patients with coronary disease as assessed by intravascular ultrasound examination.[36]

Cumulatively, these major trials questioned the validity of the HDL-C hypothesis and changed our view of the causal role of HDL-C plasma levels for the progression of coronary disease. Moreover, the results encouraged investigating the more detailed functional aspects of HDL and the composition of HDL particles as potential HDL-related aspects relevant for cardiovascular physiology and risk stratification.

DYSFUNCTIONAL HIGH-DENSITY LIPOPROTEIN IN PATIENTS WITH CARDIOVASCULAR DISEASE

An important finding of the Dal-Outcome trial was that the baseline HDL-C levels of the patients were not associated with the patients' outcomes,[33] suggesting a dissolution of protective effects of HDL in the secondary prevention setting in patients with established coronary disease.

Indeed, unlike the protective vascular effects of HDL obtained from healthy subjects, HDL from patients with cardiovascular disease, such as coronary artery disease (CAD), acute coronary syndrome, or chronic kidney diseases undergoes alterations of its protein composition or biochemical modifications, resulting in a loss or reversal of its physiologic functions. For example, it loses its suppressive effect on endothelial vascular cell adhesion molecule 1 expression resulting in increased adhesion of leukocytes to activated endothelial cells.[7,37] Similarly, antiapoptotic effects of HDL from patients with CAD or acute coronary syndrome have been reported to be abolished, because dysfunctional HDL fails to activate endothelial Bcl-xL, while promoting endothelial proapoptotic pathways, such as p38-mitogen-activated protein kinase–mediated activation of the proapoptotic Bcl-2 protein tBid. Finally, dysfunctional HDL loses its ability to stimulate NO release and NO-associated beneficial effects in endothelial cells.[7]

ALTERATION AND MODIFICATION OF HIGH-DENSITY LIPOPROTEIN PROTEIN CARGO: A DETERMINANT OF ITS FUNCTIONAL VASCULAR PROPERTIES

Exchangeable apos, in particular apoA-I, constitute the major structural proteins within HDL.[38] Furthermore, the HDL particle contains a complex and highly heterogeneous proteome, including a broad array of proteins with multiple regulatory functions in the immune and complement systems, hemostasis, and thrombosis.[7] It also contains a number of growth factors, receptors, and hormone-associated proteins.[39]

On the molecular levels, several mechanisms have been suggested to exert detrimental effects of dysfunctional HDL, among which imbalanced redox signaling seems to be of high relevance for the vasculature. One of the molecular mechanisms of dysfunctional HDL in patients with CAD is reduced activity of HDL-associated paraoxanase-1 (PON1) that, under healthy conditions, prevents HDL from oxidative modification. Reduced activity of PON1 leads to formation of advanced lipid oxidation products, such as malondialdehyde.[6,7] Consequently, reduced HDL-associated activity of PON1 results in enhanced oxidation of HDL, in particular its apoA-I, and formation of malondialdehyde, which in turn activates endothelial lectin-type oxidized LDL receptor 1. Activation of endothelial lectin-type oxidized LDL receptor 1 by oxidized HDL stimulates protein kinase C βII (PKCβII) in endothelial cells.[7] In turn, activation of PKCβII in endothelial cells inhibits eNOS-dependent NO production and eNOS-associated protective signaling pathways. In particular, increased endothelial PKCβII activation by oxidized HDL inhibits Akt-dependent eNOS-activating phosphorylation at Ser1177 and increases the phosphorylation of eNOS at Thr495, which inhibits eNOS activity.[7]

Taken together, these studies demonstrate that HDL from patients with cardiovascular diseases loses its ability to promote endothelial eNOS-activating pathways and NO production. Consequently, this results to impaired endothelial antiinflammatory and endothelial repair capacities of HDL.

ALTERED PROPERTIES OF HIGH-DENSITY LIPOPROTEIN UNDER INFLAMMATORY CONDITIONS

Under inflammatory conditions, HDL composition is affected.[40] Particularly, increased amounts of endothelial lipase[41] and secretory phospholipase A2[42] have been found, whereas decreased levels of CETP and lecithin–cholesterol acyltransferase in HDL particles have been reported.[41] Moreover, HDL is enriched with the acute phase proteins serum amyloid A, which causes increased apoA-I catabolism in the liver and kidney.[43,44] Additionally, decreased content of PON1 and increased amounts of platelet-activating factor acetylhydrolase are found in modified HDL under increased inflammatory conditions. Another protein within the HDL particle with antiapoptotic and antiinflammatory features is apoM, which physiologically binds to S1P and, thereby, mediates a number of protective effects of S1P. However, apoM levels are found to be reduced upon inflammatory responses[45] with impaired signaling by the apoM–S1P axis and, consequently, reduced protective properties of HDL. Altogether, these modifications lead to the loss of protective HDL functional properties and convert HDL into a detrimental and overall proatherogenic lipoprotein upon inflammation.[46]

THE SHIFT IN HIGH-DENSITY LIPOPROTEIN FUNCTION IS LINKED TO INFLAMMATORY PATHWAYS

A major cause of altered HDL function with detrimental vascular effects are inflammatory processes, which occur in chronic cardiovascular disease, such as ischemic heart disease and chronic heart failure, as well as chronic kidney disease. The response to inflammation in turn causes HDL dysfunction creating a vicious cycle that potentiates proatherogenic pathways.

Accumulating data suggest that the opposing effects of HDL-C on vascular cells is reflected by a shift of the composition of HDL-associated proteins or their chemical modification in patients with established cardiovascular disease as compared with healthy subjects (Fig. 2).[47–49] In particular, it is believed that distinct clusters of specific HDL-associated proteins mediate specific biological

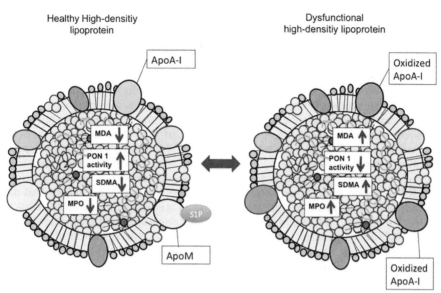

Fig. 2. Simplified model of a high-density lipoprotein with the most abundant apolipoptoteins apoA-I and apoM under healthy condition (*left scheme*). HDL displays increased chemical modification (*right scheme*) with symmetric dimethylarginine (SDMA), has reduced paraoxonase-1 (PON-1) and increased myeloperoxidase activity and increased oxidation of particularly apoA-I and apoM under diseased conditions, such as coronary artery disease or chronic kidney disease (dysfunctional HDL).

functions[48] with potential atheroprotective or atherogenic properties. One of the best studies atheroprotective proteins in HDL particles is PON1,[50] which mediates antioxidative and antiinflammatory functions of HDL.[51] PON1 is an esterase/lipolactonase that has been suggested to counteract the oxidation of phospholipids, enhance HDL-mediated eNOS-dependent NO production, and promote cholesterol efflux from macrophages.[7,51] These PON1-related properties of HDL have been supported by experimental studies with PON1 KO mice that demonstrate increased atherosclerotic lesions,[52] whereas Pon1 transgenic mice show reduced systemic measures of oxidation and seem to be protected from atherosclerosis.[53] The antioxidative properties of PON1 have also been derived from clinical studies demonstrating a significant inverse correlation between serum PON1 activity and multiple systemic measures of oxidant stress.[54] Conversely, reduced systemic PON1 activity has been linked to increased cardiovascular risk.[55] Among proatherogenic proteins identified in HDL particles is myeloperoxidase (MPO), a leukocyte-derived heme protein that, in contrast with PON1, is a major enzymatic source of protein and lipid oxidation and thereby promotes atherosclerosis.[56,57] Under physiologic conditions, MPO is typically found at very low levels in the plasma. However, in patients at high cardiovascular risk or in patients with acute coronary syndrome, increased levels of MPO can be measured in the plasma.[58] Notably, the expression and enzymatic activity of MPO is increased under inflammatory conditions.[56,59]

In fact, the major source of MPO expression and release are activated leukocytes. Notably, binding of MPO to HDL particles may occur both in the circulation and within human atherosclerotic plaque, with subsequent oxidative modification.[60–62]

In particular, MPO-mediated site-specific oxidation of apoA-I of HDL has been associated with impairment in functional properties, such as cholesterol efflux and lecithin–cholesterin–acyltransferase activation, as well as inhibition of the antiinflammatory and antiapoptotic properties of HDL.[39] Recently, the existence of an HDL–MPO–PON1 ternary complex has been identified, in which MPO and PON1 may reciprocally modulate the other's activity, and thereby regulate oxidant stress and lipid peroxidation, for example, under inflammatory conditions. This direct interaction of MPO–PON is an example of functional clusters of HDL-bound proteins,[63] demonstrating the complexity of how HDL function may be manipulated.

MODIFICATIONS OF HIGH-DENSITY LIPOPROTEIN CONTRIBUTING TO THE SHIFT IN HIGH-DENSITY LIPOPROTEIN FUNCTION IN RESPONSE TO INFLAMMATION: ROLE FOR TOLL-LIKE RECEPTOR-2

Recently, chemical modification of HDL upon binding with a methylated derivative of the amino acid L-arginine, the symmetric dimethylarginine (SDMA) to form HDL_{SDMA} has been shown to convert HDL into a noxious particle.[64] This modulation of HDL has been particularly demonstrated in patients with chronic kidney disease leading to endothelial dysfunction with reduced NO production, increased reactive oxygen species production, and increased blood pressure. However, increased serum SDMA has also been demonstrated in several cardiovascular diseases, such as coronary disease and pulmonary arterial hypertension,[65–67] suggesting a broad clinical implication of this bioamine.

Mechanistically, this abnormal HDL activates endothelial TLR-2, resulting in increased endothelial inflammation and impairment of endothelial repair capacity. Importantly, TLR-2 is expressed on endothelial cells[68] and is typically activated by microbial lipoproteins. Thus, modulation of HDL by SDMA seems to link dysfunctional HDL with the innate immune system.

Among the underlying mechanisms of how HDL_{SDMA} impacts on NO bioavailability and endothelial redox signaling is a TLR-2–mediated reduction in Akt phosphorylation at Ser473 and, consequently, a reduction in eNOS-activating phosphorylation at Ser1177.[64] Furthermore, activated TLR-2 also stimulates nicotinamide adenine dinucleotide phosphate oxidase in endothelial cells, leading to increased reactive oxygen species production.[69] Activation of TLR-2 by HDL_{SDMA} also induced phosphorylation of c-Jun *N*-terminal kinase, which in turn increases NADPH oxidase activity[70] with further adding to increased endothelial superoxide production.[64]

Notably, in a recent clinical study with 2 independent cohorts of patients with coronary disease, the combination of low SDMA levels and high HDL-C were associated with a significantly lower mortality, whereas high HDL_{SDMA} levels was were with greater mortality, linking SDMA with HDL dysfunction.[71]

These observations suggest a novel mechanism of HDL modification by bioactive amino acid derivatives, such as SDMA, which is increased in the plasma of patients with various cardiovascular conditions. Upon this modification, HDL is converted into a noxious particle that activates circuits related to the innate immune system in endothelial cells, ultimately leading to increased endothelial inflammation and impaired endothelial function. It remains to be elucidated whether therapeutic strategies aiming at reducing circulating SDMA levels would improve HDL function and, thus, have beneficial effects on vascular physiology.

SUMMARY

The negative pharmacotherapeutic trials aiming at increasing HDL-C levels cumulatively argue against a simple, causal relationship between HDL-C levels and cardiovascular risk as observed in early classic epidemiologic studies. The missing casual relationship is also supported by a recent Mendelian randomization study that showed that a single nucleotide polymorphism in the endothelial lipase gene, which increased HDL-C levels by about 12% in carriers, was not associated with reduced risk of experiencing myocardial infarction.[72] Moreover, 14 other gene polymorphisms associated with lifetime increases of HDL-C were not linked with a lower risk of myocardial infarction. Instead, some studies suggest that functional aspects of HDL are more relevant for risk stratification purposes and potentially therapeutic strategies. In this regard, the cholesterol efflux capacity of HDL has been associated inversely with the likelihood of angiographic CAD[73] and incident cardiovascular events independent of the HDL-C level,[74] although further validation studies are warranted to confirm the prognostic relevance of cholesterol efflux capacity.[75]

Conclusively, in view of the results from clinical trials aimed at raising HDL-C plasma levels and the findings from basic research the initial HDL hypothesis seems to be too simple and HDL-C alone can no longer be considered as a proper surrogate marker for risk prediction. The effects of HDL-C on the vasculature and its efflux capacity depend on many factors, including the protein composition of the HDL particle, its functional effects on vascular cells, and its efflux capacity, which all in all determine the prognostic value of HDL-C.

Thus, unlike the global inverse relation between LDL-C and cardiovascular risk both in primary and secondary prevention,[76,77] a causal relationship between HDL-C and cardiovascular risk has not been established. As described herein, HDL may serve important functions in the immune responses, and these effects may not necessarily be related to HDL-C plasma levels.

ACKNOWLEDGMENTS

Dr Arash Haghikia was supported by Deutsche Stiftung für Herzforschung and Else Kröner-Fresenius-Stiftung.

REFERENCES

1. Castelli WP, Garrison RJ, Wilson PWF, et al. Incidence of coronary heart disease and lipoprotein cholesterol levels. JAMA 1986;256(20):2835.
2. Emerging Risk Factors Collaboration, Di Angelantonio E, Sarwar N, Perry P, et al. Major lipids, apolipoproteins, and risk of vascular disease. JAMA 2009;302(18): 1993–2000.

3. Besler C, Luscher TF, Landmesser U. Molecular mechanisms of vascular effects of High-density lipoprotein: alterations in cardiovascular disease. EMBO Mol Med 2012;4(4):251–68.

4. Aron-Wisnewsky J, Julia Z, Poitou C, et al. Effect of bariatric surgery-induced weight loss on SR-BI-, ABCG1-, and ABCA1-mediated cellular cholesterol efflux in obese women. J Clin Endocrinol Metab 2011;96(4):1151–9.

5. Westerterp M, Murphy AJ, Wang M, et al. Deficiency of ABCA1 and ABCG1 in macrophages increases inflammation and accelerates atherosclerosis in mice. Circ Res 2013. https://doi.org/10.1161/CIRCRESAHA.113.301086.

6. Lüscher TF, Landmesser U, Von Eckardstein A, et al. High-density lipoprotein: vascular protective effects, dysfunction, and potential as therapeutic target. Circ Res 2014;114(1):171–82.

7. Besler C, Heinrich K, Rohrer L, et al. Mechanisms underlying adverse effects of HDL on eNOS-activating pathways in patients with coronary artery disease. J Clin Invest 2011;121(7):2693–708.

8. Nicholls SJ, Dusting GJ, Cutri B, et al. Reconstituted high-density lipoproteins inhibit the acute pro-oxidant and proinflammatory vascular changes induced by a periarterial collar in normocholesterolemic rabbits. Circulation 2005;111(12):1543–50.

9. Viswambharan H, Ming XF, Zhu S, et al. Reconstituted high-density lipoprotein inhibits thrombin-induced endothelial tissue factor expression through inhibition of RhoA and Stimulation of phosphatidylinositol 3-kinase but not akt/endothelial nitric oxide synthase. Circ Res 2004;94(7):918–25.

10. Yuhanna IS, Zhu Y, Cox BE, et al. High-density lipoprotein binding to scavenger receptor-BI activates endothelial nitric oxide synthase. Nat Med 2001;7(7):853–7.

11. Gong M, Wilson M, Kelly T, et al. HDL-associated estradiol stimulates endothelial NO synthase and vasodilation in an SR-BI-dependent manner. J Clin Invest 2003;111(10):1579–87.

12. Nofer JR, Van Der Giet M, Tölle M, et al. HDL induces NO-dependent vasorelaxation via the lysophospholipid receptor S1P3. J Clin Invest 2004;113(4):569–81.

13. Terasaka N, Yu S, Yvan-Charvet L, et al. ABCG1 and HDL protect against endothelial dysfunction in mice fed a high-cholesterol diet. J Clin Invest 2008;118(11):3701–13.

14. Guo L, Ai J, Zheng Z, et al. High density lipoprotein protects against polymicrobe-induced sepsis in mice. J Biol Chem 2013;288(25):17947–53.

15. Vishnyakova TG, Bocharov AV, Baranova IN, et al. Binding and internalization of lipopolysaccharide by Cla-1, a human orthologue of rodent scavenger receptor B1. J Biol Chem 2003;278(25):22771–80.

16. Wendel M, Paul R, Heller AR. Lipoproteins in inflammation and sepsis. II. Clinical aspects. Intensive Care Med 2007;33(1):25–35.

17. Wilhelm AJ, Zabalawi M, Grayson JM, et al. Apolipoprotein A-I and its role in lymphocyte cholesterol homeostasis and autoimmunity. Arterioscler Thromb Vasc Biol 2009;29(6):843–9.

18. Feng H, Guo L, Wang D, et al. Deficiency of scavenger receptor BI leads to impaired lymphocyte homeostasis and autoimmune disorders in mice. Arterioscler Thromb Vasc Biol 2011;31(11):2543–51.

19. Catapano AL, Pirillo A, Bonacina F, et al. HDL in innate and adaptive immunity. Cardiovasc Res 2014;103(3):372–83.

20. Fessler MB, Parks JS. Intracellular lipid flux and membrane microdomains as organizing principles in inflammatory cell signaling. J Immunol 2011;187(4):1529–35.

21. Kabouridis PS, Jury EC. Lipid rafts and T-lymphocyte function: implications for autoimmunity. FEBS Lett 2008;582(27):3711–8.

22. Gupta N, DeFranco AL. Lipid rafts and B cell signaling. Semin Cell Dev Biol 2007;18(5):616–26.

23. Murphy AJ, Woollard KJ, Hoang A, et al. High-density lipoprotein reduces the human monocyte inflammatory response. Arterioscler Thromb Vasc Biol 2008;28(11):2071–7.

24. Feig JE, Rong JX, Shamir R, et al. HDL promotes rapid atherosclerosis regression in mice and alters inflammatory properties of plaque monocyte-derived cells. Proc Natl Acad Sci U S A 2011;108(17):7166–71.

25. Mandala S. Alteration of lymphocyte trafficking by sphingosine-1-phosphate receptor agonists. Science 2002;296(5566):346–9.

26. Liu G, Yang K, Burns S, et al. The S1P1-mTOR axis directs the reciprocal differentiation of TH1 and Treg cells. Nat Immunol 2010;11(11):1047–56.

27. Rubin EM, Krauss RM, Spangler EA, et al. Inhibition of early atherogenesis in transgenic mice by human apolipoprotein AI. Nature 1991;353(6341):265–7.

28. Elam MB, Hunninghake DB, Davis KB, et al. Effect of niacin on lipid and lipoprotein levels and glycemic control in patients with diabetes and peripheral arterial disease. JAMA 2000;284(10):1263–70. Available at: http://jama.ama-assn.org/content/284/10/1263.short%5Cnpapers2://publication/uuid/0A1DC97C-B66E-4B27-A7A6-496D2250F807.

29. Brown BG, Zhao XQ, Chait A, et al. Simvastatin and niacin, antioxidant vitamins, or the combination for the prevention of coronary disease. N Engl J Med 2001;345(22):1583–92.

30. AIM-HIGH Investigators, Boden WE, Probstfield JL, Anderson T, et al. Niacin in patients with low HDL cholesterol levels receiving intensive statin therapy. N Engl J Med 2011;365(24):2255–67.

31. Parish S, Tomson J, Wallendszus K, et al. Effects of extended-release niacin with laropiprant in high-risk patients. N Engl J Med 2014;371(3):203–12.

32. Barter PJ, Caulfield M, Eriksson M, et al. Effects of torcetrapib in patients at high risk for coronary events. N Engl J Med 2007;357(21):2109–22.

33. Schwartz GG, Olsson AG, Abt M, et al. Effects of dalcetrapib in patients with a recent acute coronary syndrome. N Engl J Med 2012;367(22):2089–99.

34. Lincoff AM, Nicholls SJ, Riesmeyer JS, et al. Evacetrapib and cardiovascular outcomes in high-risk vascular disease. N Engl J Med 2017;376(20):1933–42.

35. HPS3/TIMI55-REVEAL Collaborative Group. Effects of anacetrapib in patients with atherosclerotic vascular disease. N Engl J Med 2017. https://doi.org/10.1056/NEJMoa1706444.

36. Bailey D, Jahagirdar R, Gordon A, et al. RVX-208. A small molecule that increases apolipoprotein A-I and high-density lipoprotein cholesterol in vitro and in vivo. J Am Coll Cardiol 2010;55(23):2580–9.

37. Sorrentino SA, Besler C, Rohrer L, et al. Endothelial-vasoprotective effects of high-density lipoprotein are impaired in patients with type 2 diabetes mellitus but are improved after extended-release niacin therapy. Circulation 2010;121(1):110–22.

38. Berrougui H, Isabelle M, Cloutier M, et al. Age-related impairment of HDL-mediated cholesterol efflux. J Lipid Res 2006;48(2):328–36.

39. Huang Y, Wu Z, Riwanto M, et al. Myeloperoxidase, paraoxonase-1, and HDL form a functional ternary complex. J Clin Invest 2013;123(9):3815–28.

40. Khovidhunkit W, Kim M-S, Memon RA, et al. Effects of infection and inflammation on lipid and lipoprotein metabolism: mechanisms and consequences to the host. J Lipid Res 2004;45(7):1169–96.

41. Badellino KO, Wolfe ML, Reilly MP, et al. Endothelial lipase is increased in vivo by inflammation in humans. Circulation 2008;117(5):678–85.

42. de la Llera Moya M, McGillicuddy FC, Hinkle CC, et al. Inflammation modulates human HDL composition and function in vivo. Atherosclerosis 2012;222(2):390–4.

43. Van Lenten BJ, Hama SY, De Beer FC, et al. Anti-inflammatory HDL becomes pro-inflammatory during the acute phase response. Loss of protective effect of HDL against LDL oxidation in aortic wall cell cocultures. J Clin Invest 1995;96(6):2758–67.

44. Graversen JH, Castro G, Kandoussi A, et al. A pivotal role of the human kidney in catabolism of HDL protein components apolipoprotein A-I and A-IV but not of A-II. Lipids 2008;43(5):467–70.

45. Feingold KR, Shigenaga JK, Chui LG, et al. Infection and inflammation decrease apolipoprotein M expression. Atherosclerosis 2008;199(1):19–26.

46. Christoffersen C, Obinata H, Kumaraswamy SB, et al. Endothelium-protective sphingosine-1-phosphate provided by HDL-associated apolipoprotein M. Proc Natl Acad Sci U S A 2011;108(23):9613–8.

47. Alwaili K, Bailey D, Awan Z, et al. The HDL proteome in acute coronary syndromes shifts to an inflammatory profile. Biochim Biophys Acta 2012;1821(3):405–15.

48. Davidson WS, Silva RAGD, Chantepie S, et al. Proteomic analysis of defined HDL subpopulations reveals particle-specific protein clusters: relevance to antioxidative function. Arterioscler Thromb Vasc Biol 2009;29(6):870–6.

49. Vaisar T, Pennathur S, Green PS, et al. Shotgun proteomics implicates protease inhibition and complement activation in the antiinflammatory properties of HDL. J Clin Invest 2007;117(3):746–56.

50. Shih DM, Gu L, Hama S, et al. Genetic-dietary regulation of serum paraoxonase expression and its role in atherogenesis in a mouse model. J Clin Invest 1996;97(7):1630–9.

51. Aviram M, Rosenblat M, Bisgaier CL, et al. Paraoxonase inhibits high-density lipoprotein oxidation and preserves its functions: a possible peroxidative role for paraoxonase. J Clin Invest 1998;101(8):1581–90.

52. Shih DM, Gu L, Xia YR, et al. Mice lacking serum paraoxonase are susceptible to organophosphate toxicity and atherosclerosis. Nature 1998;394:284–7.

53. Tward A, Xia Y-R, Wang X-P, et al. Decreased atherosclerotic lesion formation in human serum paraoxonase transgenic mice. Circulation 2002;106(4):484–90.

54. Bhattacharyya T, Nicholls SJ, Topol EJ, et al. Relationship of paraoxonase 1 (PON1) gene polymorphisms and functional activity with systemic oxidative stress and cardiovascular risk. JAMA 2008;299(11):1265–76.

55. Tang WHW, Hartiala J, Fan Y, et al. Clinical and genetic association of serum paraoxonase and arylesterase activities with cardiovascular risk. Arterioscler Thromb Vasc Biol 2012;32(11):2803–12.

56. Wang Z, Nicholls SJ, Rodriguez ER, et al. Protein carbamylation links inflammation, smoking, uremia and atherogenesis. Nat Med 2007;13(10):1176–84.

57. Rudolph TK, Wipper S, Reiter B, et al. Myeloperoxidase deficiency preserves vasomotor function in humans. Eur Heart J 2012;33(13):1625–34.

58. Brennan M-L, Penn MS, Van Lente F, et al. Prognostic value of myeloperoxidase in patients with chest pain. N Engl J Med 2003;349(17):1595–604.

59. Zhang R, Brennan ML, Shen Z, et al. Myeloperoxidase functions as a major enzymatic catalyst for initiation of lipid peroxidation at sites of inflammation. J Biol Chem 2002;277(48):46116–22.

60. Urundhati A, Huang Y, Lupica JA, et al. Modification of high density lipoprotein by myeloperoxidase generates a pro-inflammatory particle. J Biol Chem 2009;284(45):30825–35.

61. Zheng L, Nukuna B, Brennan ML, et al. Apolipoprotein A-I is a selective target for myeloperoxidase-catalyzed

oxidation and function impairment in subjects with cardiovascular disease. J Clin Invest 2004;114(4):529–41.

62. Zheng L, Settle M, Brubaker G, et al. Localization of nitration and chlorination sites on apolipoprotein A-I catalysed by myeloperoxidase in human atheroma and associated oxidative impairment in ABCA1-dependent cholesterol efflux from macrophages. J Biol Chem 2005;280(1):38–47.

63. Shiflett AM, Bishop JR, Pahwa A, et al. Human high density lipoproteins are platforms for the assembly of multi-component innate immune complexes. J Biol Chem 2005;280(38):32578–85.

64. Speer T, Rohrer L, Blyszczuk P, et al. Abnormal high-density lipoprotein induces endothelial dysfunction via activation of toll-like receptor-2. Immunity 2013;38(4):754–68.

65. Kielstein JT, Salpeter SR, Bode-Boeger SM, et al. Symmetric dimethylarginine (SDMA) as endogenous marker of renal function - a meta-analysis. Nephrol Dial Transplant 2006;21(9):2446–51.

66. Pullamsetti S, Kiss L, Ghofrani HA, et al. Increased levels and reduced catabolism of asymmetric and symmetric dimethylarginines in pulmonary hypertension. FASEB J 2005;19(9):1175–7.

67. Schepers E, Barreto DV, Liabeuf S, et al. Symmetric dimethylarginine as a proinflammatory agent in chronic kidney disease. Clin J Am Soc Nephrol 2011;6(10):2374–83.

68. Edfeldt K, Swedenborg J, Hansson GK, et al. Expression of toll-like receptors in human atherosclerotic lesions: a possible pathway for plaque activation. Circulation 2002;105:1158–61.

69. Beaulieu LM, Lin E, Morin KM, et al. Regulatory effects of TLR2 on megakaryocytic cell function. Blood 2011;117(22):5963–74.

70. Cabanski M, Steinmüller M, Marsh LM, et al. PKR regulates TLR2/TLR4-dependent signaling in murine alveolar macrophages. Am J Respir Cell Mol Biol 2008;38(1):26–31.

71. Zewinger S, Kleber ME, Rohrer L, et al. Symmetric dimethylarginine, high-density lipoproteins and cardiovascular disease. Eur Heart J 2017. https://doi.org/10.1093/eurheartj/ehx118.

72. Voight BF, Peloso GM, Orho-Melander M, et al. Plasma HDL cholesterol and risk of myocardial infarction: a mendelian randomisation study. Lancet 2012;380(9841):572–80.

73. Khera AV, Cuchel M, de la Llera-Moya M, et al. Cholesterol efflux capacity, high-density lipoprotein function, and atherosclerosis. N Engl J Med 2011;364(2):127–35.

74. Rohatgi A, Khera A, Berry JD, et al. HDL cholesterol efflux capacity and incident cardiovascular events. N Engl J Med 2014;371(25):2383–93.

75. Li XM, Tang WHW, Mosior MK, et al. Paradoxical association of enhanced cholesterol efflux with increased incident cardiovascular risks. Arterioscler Thromb Vasc Biol 2013;33(7):1696–705.

76. Sabatine MS, Giugliano RP, Keech AC, et al. Evolocumab and clinical outcomes in patients with cardiovascular disease. N Engl J Med 2017;376(18):1713–22.

77. Yusuf S, Bosch J, Dagenais G, et al. Cholesterol lowering in intermediate-risk persons without cardiovascular disease. N Engl J Med 2016;374(21):2021–31.

Intravascular Ultrasound Studies of Plaque Progression and Regression
Impact of Lipid-Modifying Therapies

Daisuke Shishikura, MD, Satoshi Honda, MD,
Jordan Andrews, BS, Stephen J. Nicholls, MBBS, PhD*

KEYWORDS

- Atherosclerosis • Lipids • Clinical trials • Intravascular ultrasound

KEY POINTS

- Intravascular ultrasound (IVUS) trials are performed in patients who have presented for a clinical indicated coronary angiogram.
- Serial IVUS imaging has provided important insights into the factors that are associated with progression of coronary atherosclerosis.
- When integrated into clinical trials, serial vascular imaging has permitted the assessment of the effect of medical therapies on disease progression.

INTRODUCTION

Over the course of the last 25 years, clinical trials have consistently demonstrated that lowering levels of low-density lipoprotein cholesterol (LDL-C) reduces cardiovascular events in high-risk patients.[1–3] This has led to widespread use of statins and increasing prescription of additional lipid-lowering agents in patients who are unable to achieve treatment targets.[4,5] There remains, however, a considerable residual risk of clinical events, suggesting the need to identify more effective strategies to achieve greater reductions in cardiovascular risk.[6] In parallel to these studies, technological advances in arterial wall imaging have enabled study of the factors associated with the natural history of progression of atherosclerosis.[7] When integrated into clinical trials, serial vascular imaging has permitted the assessment of the effect of medical therapies on disease progression.

EARLY IMAGING CLINICAL TRIALS

Coronary angiography generates a 2-D silhouette of the artery lumen, with the ability to quantify the extent of obstructive disease. This technique is widely used in clinical practice, with early evidence that the severity of angiographic disease associates with adverse clinical outcomes.[8,9] Early studies using serial quantitative coronary angiography demonstrated a favorable impact of statin therapy on progression of obstructive disease, with evidence of a direct relationship between the degree of lipid lowering and degree of

Disclosure: Nicholls disclosures are research support from AstraZeneca, Amgen, Anthera, Eli Lilly, Esperion, Novartis, Cerenis, The Medicines Company, Resverlogix, InfraReDx, Roche, Sanofi-Regeneron and LipoScience and a consultant for AstraZeneca, Eli Lilly, Anthera, Omthera, Merck, Takeda, Resverlogix, Sanofi-Regeneron, CSL Behring, Esperion, Boehringer Ingelheim. Other authors have no disclosures.
South Australian Health and Medical Research Institute, University of Adelaide, PO Box 11060, Adelaide, SA 5001, Australia
* Corresponding author.
E-mail address: stephen.nicholls@sahmri.com

cardiology.theclinics.com

angiographic benefit.[10–12] Extending beyond these benefits of LDL-C lowering, other studies have demonstrated that administration of fenofibrate in patients with diabetes can slow progression of obstructive disease[13] and that addition of niacin to background statin therapy produces regression of angiographic disease.[14] These later findings suggested that potentially targeting additional lipid parameters, beyond LDL-C, may provide further benefit for high-risk patients. A fundamental limitation of angiography is its inability to directly image the vessel wall.[15] Accordingly, it is unable to provide a comprehensive evaluation of the impact of medical therapies on the full burden of atherosclerotic disease.

Noninvasive B-mode ultrasound imaging of the carotid artery permits measurement of carotid intima-medial thickness (cIMT), representing an early change within the artery wall that correlates with cardiovascular risk factors, atherosclerotic disease burden and adverse cardiovascular outcomes.[16] Clinical trials have demonstrated a direct relationship between the degree of LDL-C lowering with statins and slowing of cIMT progression.[17] Later studies observed cIMT regression with use of high-intensity statin agents.[18,19] These findings provided insights into the impact of statin therapy on early changes in the artery wall.

INTRAVASCULAR ULTRASOUND

The ability to place high-frequency ultrasound transducers within the coronary artery lumen permits intravascular ultrasound (IVUS) to generate high-resolution imaging of the full thickness of the artery wall.[20] This enables visualization of the full burden of atherosclerotic plaque within the vessel wall, with quantitative techniques able to measure the area of plaque within each cross-sectional image. Continuous imaging during catheter withdrawal produces a series of cross-sectional images throughout a length of artery extending the quantitation of plaque burden to a volumetric measure. Comparison of imaging in anatomically matched segments, defined by the presence of proximal and distal side branches, permits measurement of changes in plaque volume over time.[21] This provides a unique opportunity to characterize the factors associated with plaque progression and to determine whether medical therapies can slow disease progression or promote regression of atherosclerotic plaque.[22–27] Subsequent studies have demonstrated that the burden and progression of coronary atherosclerosis are associated with the subsequent incidence of cardiovascular death, myocardial infarction, or coronary revascularization.[28,29]

Several clinical trials have demonstrated important insights into the role of medical therapies modifying plasma lipoproteins and their impact on atherosclerotic plaque within the coronary vasculature.

STATIN ADMINISTRATION

An early study using serial IVUS imaging demonstrated no impact of intensive statin therapy on plaque progression yet reported a favorable impact on plaque characteristics, suggesting a potentially beneficial effect on plaque composition.[30] Subsequent studies, however, have consistently demonstrated that intensive statin therapy exerts a protective effect on disease progression.[25–27] The Reversal of Atherosclerosis with Aggressive Lipid Lowering (REVERSAL) study compared the effects of atorvastatin (80 mg) and pravastatin (40 mg) on progression of coronary atherosclerosis in 502 patients. Greater lowering of LDL-C (79 mg/dL vs 110 mg/dL) with intensive atorvastatin was associated with halting of plaque progression.[25] Subsequent analyses reported a direct relationship between slowing of disease progression with both lowering of LDL-C and the inflammatory marker, C-reactive protein (CRP).[31] The finding of an independent relationship between CRP lowering and slowing disease progression supported claims that statins may exert anti-inflammatory effects in vivo.

A Study to evaluate the Effect of Rosuvastatin On Intravascular Ultrasound-Derived Coronary Atheroma Burden (ASTEROID) subsequently evaluated the impact of high-dose rosuvastatin for 24 months on coronary plaque burden.[26] Lowering LDL-C to 60 mg/dL and raising high-density lipoprotein cholesterol (HDL-C) by approximately 15% with rosuvastatin was associated with plaque regression. Although this study reinforced the direct relationship between LDL-C lowering and changes in plaque burden, further analyses also reported a direct relationship between HDL-C raising and slowing disease progression with statins.[32] The change in the ratio of apolipoprotein B/apolipoprotein A-I, reflecting the proportion of atherogenic to protective lipoproteins, emerged as the strongest predictor of disease progression in the setting of statin therapy.

These findings provided the impetus to perform the largest serial IVUS study of plaque progression. The Study of Coronary Atheroma by inTravascular Ultrasound: Effect of Rosuvastatin versus AtorvastatiN (SATURN) directly compared the impact of the 2 most intensive statins (atorvastatin 80 mg and rosuvastatin 40 mg) for

24 months.[27] Achieving low levels of LDL-C (70 mg/dL with atorvastatin and 61 mg/dL with rosuvastatin) and higher HDL-C levels (greater than 48 mg/dL) was associated with marked plaque regression with both agents, although no difference was observed between the groups. These findings contributed to the consistent relationship between LDL-C lowering and favorable effects on disease progression, with the observation that achieving an LDL-C below LDL-C was typically associated with plaque regression. Approximately one-third of patients achieving an LDL-C less than 70 mg/dL, however, continue to demonstrate plaque progression. Associated with an ongoing propensity of progression, despite achieving low LDL-C levels, are the presence of additional risk factors and increases in levels of apolipoprotein B. The latter observation highlights the potential to continue targeting atherogenic lipoproteins, even when a patient's LDL-C is at target levels.[33]

LOW-DENSITY LIPOPROTEIN LOWERING BEYOND STATINS

Several subsequent trials have investigated the impact of adding alternative LDL-C–lowering agents to statin therapy on coronary atherosclerosis.[34,35] In the Plaque Regression With Cholesterol Absorption Inhibitor or Synthesis Inhibitor Evaluated by Intravascular Ultrasound (PRECISE-IVUS) trial, patients were treated with a combination of atorvastatin and the cholesterol absorption inhibitor, ezetimibe, or atorvastatin monotherapy for 12 months.[34] Achieving a lower LDL-C with combination therapy (63 mg/dL vs 73 mg/dL) was associated with incremental regression of atherosclerotic plaque. The Global Assessment of Plaque Regression With a PCSK9 Antibody as Measured by Intravascular Ultrasound (GLAGOV) trial evaluated the impact of use of the proprotein convertase subtilisin kexin type 9 (PCSK9) inhibitor, evolocumab, versus placebo in patients treated with background statin therapy for at least 4 weeks. After 18 months of treatment, achieving a lower LDL-C with the combination of evolocumab and statin (37 mg/dL vs 92 mg/dL) was associated with regression of coronary atherosclerosis and a greater proportion of individual patients demonstrating any degree of plaque regression.[35] A direct relationship was observed between achieved LDL-C levels and disease progression, with no evidence of lack of incremental benefit at very low LDL-C levels. In patients already at target LDL-C goal (<70 mg/dL) at baseline, greater regression was observed with the combination of evolocumab and statin therapy, suggesting potentially greater modifiability of their atherosclerotic plaque.

ADDITIONAL ATHEROGENIC LIPID TARGETS

As increasingly intensive lipid-lowering strategies are used in clinical practice, there has been a renewal of interest in targeting other atherogenic lipid parameters. In statin-treated patients, elevated achieved levels of non–HDL-C, triglycerides, or remnant cholesterol, each reflecting a broader population of atherogenic lipoproteins, is associated with greater plaque progression rates at all LDL-C levels. This suggests that targeting triglyceride-rich lipoproteins may produce incremental benefit in statin-treated patients. In patients with type 2 diabetes mellitus, favorable modification of the triglyceride/HDL-C ratio was the strongest predictor of slowing disease progression, underscoring the potential benefit of the peroxisome proliferator activated receptor gamma agonist, pioglitazone, in serial imaging studies.[36] In a similar fashion, lipoprotein (a) (Lp[a]) is an independent predictor of cardiovascular risk, but has not been well investigated in serial IVUS trials. In statin-treated patients, Lp(a) has not to date been demonstrated to be associated with disease progression, although the prevalence of elevated Lp(a) levels has been relatively small in these studies.[37] An alternative approach to targeting atherogenic lipoproteins in patients with coronary artery disease has been to inhibit cholesterol esterification within the artery wall. Although preclinical studies of acyl-CoA:cholesterol actyltransferase inhibitors demonstrated reduction in foam cell formation and antiatherosclerotic effects in animal models,[38] they did not prove favorable in humans. Administration of pactimibe was reported to potentially accelerate plaque progression, which may reflect a proapoptotic effect of increasing free cholesterol levels within the artery wall.[39]

HIGH-DENSITY LIPOPROTEIN AS A THERAPEUTIC TARGET

Epidemiology and preclinical studies have suggested that high-density lipoprotein (HDL) exerts a protective effect on cardiovascular risk.[40,41] In statin-treated patients, modest increases in HDL-C independently were associated with slowing of disease progression, supporting a potential therapeutic role for targeting HDL functionality in patients with coronary disease. The studies to date, however, have been generally disappointing. Although an early study demonstrated that short-term intravenous infusions of an HDL mimetic containing apolipoprotein A-I$_{Milano}$ produced rapid regression of coronary atherosclerosis in patients after an acute coronary syndrome,[42] more recent trials have failed to report benefit using either a similar mimetic or those containing wild-type apolipoprotein A-I. Whether this reflects challenges in administering HDL in addition to intensive statin therapy in the modern era or variability of response in the proinflammatory state after an acute coronary syndrome remains to be determined. Apabetalone is a selective bromodomain and extraterminal (BET) protein inhibitor, initially developed due to its ability to up-regulate endogenous synthesis of apolipoprotein A-I and enhance systemic cholesterol efflux capacity. A proof-of-concept study, however, demonstrated that modest raising of HDL-C did not produce incremental plaque regression compared with background medical therapy.[43] The complex role of BET proteins in regulation of inflammatory and calcifying pathways implicated in cardiovascular disease has supported its ongoing clinical development. Cholesteryl ester transfer protein (CETP) inhibitors were originally developed on the basis of their ability to substantially raise HDL-C levels. A serial IVUS study of torcetrapib demonstrated an inability to slow disease progression.[44] Subsequent analyses reported plaque regression in the torcetrapib-treated patients achieving the highest HDL-C levels, suggesting no adverse effects on HDL functionality.[45] Such reports supported ongoing development of other CETP inhibitors in clinical trials.

IMPLICATIONS AND FUTURE STEPS

The ultimate impact of the finding of these studies is determined by their ability for their results to be associated with cardiovascular outcomes. Pooled analyses of serial IVUS trials has demonstrated that both the burden and degree of progression of coronary atherosclerosis are associated with adverse cardiovascular events.[28] Similarly, the ability of agents to exert complementary effects on both plaque progression and cardiovascular events is important. High-intensity statin agents favorably modify disease progression and cardiovascular events, with lowering of both LDL-C and CRP independently associated with their benefit. More recently, evolocumab had beneficial effects in both imaging and cardiovascular event trials with similar patient characteristics and achieved LDL-C levels.[35] Finally, the finding that modest HDL-C raising was associated with statin benefits and substantial HDL-C raising with torcetrapib benefits on atherosclerotic plaque complements reports of similar associations from clinical event trials.

Beyond evaluating the impact of medical therapies on disease progression, there is considerable interest in determining their effects on plaque composition. Gray-scale IVUS imaging is limited by its ability to distinguish individual plaque components. Spectral analysis of its radiofrequency backscatter, however, has been reported to distinguish fibrotic, fibrofatty, necrotic, and calcific plaque components. Substudies of IVUS trials have demonstrated that plaque regression observed with both high-intensity statins and evolocumab are associated with a reduction in fibrofatty and increase in plaque calcium.[46] Whether other emerging imaging modalities, such as optical coherence tomography, near-infrared spectroscopy, CT coronary angiography, and radioisotope molecular imaging, will provide incremental information remains to be determined.

Given the need for invasive coronary imaging, IVUS trials are performed in patients who have presented for a clinical indicated coronary angiogram. It is unknown whether the findings of these studies apply to asymptomatic patients at an earlier stage of the disease process. The ongoing evolution of noninvasive imaging may permit these studies.

SUMMARY

Serial IVUS imaging has provided important insights into the factors that are associated with progression of coronary atherosclerosis. In particular, they have reported that intensive LDL-C lowering with high-intensity statins administered as monotherapy or in combination with other lipid-lowering agents produces disease regression. These findings have provided important insights, giving a biological rationale for the effects of these therapeutic approaches in high-cardiovascular-risk patients.

REFERENCES

1. Cholesterol Treatment Trialists (CTT) Collaboration, Baigent C, Blackwell L, Emberson J, et al. Efficacy and safety of more intensive lowering of LDL cholesterol: a meta-analysis of data from 170,000 participants in 26 randomised trials. Lancet 2010;376: 1670–81.
2. Cannon CP, Blazing MA, Giugliano RP, et al. Ezetimibe added to statin therapy after acute coronary syndromes. N Engl J Med 2015;372:2387–97.
3. Sabatine MS, Giugliano RP, Keech AC, et al. Evolocumab and clinical outcomes in patients with cardiovascular disease. N Engl J Med 2017;376:1713–22.
4. Rosenson RS, Farkouh ME, Mefford M, et al. Trends in use of high-intensity statin therapy after

myocardial infarction, 2011 to 2014. J Am Coll Cardiol 2017;69:2696–706.

5. Writing C, Lloyd-Jones DM, Morris PB, et al. 2016 ACC expert consensus decision pathway on the role of non-statin therapies for LDL-cholesterol lowering in the management of atherosclerotic cardiovascular disease risk: a report of the American College of Cardiology task force on clinical expert consensus documents. J Am Coll Cardiol 2016;68:92–125.

6. Sampson UK, Fazio S, Linton MF. Residual cardiovascular risk despite optimal LDL cholesterol reduction with statins: the evidence, etiology, and therapeutic challenges. Curr Atheroscler Rep 2012;14:1–10.

7. Tarkin JM, Dweck MR, Evans NR, et al. Imaging atherosclerosis. Circ Res 2016;118:750–69.

8. Burggraf GW, Parker JO. Prognosis in coronary artery disease. Angiographic, hemodynamic, and clinical factors. Circulation 1975;51:146–56.

9. Harris PJ, Lee KL, Harrell FE Jr, et al. Outcome in medically treated coronary artery disease. Ischemic events: nonfatal infarction and death. Circulation 1980;62:718–26.

10. Jukema JW, Bruschke AV, van Boven AJ, et al. Effects of lipid lowering by pravastatin on progression and regression of coronary artery disease in symptomatic men with normal to moderately elevated serum cholesterol levels. The Regression Growth Evaluation Statin Study (REGRESS). Circulation 1995;91:2528–40.

11. Effect of simvastatin on coronary atheroma: the Multicentre Anti-Atheroma Study (MAAS). Lancet 1994; 344:633–8.

12. Blankenhorn DH, Azen SP, Kramsch DM, et al. Coronary angiographic changes with lovastatin therapy. The Monitored Atherosclerosis Regression Study (MARS). Ann Intern Med 1993;119: 969–76.

13. Effect of fenofibrate on progression of coronary-artery disease in type 2 diabetes: the Diabetes Atherosclerosis Intervention Study, a randomised study. Lancet 2001;357:905–10.

14. Brown BG, Zhao XQ, Chait A, et al. Simvastatin and niacin, antioxidant vitamins, or the combination for the prevention of coronary disease. N Engl J Med 2001;345:1583–92.

15. Mintz GS, Painter JA, Pichard AD, et al. Atherosclerosis in angiographically "normal" coronary artery reference segments: an intravascular ultrasound study with clinical correlations. J Am Coll Cardiol 1995;25:1479–85.

16. Peters SA, Grobbee DE, Bots ML. Carotid intima-media thickness: a suitable alternative for cardiovascular risk as outcome? Eur J Cardiovasc Prev Rehabil 2011;18:167–74.

17. Espeland MA, O'Leary DH, Terry JG, et al. Carotid intimal-media thickness as a surrogate for cardiovascular disease events in trials of HMG-CoA reductase inhibitors. Curr Control Trials Cardiovasc Med 2005;6:3.

18. Taylor AJ, Kent SM, Flaherty PJ, et al. ARBITER: arterial biology for the investigation of the treatment effects of reducing cholesterol: a randomized trial comparing the effects of atorvastatin and pravastatin on carotid intima medial thickness. Circulation 2002;106:2055–60.

19. Smilde TJ, van Wissen S, Wollersheim H, et al. Effect of aggressive versus conventional lipid lowering on atherosclerosis progression in familial hypercholesterolaemia (ASAP): a prospective, randomised, double-blind trial. Lancet 2001;357:577–81.

20. Mintz GS, Nissen SE, Anderson WD, et al. American College of Cardiology clinical expert consensus document on standards for acquisition, measurement and reporting of intravascular ultrasound studies (IVUS). A report of the American College of Cardiology task force on clinical expert consensus documents. J Am Coll Cardiol 2001;37:1478–92.

21. Nicholls SJ, Sipahi I, Schoenhagen P, et al. Application of intravascular ultrasound in anti-atherosclerotic drug development. Nat Rev Drug Discov 2006;5:485–92.

22. Nicholls SJ, Tuzcu EM, Sipahi I, et al. Effects of obesity on lipid-lowering, anti-inflammatory, and antiatherosclerotic benefits of atorvastatin or pravastatin in patients with coronary artery disease (from the REVERSAL Study). Am J Cardiol 2006;97: 1553–7.

23. Chhatriwalla AK, Nicholls SJ, Wang TH, et al. Low levels of low-density lipoprotein cholesterol and blood pressure and progression of coronary atherosclerosis. J Am Coll Cardiol 2009;53:1110–5.

24. Nicholls SJ, Tuzcu EM, Kalidindi S, et al. Effect of diabetes on progression of coronary atherosclerosis and arterial remodeling: a pooled analysis of 5 intravascular ultrasound trials. J Am Coll Cardiol 2008; 52:255–62.

25. Nissen SE, Tuzcu EM, Schoenhagen P, et al. Effect of intensive compared with moderate lipid-lowering therapy on progression of coronary atherosclerosis: a randomized controlled trial. JAMA 2004;291:1071–80.

26. Nissen SE, Nicholls SJ, Sipahi I, et al. Effect of very high-intensity statin therapy on regression of coronary atherosclerosis: the ASTEROID trial. JAMA 2006;295:1556–65.

27. Nicholls SJ, Ballantyne CM, Barter PJ, et al. Effect of two intensive statin regimens on progression of coronary disease. N Engl J Med 2011;365:2078–87.

28. Nicholls SJ, Hsu A, Wolski K, et al. Intravascular ultrasound-derived measures of coronary atherosclerotic plaque burden and clinical outcome. J Am Coll Cardiol 2010;55:2399–407.

29. Puri R, Wolski K, Uno K, et al. Left main coronary atherosclerosis progression, constrictive remodeling,

and clinical events. JACC Cardiovasc Interv 2013;6: 29–35.

30. Schartl M, Bocksch W, Koschyk DH, et al. Use of intravascular ultrasound to compare effects of different strategies of lipid-lowering therapy on plaque volume and composition in patients with coronary artery disease. Circulation 2001;104:387–92.

31. Nissen SE, Tuzcu EM, Schoenhagen P, et al. Statin therapy, LDL cholesterol, C-reactive protein, and coronary artery disease. N Engl J Med 2005;352: 29–38.

32. Nicholls SJ, Tuzcu EM, Sipahi I, et al. Statins, high-density lipoprotein cholesterol, and regression of coronary atherosclerosis. JAMA 2007;297:499–508.

33. Bayturan O, Kapadia S, Nicholls SJ, et al. Clinical predictors of plaque progression despite very low levels of low-density lipoprotein cholesterol. J Am Coll Cardiol 2010;55:2736–42.

34. Tsujita K, Sugiyama S, Sumida H, et al. Impact of dual lipid-lowering strategy with ezetimibe and atorvastatin on coronary plaque regression in patients with percutaneous coronary intervention: the multicenter randomized controlled PRECISE-IVUS Trial. J Am Coll Cardiol 2015;66:495–507.

35. Nicholls SJ, Puri R, Anderson T, et al. Effect of evolocumab on progression of coronary disease in statin-treated patients: the GLAGOV randomized clinical trial. JAMA 2016;316:2373–84.

36. Nicholls SJ, Tuzcu EM, Wolski K, et al. Lowering the triglyceride/high-density lipoprotein cholesterol ratio is associated with the beneficial impact of pioglitazone on progression of coronary atherosclerosis in diabetic patients: insights from the PERISCOPE (Pioglitazone Effect on Regression of Intravascular Sonographic Coronary Obstruction Prospective Evaluation) study. J Am Coll Cardiol 2011;57:153–9.

37. Nissen SE, Nicholls SJ, Wolski K, et al. Effect of rimonabant on progression of atherosclerosis in patients with abdominal obesity and coronary artery disease: the STRADIVARIUS randomized controlled trial. JAMA 2008;299:1547–60.

38. Bocan TM, Mueller SB, Uhlendorf PD, et al. Inhibition of acyl-CoA cholesterol O-acyltransferase reduces the cholesteryl ester enrichment of atherosclerotic lesions in the Yucatan micropig. Atherosclerosis 1993;99:175–86.

39. Nissen SE, Tuzcu EM, Brewer HB, et al. Effect of ACAT inhibition on the progression of coronary atherosclerosis. N Engl J Med 2006;354:1253–63.

40. Castelli WP. Cholesterol and lipids in the risk of coronary artery disease–the Framingham Heart Study. Can J Cardiol 1988;4(Suppl A):5A–10A.

41. Barter P, Gotto AM, LaRosa JC, et al. HDL cholesterol, very low levels of LDL cholesterol, and cardiovascular events. N Engl J Med 2007;357:1301–10.

42. Nissen SE, Tsunoda T, Tuzcu EM, et al. Effect of recombinant ApoA-I Milano on coronary atherosclerosis in patients with acute coronary syndromes: a randomized controlled trial. JAMA 2003;290: 2292–300.

43. Nicholls SJ, Puri R, Wolski K, et al. Effect of the BET protein inhibitor, RVX-208, on progression of coronary atherosclerosis: results of the phase 2b, randomized, double-blind, multicenter, ASSURE trial. Am J Cardiovasc Drugs 2016;16:55–65.

44. Nissen SE, Tardif JC, Nicholls SJ, et al. Effect of torcetrapib on the progression of coronary atherosclerosis. N Engl J Med 2007;356:1304–16.

45. Nicholls SJ, Tuzcu EM, Brennan DM, et al. Cholesteryl ester transfer protein inhibition, high-density lipoprotein raising, and progression of coronary atherosclerosis: insights from ILLUSTRATE (Investigation of Lipid Level Management Using Coronary Ultrasound to Assess Reduction of Atherosclerosis by CETP Inhibition and HDL Elevation). Circulation 2008;118:2506–14.

46. Puri R, Libby P, Nissen SE, et al. Long-term effects of maximally intensive statin therapy on changes in coronary atheroma composition: insights from SATURN. Eur Heart J Cardiovasc Imaging 2014; 15:380–8.

Moving?

Printed and bound by CPI Group (UK) Ltd, Croydon, CR0 4YY

12/10/2024

01773428-0001